Instructor Manual for Neonatal Resuscitation

Editor
Jeanette Zaichkin, RN, MN, NNP-BC

Associate Editors
Gary Weiner, MD, FAAP
Cheryl Major, RNC-NIC, BSN

NRP Steering Committee Members
Christopher Colby, MD, FAAP
Marilyn Escobedo, MD, FAAP
Karen D. Fairchild, MD, FAAP
Louis P. Halamek, MD, FAAP
George A. Little, MD, FAAP
Jane E. McGowan, MD, FAAP
Steven Ringer, MD, PhD, FAAP
Gary M. Weiner, MD, FAAP
Myra H. Wyckoff, MD, FAAP

NRP Steering Committee Liaison Representatives
Praveen Kumar, MD, FAAP
   AAP Committee on Fetus and Newborn
Mildred Ramirez, MD, FACOG
   American College of Obstetricians and Gynecologists
Khalid Aziz, MD, FRCPC
   Canadian Paediatric Society
Barbara Nightengale, RN, MSN, NNP-BC
   National Association of Neonatal Nurses
John Gallagher, RRT-NPS
   American Association for Respiratory Care

Managing Editor
Rachel Poulin, MPH
Wendy Marie Simon, MA, CAE

The committee would like to express thanks to the following reviewers and contributors:
Susan Amundsen
Jodee Anderson, MD, FAAP
Julie Arafeh, RN, MSN
Denise Dubuque, RN
Leslee Goetz, MN, RNC-OB
Cynthia Jensen, RN, MS, CNS
Sarah A. Korkowski, MSN, NNP-BC
Terrie Lockridge, MSN, RNC-NIC
Lori A. Markham, MSN, MBA, NNP-BC, CCRN

Linda McCarney, MSN, RN, NNP-BC, EMT-P
Karen Menghini, RN, MSN, NNP-BC
Kathy O'Connell, MN, RN
Webra Price-Douglas, PhD, CRNP, IBCLC
Brian K. Ross, PhD, MD
Frances E. Rushton, MD, FAAP, AAP Board-appointed Reviewer
Sharyl Sadowski, MS, RNC, AP, NNP-BC
Theodora (Lola) Stavroudis, MD, FAAP
Laura A. Stokowski, MS, RN
Lauren Thorngate, PhC, RN, CCRN
Kim Watkins, RRT-NPS

AAP Life Support Staff
Wendy Marie Simon, MA, CAE
Rory Hand, EdM
Rachel Poulin, MPH
Kristy Crilly
Nancy Gardner
Melissa Marx

AAP Marketing and Production Staff
Theresa Wiener

Copyeditor
Jill Rubino

American Heart Association Emergency Cardiovascular Care Leadership
Leon Chameides, MD, FAAP
Brian Eigel, PhD
Mary Fran Hazinski, RNC
Robert Hickey, MD, FAAP
Vinay Nadkarni, MD, FAAP

American Heart Association Emergency Cardiovascular Care Pediatric Subcommittee
Marc D. Berg, MD, FAAP, Chair, 2009-2011
Monica E. Kleinman, MD, FAAP, *Immediate Past Chair, 2007-2009*
Dianne L. Atkins, MD, FAAP
Jeffrey M. Berman, MD
Kathleen Brown, MD, FAAP
Adam Cheng, MD
Laura Conley, BS, RRT, RCP, NPS
Allan R. de Caen, MD
Aaron Donoghue, MD, FAAP, MSCE
Melinda L. Fiedor Hamilton, MD, MSc
Ericka L. Fink, MD, FAAP

Eugene B. Freid, MD, FAAP
Cheryl K. Gooden, MD, FAAP
John Gosford, BS, EMT-P
Patricia Howard
Kelly Kadlec, MD, FAAP
Sharon E. Mace, MD, FAAP
Bradley S. Marino, MD, FAAP, MPP, MSCE
Reylon Meeks, RN, BSN, MS, MSN, EMT, PhD
Vinay Nadkarni, MD, FAAP
Jeffrey M. Perlman, MB, ChB, FAAP
Lester Proctor, MD, FAAP
Faiqa A. Qureshi, MD, FAAP
Kennith Hans Sartorelli, MD, FAAP
Wendy M. Simon, MA, CAE
Mark A. Terry, MPA, NREMT-P
Alexis Topjian, MD, FAAP
Elise W. van der Jagt, MD, FAAP, MPH
Arno Zaritsky, MD, FAAP

Associated Education Materials for the *Instructor Manual for Neonatal Resuscitation, 6th Edition*

Textbook of Neonatal Resuscitation, 6th Edition, John Kattwinkel, MD, FAAP, Editor; Jane McGowan, MD, FAAP, and Jeanette Zaichkin, RN, MN, NNP-BC, Associate Editors

NRP Instructor DVD: An Interactive Tool for Facilitation of Simulation-based Learning, Louis P. Halamek, MD, FAAP, and Jeanette Zaichkin, RN, MN, NNP-BC, Editors

NRP Online Examination, Steven Ringer, MD, PhD, FAAP, and Jerry Short, PhD, Editors

NRP Reference Chart, Code Cart Cards, and Pocket Cards, Karen D. Fairchild, MD, FAAP, Editor

NRP Simulation Poster, Louis P. Halamek, MD, FAAP, Editor

Simply NRP, Gary Weiner, MD, FAAP, and Jeanette Zaichkin, RN, MN, NNP-BC, Editors

Neonatal Resuscitation Scenarios, Gary Weiner, MD, FAAP, and Jeanette Zaichkin, RN, MN, NNP-BC, Editors

Fifth edition, 2011
Fourth edition, 2006
Third edition, 2000
Second edition, 1995
First edition, 1987

ISBN-13: 978-1-58110-501-8

NRP303

Contents

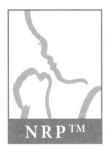

Contents

APPENDIX G:

Instructor Courses 337

APPENDIX H:

Neonatal Code Forms and Documentation 351

Foreword

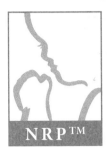

Five years ago, the Neonatal Resuscitation Program (NRP) Steering Committee started a serious discussion about the quality of NRP learning. After 20 years, the NRP was due for a change. Our slide and lecture format was lagging behind adult learning theory, and our curriculum did not adequately address teamwork and communication. Neonatal Resuscitation Program instructors were doing such a great job teaching every lesson of the NRP textbook and helping students through their Megacode that students needed to do nothing to prepare. Some students would show up to their NRP course with the textbook still in its plastic wrapper, and NRP veterans did not expect to learn much new. With so many people needing NRP provider status as a requirement of employment or credentialing, we were losing our focus on quality learning and instead, measuring our success by how fast we could get learners through a Megacode check-off. This was efficient and well intentioned, but not in the best interests of our learners or the babies in need of resuscitation. In addition, we knew that not every instructor was committed to NRP excellence, and some participated in a very small way to maintain their instructor status only to avoid any type of evaluation.

Just over 2 years ago, in a trial attempt of the proposed 6th edition course format, I led my first NRP Provider Course using a simulation-based curriculum. I was nervous, and couldn't do every single thing I wanted to do (we didn't film the scenarios), but it was a start. It marked the first time I had asked students to read the textbook and take the online examination before coming to the course. Would they feel resentful about this pre-course preparation and feel I was slacking off as their NRP instructor? Would they know the information? Would I end up lecturing lesson-by-lesson anyway? I was surprised when every student handed in their examination verification for the online examination and, when questioned, had no complaints about the process. No one missed the slides and lecture. They just wanted to get to work.

I explained the new methodology and confessed that they were my first students of simulation-based learning. They were happy to help with this experiment. Some of my ideas worked, and some were not successful. At this first course, we kind of bumbled through it together, and we learned a lot. We covered the manikin with fake blood and pureed green bean meconium and probably laughed too much during those first scenarios. After the course, 2 of the participants told me it was the best NRP class they had ever taken. It was certainly the best NRP class I had ever experienced. It was scary, it was more work than the old way of teaching, and, at first, it took more time, but it was great fun. Two years later, we're still refining and tweaking the course, but we're pretty good at it now.

And students are still telling us that our courses offer the best learning environment and the most engaging NRP experience they have ever had.

We are lucky to be NRP instructors at this moment in NRP development. This is a landmark edition and marks the most significant changes made to the teaching methodology since the inception of the course in 1987. You may need some time to learn the new methods, but it will be worth it in the end because these will be the finest courses you have ever taught. With your skills and guidance, your students will come to you after their course and say, "That was the best NRP course ever."

If simulation-based learning is new to you, don't feel as though you must be an expert at the beginning. Read and watch the new materials and take the first steps with an open mind and a sense of adventure. As you gain experience, you will find your own style within these concepts, and soon you will appreciate major improvements in team performance. The real payoff will come when a team identifies something during a debriefing that needs improvement and will result in a better outcome for newborns.

This is my third edition as editor of the *Instructor Manual for Neonatal Resuscitation*. More than any previous edition, I needed input from many people to make our manual practical and understandable. My goal is to keep the Neonatal Resuscitation Program useful for all health care professionals in many different birth settings, and I believe our team has accomplished this goal.

I especially wish to thank Dr. Gary Weiner for his incredible knowledge of neonatal resuscitation and the best ways to learn it, and for his humor, encouragement, and optimism when things got discouraging.

I also wish to thank Dr John Kattwinkel for his patience and leadership as we ensured that the textbook, the Instructor DVD, the Instructor Webinars, *Simply NRP*, and the Instructor Manual presented consistent information in all formats. Thank you to Dr Louis Halamek who taught me most of what I know about simulation and debriefing. A special thanks to Wendy Marie Simon, Rachel Poulin, and Rory Hand at the American Academy of Pediatrics, who have worked with me on an almost daily basis for the past 2 years to get all these projects pulled together on time and in great shape.

I hope you will embrace these changes and enjoy renewed enthusiasm as an NRP instructor. Not only will your students have a chance to grow professionally with each course, so will you.

Jeanette Zaichkin, RN, MN, NNP-BC

Neonatal Resuscitation Program (NRP) 2011
A Brief Summary for Busy People

NRP 2006, 5th Edition	NRP 2011, 6th Edition
Lessons in the Program	**Lessons in the Program**
Minimal Requirement: Lessons 1-4 and 9	Minimal Requirement: Lessons 1-4 and 9
Lesson 1: Overview and Principles of Resuscitation	Lesson 1: Overview and Principles of Resuscitation* (new Performance Skills Station)
Lesson 2: Initial Steps in Resuscitation*	Lesson 2: Initial Steps of Resuscitation*
Lesson 3: Use of Resuscitation Devices for Positive-Pressure Ventilation*	Lesson 3: Use of Resuscitation Devices for Positive-Pressure Ventilation*
Lesson 4: Chest Compressions*	Lesson 4: Chest Compressions*
Lesson 5: Endotracheal Intubation*	Lesson 5: Endotracheal Intubation and Laryngeal Mask Airway Insertion* (new Performance Skills Station)
Lesson 6: Medications*	Lesson 6: Medications*
Lesson 7: Special Considerations	Lesson 7: Special Considerations
Lesson 8: Resuscitation of Babies Born Preterm	Lesson 8: Resuscitation of Babies Born Preterm
Lesson 9: Ethics and Care at the End of Life	Lesson 9: Ethics and Care at the End of Life
NRP Course Options	**NRP Course Options**
Provider Course	No more Renewal Course. Everyone takes a Provider Course tailored to the needs of the learners.
Renewal Course	
Written Evaluation	Online Examination required. No more hard-copy examination after December 2011.
Online Evaluation (optional)	
NRP provider status should be renewed every 2 years by taking an NRP Renewal Course prior to the expiration date on the NRP card. If Provider status expires, the learner must take the full NRP Provider Course.	NRP provider status is maintained by taking an NRP Provider Course every 2 years. Each institution determines its own policy regarding what happens if a person's NRP provider status expires.
Provider Course Components	**Provider Course Components**
Most Provider Courses use slide/lecture format.	Learners self-study the *Textbook of Neonatal Resuscitation, 6th Edition,* and take the online examination prior to the Provider Course.
Evaluative components: written evaluation, Performance Skills Stations, and Megacode evaluation.	
	Provider Course includes little or no lecture, and uses course time for hands-on learning, immersive simulations, and constructive debriefings.
	The Performance Skills Stations are optional and used for learning, review, and practice.
	The NRP online examination and Integrated Skills Station are required and used for evaluation.
	The Simulation and Debriefing component is required and used to improve teamwork and communication.

*Performance Checklist in addition to written examination

Neonatal Resuscitation Program (NRP) 2011
A Brief Summary for Busy People

NRP 2006, 5th Edition	NRP 2011, 6th Edition
Factors Associated With the Need for Resuscitation Persistent fetal bradycardia Uterine hyperstimulation Age <16 or >35 years	**Factors Associated With the Need for Resuscitation** 6th edition presents many changes in OB terminology, such as • Category 2 or 3 fetal heart rate (HR) patterns • Uterine tachysystole with fetal HR changes Mother older than 35 years Deleted: Prolonged second stage of labor (>2 hours) Deleted: Non-reassuring fetal HR patterns
Equipment The 5th edition of the textbook does not include a Performance Checklist to help participants learn about ensuring presence and function of resuscitation supplies and equipment.	**Equipment** "Equipment Check" is a new Performance Skills Station in Lesson 1. "Quick Pre-resuscitation Checklist" is a new tool that enables you to check the presence and function of the most essential equipment and supplies at the radiant warmer in the same order as they are used according to the NRP flow diagram. No longer listed as "optional" in the birth setting: • Compressed air source • Oxygen blender to mix oxygen and compressed air with flowmeter • Pulse oximeter and oximeter probe • Laryngeal mask airway Added: Laryngoscope blade size 00 (optional) Deleted: Sodium bicarbonate 4.2% from the list of items needed for immediate resuscitation Deleted: Naloxone hydrochloride 0.4 mg/mL from the list of items needed for immediate resuscitation The Equipment Check procedure is demonstrated on the DVD that accompanies the 6th edition of the textbook.
Personnel There is no special focus on teamwork and communication in the 5th edition of the textbook.	**Personnel** Behavioral skills such as teamwork, leadership, and effective communication are critical to successful resuscitation of the newborn. NRP Key Behavioral Skills: • Know your environment. • Anticipate and plan. • Assume the leadership role. • Communicate effectively. • Delegate workload optimally. • Allocate attention wisely • Use all available information. • Use all available resources • Call for help when needed. • Maintain professional behavior.

Neonatal Resuscitation Program (NRP) 2011
A Brief Summary for Busy People

NRP 2006, 5th Edition	NRP 2011, 6th Edition
Post-resuscitation Care (3 levels) Routine care (standard observation) Observational care (frequent evaluation) Post-resuscitation care (continuing evaluation and monitoring in a nursery environment)	**Post-resuscitation Care (2 levels)** Routine Care: For vigorous term babies with no risk factors and babies who have responded to the initial steps. Babies who required initial steps may not need to be separated from their mothers after birth to receive close monitoring and further stabilization. Post-resuscitation care: For babies who have depressed breathing or activity, and/or require supplemental oxygen. Require frequent evaluation. Some may transition to routine care; others will require ongoing support. Transfer to an intensive care nursery may be necessary.
The NRP Flow Diagram (overview) At birth, answer 4 questions to determine the need for initial steps: • Is the newborn term? • Is the fluid clear? • Is the newborn breathing or crying? • Does the newborn have good muscle tone?	**The NRP Flow Diagram (overview)** Prior to beginning the steps in the NRP flow diagram, ask the OB provider for relevant perinatal history, including these questions: • What is the gestational age? • Is the fluid clear? • How many babies are expected? • Are there any additional risk factors? At birth, answer 3 questions to determine the need for initial steps at the radiant warmer: • Is the newborn term? • Is the newborn breathing or crying? • Does the newborn have good muscle tone? If any answer is "no," the newborn should receive initial steps at the radiant warmer. Deleted: At birth, answer the question, "Is the fluid clear?" to determine the need for initial steps at the radiant warmer. Note: The vigorous meconium-stained newborn need not receive initial steps at the radiant warmer, but may receive routine care (with appropriate monitoring) with his mother. Routine care of newborn staying with mother: Warm (skin-to-skin contact is recommended), clear airway by wiping the baby's mouth and nose if necessary, dry the newborn, and provide ongoing evaluation of breathing, activity, and color. Suctioning following birth (including bulb suctioning with a bulb syringe) should be reserved for babies who have obvious obstruction to spontaneous breathing or who require positive-pressure ventilation.

Neonatal Resuscitation Program (NRP) 2011

A Brief Summary for Busy People

NRP 2006, 5th Edition	NRP 2011, 6th Edition
	Initial Steps and additional interventions:
	Position head to open airway; clear the airway as necessary (non-vigorous meconium-stained newborn requires intubation and suctioning).
	Dry, stimulate, reposition to open airway.
Simultaneously evaluate respirations, HR, and color. Interventions are based on these 3 indicators.	Evaluate respirations and heart rate. If HR is less than 100 beats per minute (bpm), or if newborn is apneic or gasping, begin positive-pressure ventilation. If HR is more than 100 bpm and respirations are labored, consider continuous positive airway pressure (CPAP), especially for preterm newborns.
	Subsequently, evaluation and decision making are based on respirations, HR, and oxygenation (per pulse oximetry).
Chest compressions are indicated when the heart rate remains less than 60 bpm despite 30 seconds of effective positive-pressure ventilation.	After ensuring effective ventilation, if heart rate remains below 60 bpm, despite 30 seconds of effective ventilation, provide chest compressions and continue assisted ventilation.
	Note: the flow diagram timeline stops at 60 seconds and adds an extra step (take ventilation corrective steps) to ensure effective ventilation, recognizing that many factors may influence the time required to achieve effective ventilation.
	Intubation is strongly recommended when chest compressions begin, if not already done.
	Increase oxygen concentration to 100% when chest compressions begin.
Continue chest compressions coordinated with ventilation for 30 seconds before assessing heart rate.	Continue chest compressions coordinated with effective ventilation for at least 45 to 60 seconds before assessing heart rate.
	Note: The time for heart rate assessment has been increased from 30 seconds to 45 to 60 seconds because coronary perfusion drops every time compressions are interrupted.
	If heart rate remains <60 bpm after at least 45 to 60 seconds of chest compressions coordinated with effective ventilation, administer epinephrine.
	Insert emergency umbilical venous catheter for administration of epinephrine.
	The intratracheal route of epinephrine results in lower and less predictable blood levels that are often not effective, but this route is acceptable while the umbilical venous line is being placed.
	If the newborn appears to be in shock and is not responding to resuscitation, administration of a volume expander may be indicated.

Neonatal Resuscitation Program (NRP) 2011
A Brief Summary for Busy People

NRP 2006, 5th Edition	NRP 2011, 6th Edition
Use of Oxygen and Pulse Oximetry	**Use of Oxygen and Pulse Oximetry**
Use an oxygen blender and pulse oximeter when resuscitating babies less than approximately 32 weeks.	A compressed air source, an oxygen blender, and a pulse oximeter should be available in the immediate delivery area for every birth.
	There is ongoing controversy about how much oxygen to use during neonatal resuscitation.
For babies born at term, the NRP recommends 100% oxygen for cyanosis or when positive-pressure ventilation is required. Resuscitation with something less than 100% oxygen may be just as successful.	Resuscitation of term newborns may begin with 21% oxygen; resuscitation of preterm newborns may begin with a somewhat higher oxygen concentration.
If supplemental oxygen is unavailable, use room air to deliver positive-pressure ventilation.	Use pulse oximetry when
	• Resuscitation is anticipated
	• Positive-pressure ventilation is required for more than a few breaths
	• Central cyanosis is persistent, or you need to confirm your perception of central cyanosis
	• Supplemental oxygen is administered
	Oximetry can be helpful to assist in judging the accuracy of your assessment, but should not delay your resuscitation actions. Stabilization of ventilation, heart rate, and oxygenation should remain priorities.
	Place the oximeter probe on the newborn's right hand or wrist (measure pre-ductal saturation) and then connect it to the instrument.
	Using pulse oximetry, supplemental oxygen concentration should be adjusted to achieve the target values for pre-ductal saturations summarized in the table on the NRP flow diagram. The table is used for both term and preterm babies.
Using pulse oximetry for preterm newborns, target oxygen saturation is >95%.	Care should be taken to avoid oxygen saturation exceeding 95%.
If baby is breathing at birth, HR is >100 bpm, but cyanotic, give supplemental oxygen.	It may take up to 10 minutes for a healthy newborn to increase saturation to the normal range of over 90%. If persistent cyanosis is visible, confirm a low oxygen saturation with pulse oximetry and adjust the supplemental oxygen concentration to achieve the target values for pre-ductal saturations summarized in the table on the NRP flow diagram.
	Deleted: If the heart rate does not respond by increasing rapidly to >100 bpm, correct any ventilation problem and use 100% oxygen.
	Deleted: If there is no appreciable improvement within 90 seconds following birth, up to 100% supplemental oxygen should be administered.

Neonatal Resuscitation Program (NRP) 2011
A Brief Summary for Busy People

NRP 2006, 5th Edition	NRP 2011, 6th Edition
CPAP For preterm newborns, consider giving CPAP if the baby is breathing spontaneously and has a heart rate above 100 bpm, but appears to have labored respirations or is cyanotic or having low oxygen saturation.	**CPAP** Consider giving CPAP if a baby is breathing spontaneously and has a heart rate above 100 bpm, but has labored respirations, is cyanotic, or has low oxygen saturation (does not meet target saturation levels on the table in the NRP flow diagram). CPAP cannot be given with a self-inflating bag. CPAP skills are demonstrated on the DVD that accompanies the 6th edition of the textbook.
Positive-pressure ventilation Indications for positive-pressure ventilation <ul><li>Apnea/gasping</li><li>Heart rate less than 100 bpm, even if breathing</li><li>Persistent central cyanosis despite 100% free-flow oxygen</li></ul>	**Positive-pressure ventilation** Indications for positive-pressure ventilation: <ul><li>Apnea/gasping</li><li>Heart rate below 100 bpm, even if breathing</li><li>Persistent central cyanosis and low oxygen saturation, despite free-flow oxygen increased to 100%</li></ul>All positive-pressure devices, including the self-inflating bag, should have an integral pressure gauge, or if there is a site for attaching a pressure gauge (manometer), it should be attached. "Effective ventilation" is defined by the presence of <ul><li>Bilateral breath sounds</li><li>Chest movement (heart rate may rise without visible chest movement, especially in preterm newborns)</li></ul>Start with an inspiratory pressure of about 20 cm H_2O at a rate of about 40 to 60 breaths/minute. Avoid excessive chest movement. Use the lowest inflation pressure necessary to maintain a heart rate >100 bpm and a gradually improving oxygen saturation. Assess for rising heart rate and improving oxygen saturation (per pulse oximetry). If not evident (within 5 to 10 breaths), ask your assistant to assess bilateral breath sounds and chest movement. If these are not immediately evident, perform as many of the ventilation corrective steps as needed to achieve bilateral breath sounds and chest movement. The acronym "MR SOPA" may be used to remember the sequence of ventilation corrective steps. **M:** Adjust the **mask** on the face. **R: Reposition** the head to ensure an open airway.

NRP 2006, 5th Edition	NRP 2011, 6th Edition
	Re-attempt ventilation. If not effective,
	S: Suction the mouth and nose.
	O: Ventilate with the baby's mouth slightly **open** and lift the jaw forward.
	Re-attempt ventilation. If not effective,
	P: Gradually increase **pressure** every few breaths, (cautiously, and to a maximum of 40 cm H_2O), until there are bilateral breath sounds and visible chest movement.
	If ventilation attempt is still ineffective,
	A: Consider airway **alternative** (endotracheal tube or laryngeal mask airway).
	While administering effective positive-pressure ventilation, reassess respiratory effort, heart rate, and oxygen saturation continuously, or at least every 30 seconds.
	If the heart rate is more than 60 bpm but less than 100 bpm, continue to administer effective positive-pressure ventilation as long as the baby is showing steady improvement.
	If the heart rate is persistently more than 60 bpm but less than 100 bpm, ensure effective ventilation, call for additional expertise, and consider other complications such as a pneumothorax or hypovolemia.
	If heart rate is below 60 bpm despite 30 seconds of effective positive-pressure ventilation (defined by audible bilateral breath sounds and chest movement) begin chest compressions.
	Skills related to positive-pressure ventilation and MR SOPA are demonstrated on the DVD that accompanies the 6th edition of the textbook.
Chest Compressions	**Chest Compressions**
Chest compressions are indicated whenever the heart rate remains less than 60 bpm, despite 30 seconds of effective positive-pressure ventilation.	Ensure effective ventilation prior to beginning chest compressions.
	Chest compressions are indicated whenever the heart rate is below 60 bpm, despite at least 30 seconds of effective positive-pressure ventilation.
	The 2 techniques are the thumb technique and the 2-finger technique; however, the thumb technique is preferred and should be used in most situations.

Neonatal Resuscitation Program (NRP) 2011
A Brief Summary for Busy People

Neonatal Resuscitation Program (NRP) 2011
A Brief Summary for Busy People

NRP 2006, 5th Edition	NRP 2011, 6th Edition
	Use enough pressure to depress the sternum to a depth of approximately one-third of the anterior-posterior diameter of the chest.
	When the heart rate is below 60 bpm, the oximeter may not work. Increase the oxygen concentration to 100% until the oximeter is giving a reliable signal and can guide the appropriate adjustment of supplemental oxygen.
	Use 3 compressions plus 1 ventilation, resulting in approximately 120 "events" per 60 seconds (90 compressions plus 30 breaths).
Intubation when beginning chest compressions may help ensure adequate ventilation and facilitate the coordination of ventilation and chest compressions.	Intubation is strongly recommended when chest compressions begin to help ensure effective ventilation.
After 30 seconds of chest compressions and ventilation, check the heart rate.	Interruption of chest compressions to check the heart rate may result in a decrease of perfusion pressure in the coronary arteries. Therefore, continue chest compressions and coordinated ventilations *for at least 45 to 60 seconds* before stopping briefly to assess the heart rate.
	If perfusion is very low, the oximeter may not detect a consistent pulse. If the oximeter is functioning, or if you can feel the pulse easily at the base of the cord, you will not need to stop ventilation to determine the heart rate; otherwise, you will need to stop both compressions and ventilation for a few seconds to auscultate the heart rate.
	If you anticipate the need to place an emergency umbilical venous catheter, continue chest compressions by moving to the head of the bed (near the newborn's head) and continuing the thumb technique. This is most easily accomplished if the newborn is intubated.
	Discontinue chest compressions when the heart rate increases to above 60 bpm. Continue positive-pressure ventilations at 40 to 60 breaths/minute and assess heart rate, respiratory status, and oxygen saturation continuously, or at least every 30 seconds.
	When the heart rate rises >100 bpm and the newborn begins to breathe spontaneously, slow the ventilation rate and provide post-resuscitation care.
	Chest compressions being given from the head of the newborn are demonstrated on the DVD that accompanies the 6th edition of the textbook.

Neonatal Resuscitation Program (NRP) 2011
A Brief Summary for Busy People

NRP 2006, 5th Edition	NRP 2011, 6th Edition
Endotracheal Intubation	**Endotracheal Intubation**
Indications for intubation include:	Intubation Is recommended when:
• To suction the trachea in presence of meconium when the newborn is not vigorous • To improve efficacy of ventilation after several minutes of bag-and-mask ventilation or ineffective bag-and-mask ventilation • To facilitate coordination of chest compressions and ventilation and to maximize the efficiency of each ventilation • To administer epinephrine if required to stimulate the heart while IV access is being established	• Tracheal suctioning of the non-vigorous meconium-stained newborn is needed. • Positive-pressure ventilation does not result in adequate clinical improvement and ventilation with a mask is ineffective despite corrective efforts. • The need for positive-pressure ventilation lasts beyond a few minutes, to improve the efficacy and ease of assisted ventilation. • Chest compressions are necessary, to facilitate coordination of ventilations and compressions and maximize the efficiency of each positive-pressure breath. • Special indications occur, such as extreme prematurity, surfactant administration, or suspected diaphragmatic hernia.
The intubation procedure ideally should be completed within 20 seconds.	The intubation procedure ideally should be completed within 30 seconds.
The correct-sized laryngoscope blade for a term newborn is No. 1. The correct-sized blade for a preterm newborn is No. 0.	The blade of a laryngoscope should be No. 1 for term newborns, No. 0 for preterm newborns, and No. 00 for extremely preterm newborns.
	Intubation and a method for securing the tube are demonstrated on the DVD that accompanies the 6th edition of the textbook.
Laryngeal Mask Airway	**Laryngeal Mask Airway**
Laryngeal mask airway information is in an Appendix to Lesson 5 and does not include a Performance Checklist.	Laryngeal mask airway information is incorporated into the main body of Lesson 5 and included on the Lesson 5 Performance Checklist.
	The laryngeal mask airway has been shown to be an effective alternative for assisting ventilation.
	Use may be indicated when
	• Facial or upper airway malformations render ventilation by mask ineffective. • Positive-pressure ventilation with a face mask fails to achieve effective ventilation and intubation is not possible.
	The laryngeal mask airway has these limitations:
	• Currently available devices are too large for small preterm babies or those less than about 32 weeks' gestation. • The device cannot be used to suction meconium from the airway.

Neonatal Resuscitation Program (NRP) 2011
A Brief Summary for Busy People

NRP 2006, 5th Edition	NRP 2011, 6th Edition
	• An air leak at the mask-larynx interface may result in insufficient pressure to the lungs. • There is insufficient evidence to recommend using the laryngeal mask airway to administer intratracheal medications. • There is insufficient evidence to recommend the laryngeal mask airway for prolonged assisted ventilation in newborns. Before deflating the cuff and removing the laryngeal mask airway, suction secretions from the mouth and throat. Laryngeal mask airway placement is demonstrated on the DVD that accompanies the 6th edition of the textbook.
Epinephrine Epinephrine, a cardiac stimulant, is indicated when the heart rate remains below 60 bpm, despite 30 seconds of assisted ventilation followed by another 30 seconds of coordinated chest compressions and ventilations.	**Epinephrine** If the heart rate remains below 60 bpm despite ongoing ventilation and chest compressions, your first action is to ensure that ventilation and compressions are being given optimally. Epinephrine is indicated when the heart rate remains below 60 bpm after 30 seconds of effective assisted ventilation (preferably via endotracheal tube) and at least another 45 to 60 seconds of coordinated chest compressions and effective ventilation.
The endotracheal route is often faster and more accessible than placing an umbilical catheter, but is associated with unreliable absorption and may not be effective at the lower dose.	The intratracheal route is associated with unreliable absorption and is likely to be ineffective. Nevertheless, since the endotracheal route is the most readily accessible, administration of a dose of epinephrine via an endotracheal tube may be considered while the intravenous route is being established. The umbilical venous route is the preferred route of drug administration. The intraosseous approach may be a reasonable alternative route for vascular access for those trained in the technique. There are limited data regarding the delivery of medications via intraosseous lines in newborns, particularly preterm newborns. Recommended concentration: 1:10,000 (0.1 mg/mL) Recommended route: Intravenous (umbilical vein). Consider endotracheal route ONLY while IV access being obtained Give rapidly—as quickly as possible. Recommended IV dose: 0.1-0.3 mL/kg of 1:10,000 solution per umbilical vein in a 1-mL syringe.

Neonatal Resuscitation Program (NRP) 2011
A Brief Summary for Busy People

NRP 2006, 5th Edition	NRP 2011, 6th Edition
Recommended intratracheal dose: *0.3 to 1 mL/kg* of 1:10,000 solution.	Follow IV administration of epinephrine with 0.5 to 1 mL flush of normal saline.
	Recommended intratracheal dose: *0.5 to 1 mL/kg* of 1:10,000 solution per endotracheal tube in a 3- to 6-mL syringe.
	Check the newborn heart rate about 1 minute after administering epinephrine (longer if given endotracheally). Epinephrine dose may be repeated every 3 to 5 minutes.
	Administration of epinephrine is demonstrated on the DVD that accompanies the 6th edition of the textbook.
Volume Administration	**Volume Administration**
Indications for volume expansion include	Indications for volume expansion include
Baby is not responding to resuscitation AND Baby appears in shock AND There is a history of fetal blood loss	Newborn is not responding to resuscitation AND Newborn appears in shock OR There is a history of a condition associated with fetal blood loss.
	Note: Volume might be considered even if there has not been obvious blood loss, but bradycardia persists.
	Recommended volume expander
	Solution: Normal saline, Ringer's lactate, or O Rh-negative packed red blood cells Dose: 10 mL/kg Route: Umbilical vein Preparation: Correct volume in large syringe Rate: Over 5 to 10 minutes
Special Considerations	**Special Considerations**
No information regarding therapeutic hypothermia.	Therapeutic hypothermia following perinatal asphyxia should be
	Used only for babies ≥36 weeks' gestation and who meet previously defined criteria for this therapy Initiated before 6 hours after birth Used only by centers with specialized programs equipped to provide the therapy

Neonatal Resuscitation Program (NRP) 2011

A Brief Summary for Busy People

NRP 2006, 5th Edition	NRP 2011, 6th Edition
	No significant changes in the *Textbook of Neonatal Resuscitation, 6th Edition,* for resuscitation recommendations for • Choanal atresia • Robin syndrome • Pneumothorax • Diaphragmatic hernia • Persistent cyanosis and bradycardia • Post-resuscitation care • Use of sodium bicarbonate 4.2% • Use of naloxone 1.0 mg/mL solution • Resuscitation of the newborn outside the delivery room
Resuscitation of Babies Born Preterm Additional resources needed to prepare for an anticipated preterm birth include: Additional trained personnel, including intubation expertise	**Resuscitation of Babies Born Preterm** Additional resources needed to prepare for an anticipated preterm birth include: • Additional trained personnel, including someone with intubation and emergency umbilical venous catheterization expertise If your hospital does not routinely care for preterm babies who require ongoing assisted ventilation, you will need to arrange transfer to an appropriate facility.

To help keep the preterm baby warm,
 	
    Increase the temperature of the delivery room.
 	
    If the baby is born at less than 28 weeks' gestation, consider placing him, below the neck, in a recloseable polyethylene bag.
 	
    Place a portable warming pad under the layers of towels on the resuscitation table.
	To help keep the preterm baby warm,
	
	• Increase the temperature of the delivery room and the area where the baby will be resuscitated to approximately 25°C to 26°C (77°F to 79°F)
	• Use polyethylene plastic wrap for babies delivered at less than 29 weeks' gestation (or 28 weeks and less). Use a sheet of plastic food wrap, a food-grade 1-gallon plastic bag, or a commercially available sheet of polyethylene plastic.
	• Place a portable warming pad under layers of towels on the resuscitation table.
	
	Delivery room management of the extremely low birthweight (ELBW) newborn is demonstrated on the DVD that accompanies the 6th edition of the textbook.

Neonatal Resuscitation Program (NRP) 2011
A Brief Summary for Busy People

NRP 2006, 5th Edition	NRP 2011, 6th Edition
Ethics and Care at the End of Life	Ethics and Care at the End of Life
	In many states, if the mother is a minor, she is considered "emancipated" and can legally make decisions about her fetus and newborn, but not necessarily for herself. Usually, the baby's father also has specific legal rights with regard to the baby, but only if he is married to the mother, or is listed as the father on the official birth certificate. Check the regulations for your specific state.
Unless conception occurred via in vitro fertilization, techniques used for obstetrical dating are accurate only to ±1 to 2 weeks.	Unless conception occurred via in vitro fertilization, techniques used for obstetric dating are accurate to 3 to 5 days if applied in the first trimester, and only to ±1 to 2 weeks subsequently. Estimates of fetal weight are accurate only to ±15 to 20%.
Discontinuation of resuscitation efforts may be appropriate after 10 minutes of absent heart rate following complete and adequate resuscitation efforts.	Discontinuation of resuscitation efforts should be considered after 10 minutes of absent heart rate. The decision to continue resuscitation efforts beyond 10 minutes beyond this point should take into consideration factors such as the presumed etiology of the arrest, the gestational age of the baby, the presence or absence of complications, the potential role of therapeutic hypothermia, and the parents' previously expressed feelings about acceptable risk of morbidity.
	Parents should be urged to direct questions directly to the obstetric provider regarding concerns they may have about events and care before birth; providers responsible for pediatric care should be careful not to make comments that might be considered judgmental about obstetric care.

Neonatal Resuscitation Program (NRP) Revisions 2011
A Brief Summary for Busy People

Information for NRP Instructors

1. One important goal of the revised NRP education methodology is to have the majority of instructor-participant interaction focused on hands-on learning, immersive simulations, and constructive debriefings. To achieve this goal, participants self-study the *Textbook of Neonatal Resuscitation, 6th Edition,* and/or the accompanying DVD. The instructor is available to assist learners if necessary as they prepare for online testing and the NRP course. Class time is used for review and practice of technical skills and simulation training. Instructors no longer use slides and lecture during an NRP course to repeat content from the textbook that learners should have already mastered.

2. Every learner takes an NRP Provider Course. There is no longer an NRP Renewal Course. The NRP instructor tailors the core elements of each course to suit the learning objectives of the trainees.

3. Neonatal Resuscitation Program provider status is maintained by taking an NRP Provider Course every 2 years. Each institution determines its own policy regarding what happens if a person's NRP provider status expires.

4. Students may take the minimum requirements of the NRP course (Lessons 1 through 4 and Lesson 9) or take additional lessons as determined by professional responsibilities and/or hospital policy. Each learner may receive credit for practicing every skill in the course; however, the NRP course does not certify the learner to perform any resuscitation technique. Course participants should not exceed their scope of practice as defined by their professional governing body and institutional job descriptions.

5. The 5th edition written test and online evaluation may be used until December 31, 2011. After that time, the 6th edition online examination must be used. There will be no hard copy examination available after December 2011.

6. The 6th edition online NRP examination must be passed by each course participant in the 30 days *before* the NRP course. Continuing education credit is offered to nurses, physicians, respiratory therapists, and emergency medical services personnel.

7. HealthStream is the vendor for the 6th edition NRP online examination. The fee for the examination varies depending on how many examinations are purchased and how the examination is accessed. If your institution uses HealthStream as its Learning Management System, your learners may receive the examination in the same way other hospital learning programs are obtained. If your institution is not a HealthStream client, you may purchase online examinations in small- or large-volume purchases. HealthStream will set up a Web site for your use. Individuals may also purchase an online examination with a personal credit card. For more information, visit **www.aap.org/nrp** and click on "Online Examination".

8. Components of the NRP Provider Course:

   a. Self-study the textbook and pass the online examination in the 30 days before the course (required).

   b. Performance Skills Stations are an opportunity to discuss, practice, and review technical skills (optional). Most learners benefit from review and practice of technical skills such as Equipment Check, Initial Steps, Positive-pressure Ventilation, etc. After review and practice, the learner demonstrates the skill in the context of a brief scenario, starting with Equipment Check and proceeding through the target Performance Skills Station, such as Chest Compressions.

Neonatal Resuscitation Program (NRP) Revisions 2011
A Brief Summary for Busy People

Information for NRP Instructors, continued

c. The Integrated Skills station is an evaluative component of the Provider Course (required). The learner demonstrates the technical skills necessary to resuscitate a newborn using proper technique and in sequence of the NRP flow diagram, with no guidance or coaching from the instructor. The Integrated Skills Station is not formally scored. If significant errors are made, the learner returns to the Performance Skill Station for additional practice.

d. Simulation and Debriefing focuses on improving communication and teamwork (required). Simulation-based learning encourages learners to "suspend disbelief" and act as they would in an actual resuscitation. Simulation allows learners to work through high risk situations in a safe learning environment. Students to actively engage in the learning process, then reflect on the experience and critically evaluate their actions.

9. Simulation training is dependent on good methodology, not technology; therefore, sophisticated electronic simulators are not necessary.

10. You have the option of using a printer to print the student's name, course completion date, and renewal date directly on to the card, which is sent to the instructor by mail after roster approval. A print template is available online at **www.aap.org/nrp**.

11. Neonatal Resuscitation Program Instructor Maintenance Requirements (includes regional trainers)

a. Simulation and debriefing skills are new to most NRP instructors. Each current NRP instructor must own a personal copy of the *NRP Instructor DVD: An Interactive Tool for Facilitation of Simulation-based Learning* and complete the post-DVD education activity by January 1, 2012.

b. Each instructor must teach or co-teach at least 2 courses in the 2 years for which their instructor card is valid.

c. Beginning in January 2013, every NRP instructor must take the online examination (Lessons 1 through 9) prior to their instructor status renewal date. Beginning in spring 2011, every instructor may take the online examination once/calendar year if desired at no charge; however, continuing education credit may be awarded only once every 2 years.

12. Neonatal Resuscitation Program Instructor eligibility

a. Only registered nurses (including NNPs, CNMs, etc), physicians (MD or DO), respiratory therapists, and physician assistants are eligible to become NRP instructors. There are no exceptions and no waivers. Professionals who became NRP instructors by waiver in the past will maintain their instructor status as long as maintenance requirements are met.

b. Neonatal Resuscitation Program instructor candidates are required to meet prerequisites prior to their NRP Instructor Course. Instructor candidates must have current NRP provider status (Lessons 1 through 9), produce a letter of recommendation and support from their manager/hospital administrator, pass the 6th edition online examination in the 30 days before their Instructor Course (Lessons 1 through 9), and watch the NRP Instructor DVD and complete the post-DVD education activity, and should take the Instructor Self-assessment, which is included in the NRP Instructor Manual.

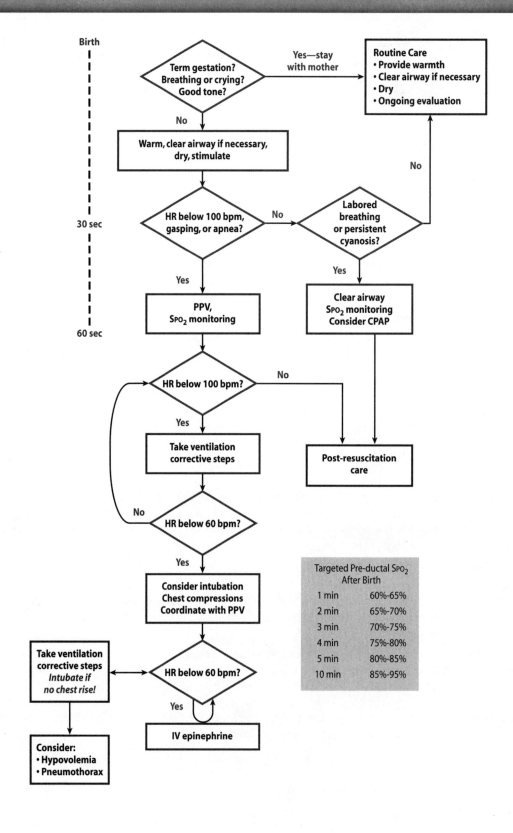

Birth

Term gestation?
Breathing or crying?
Good tone?

Yes—stay
with mother

Routine Care
• Provide warmth
• Clear airway if necessary
• Dry
• Ongoing evaluation

No

Warm, clear airway if necessary,
dry, stimulate

30 sec

HR below 100 bpm,
gasping, or apnea?

No

Labored
breathing
or persistent
cyanosis?

No

Yes

Yes

60 sec

PPV,
Spo₂ monitoring

Clear airway
Spo₂ monitoring
Consider CPAP

HR below 100 bpm?

No

Yes

**Take ventilation
corrective steps**

**Post-resuscitation
care**

No

HR below 60 bpm?

Yes

**Consider intubation
Chest compressions
Coordinate with PPV**

Targeted Pre-ductal Spo₂ After Birth	
1 min	60%-65%
2 min	65%-70%
3 min	70%-75%
4 min	75%-80%
5 min	80%-85%
10 min	85%-95%

**Take ventilation
corrective steps**
*Intubate if
no chest rise!*

HR below 60 bpm?

Yes

Consider:
• Hypovolemia
• Pneumothorax

IV epinephrine

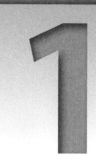

Neonatal Resuscitation Program™: Past, Present, and Future

While the mastery of knowledge and skills necessary to perform neonatal resuscitation is essential for becoming an instructor, the knowledgeable instructor also knows the historical origin of the Neonatal Resuscitation Program (NRP™), how practice guidelines originate, the philosophy behind the education methodology, and what changes are anticipated for the future.

Chapter 1 presents the opportunity to read a 2008 article by Louis Halamek, Stanford University neonatologist and past co-chairperson of the American Academy of Pediatrics (AAP) NRP Steering Committee. This succinct and thought-provoking piece lays the foundation for what NRP instructors need to know about the origin, past history, and continuing adaptations of the program that we support as the national standard for neonatal resuscitation training.

In Chapter 1 you will learn about the

- Origin and goals of the NRP

- Guiding principles of the NRP

- Changing role of the NRP instructor and learner

- Shift from passive learning to interactive learning through simulation-based training

- Evolving plans for the NRP of the future

The Genesis, Adaptation, and Evolution of the Neonatal Resuscitation Program

Louis P. Halamek, MD*

*Division of Neonatal and Developmental Medicine, Department of Pediatrics, Stanford University, Palo Alto, Calif.

educational perspectives e142 NeoReviews Vol.9 No.4 April 2008

Abstract

For more than 2 decades, the Neonatal Resuscitation Program (NRP) of the American Academy of Pediatrics (AAP) has set a national standard and international example for training in the resuscitation of the newborn. The concept of a standardized approach to neonatal resuscitation, based on the best available evidence, was revolutionary in 1987 when the NRP was officially launched. Because the NRP continues to adapt, it remains one of the most successful educational interventions in health care. This article describes its genesis, continuing adaptation, and prospects for evolution in the next decade.

Genesis

"To emphasize that in every area where a delivery might occur (delivery room, emergency department, etc.,) there be at least one person available who has acquired the basic and/or advanced resuscitation skills." (1)

As the subspecialty of neonatology grew in the 1960s and 1970s and neonatal intensive care units sprang up in hospitals across the United States, health-care professionals working in these units recognized the need to develop a consistent approach to caring for neonates transitioning from an intrauterine to an extrauterine existence. In the 1980s, the Committee on the Fetus and Newborn and the Section of Perinatal Pediatrics of the AAP made training in neonatal resuscitation a national priority and established the Resuscitation of the Newborn Task Force led by George Peckham, MD (Table 1). This task force set a goal of having at least one professional trained in neonatal resuscitation at every delivery in the country. They built on the work of Ronald Bloom, MD, and Catherine Cropley, RN, MN, who, while working at the Drew Postgraduate Medical School in Los Angeles, received a grant from the National Institutes of Health to create the Neonatal Education Program (NEP) that subsequently served as the basis for the NRP. Errol Alden, MD, then Director of Education at the AAP, spearheaded the establishment of a formal relationship with Leon Chameides, MD, John

Raye, MD, and others at the American Heart Association (AHA) and other national organizations (Table 2) to facilitate expert review of the contents of the NRP and develop a strategy for its dissemination throughout the country. After extensive discussion, planning, and preparation, NRP was officially launched in 1987.

From the very first program, it was clear that the NRP would need to be sufficiently flexible to adapt readily to the changing needs of a diverse population of trainees. Key guiding principles built into the program included:

1) *Base practice recommendations on the best available evidence.* Although many aspects of neonatal resuscitation are based on rational conjecture because of the paucity of available data, those guiding the development of the NRP always have striven to achieve consensus among experts in the field regarding clinical practice recommendations. Informal at first, this process has become international in scope through the International Liaison Committee on Resuscitation (ILCOR).

2) *Recognize the different types of skills necessary for successful neonatal resuscitation.* The various professionals caring for the newborn in the delivery room have different levels of responsibility and, therefore, must possess different skill sets. The modular nature of the NEP, which was focused on specific content knowledge and hands-on skills, was carried over in development of the NRP, which has allowed the NRP to adapt to the specific needs of individual trainees yet remain relevant to the entire resuscitation team.

3) *Understand the importance of self-education for the adult learner.* Another unique aspect of the training methodology used in NRP is its self-instructional design. Although the clinical experience of the instructors is recognized as a valuable resource for trainees, the NRP is designed so that groups or individuals may benefit from its content and trainees can use the materials during independent study to prepare for group training activities.

4) *Adequately prepare instructors.* Heavy emphasis initially was placed on establishing groups of highly trained, geographically distributed instructors. These national and regional instructors trained additional instructors, who delivered NRP to the many professionals at healthcare facilities throughout the country. Formal training materials for NRP instructors were developed to facilitate this process.

5) *Regionalize training.* The system whereby national instructors taught regional instructors, who then trained Hospital-based Instructors, allowed the NRP to be rolled out in a controlled and efficient manner. Not limiting instructors to a specific facility or training center allows them to deliver NRP to trainees throughout their region, not just at their local institution.

Since its inception in 1987, the NRP has enjoyed tremendous success: More than 2,200,000 trainees have experienced NRP, as taught by more than 27,000 instructors in the United States alone. NRP training materials have been well received and have won several awards for innovative contributions to healthcare education and training. The NRP provider manual has been translated into 25 languages, and NRP has been taught in 124 different countries around the world.* The acceptance of NRP has been so profound that the program serves as a cornerstone of the international efforts of the AAP. In fact, the AAP's Office of International Affairs is headed by William Keenan, MD, one of the founders of the NRP, who was named a "Giant of Resuscitation" by ILCOR and the AHA in 2005. (2)

Adaptation

Despite 2 decades of resounding success, the NRP has had to adapt continually to stay relevant and provide an optimal learning experience for its trainees. One of the most obvious examples of this adaptation lies in the regular re-evaluation of the clinical guidelines adopted by the NRP. Despite regional and national differences in the approach to neonatal resuscitation, it has been recognized that newborns around the world exhibit many similar pathophysiologies. ILCOR began an effort in 1992 to address the need for closer international collaboration on issues involving neonatal, pediatric, and adult cardiopulmonary resuscitation and emergency cardiovascular care. (3) It is comprised of various delegations (neonatal, pediatric, adult) representing the AHA, the Heart and Stroke Foundation of Canada, the Inter American Heart Foundation, the European Resuscitation Council, the Australian and New Zealand Committee on Resuscitation, and the Resuscitation Councils of Southern Africa. (4) Every 5 years, the neonatal delegation identifies important questions pertinent to newborn resuscitation, reviews the available evidence, reaches consensus as to the best evidence-based answers to these questions, and posts this review online. (5) Groups such as the Steering Committee of the NRP then generate nation- and region-specific guidelines for clinical care based on this review of the science and publish these in major peer-reviewed journals. (6)

Table 1. **Original Members of the Resuscitation of the Newborn Task Force**

Ronald Bloom, MD	George Peckham, MD
Frederic Burg, MD	Alan Schwartz, MD
Gregory Carroll, PhD	Kit Stahler, MD
William Fox, MD	William Taeusch, MD
Charles Gibbs, MD	

*2011 statistics: More than 2,700,000 trainees have experienced NRP, as taught by more than 28,000 instructors. The program has been translated into 26 languages and has been taught in 130 different countries.

Table 2. Founding Members of the NRP

Errol Alden, MD	John Kattwinkel, MD
Ronald Bloom, MD	William Keenan, MD
David Burchfield, MD	George Peckham, MD
Leon Chameides, MD	John Raye, MD
Catherine Cropley, RN, MN	

Of course, the mission of the NRP is not limited to simply disseminating clinical guidelines; it also provides the learning tools to facilitate acquisition of not only the content knowledge but also the technical skills required to implement the clinical guidelines. The debut of NRP in 1987 represented the first time that clinical guidelines had been listed, vetted, and delivered in a coherent, efficient, and effective manner on a national scale. Since that time, under the leadership of the NRP Steering Committee, the program has continued to be on the cutting edge of professional education and training. A number of innovative educational tools were released in its most recent iteration (2005), including:

- *The Textbook of Neonatal Resuscitation.* 5th ed

- *Textbook of Neonatal Resuscitation Multimedia* CDROM

- *Cases in Neonatal Resuscitation* DVD

- *Ethics and Care at the End of Life: Involving Parents in Ethical Decision Making* DVD

The textbook contains a wealth of content information and is liberally illustrated with line drawings and photos. (7) The CDROM accompanying the textbook contains a large number of illustrations, photographs, and videos that map to specific chapters in the textbook. Such multimedia elements create a much more immersive learning experience for trainees by allowing them to manipulate images almost as they would real physical objects. The DVD containing cases in neonatal resuscitation allows the trainee to enter a clinical scenario, choose a course of action from a list of possible interventions, and witness the results of his or her choices; each choice is followed by feedback from an on-screen virtual mentor during a short debriefing. The final DVD depicts a difficult ethical situation, that of impending delivery of a preterm neonate at the limits of viability in a community hospital, and draws the trainee into the scenario via a series of "teachable moments." In sum, these materials provide a rich source of content that can be used to enhance the learning opportunities of both individuals and groups.

Content knowledge can be assessed by completion of an online examination that can be taken at the trainee's convenience. This demands that trainees assume responsibility for their own education;

they no longer can expect instructors to "spoon feed" didactic material to them in just the right amount to allow them to complete the written examination successfully. By raising the expectations placed on trainees for thorough advance preparation (as documented by successful completion of the online examination), instructors can use their time with trainees to provide learning opportunities that are much richer and more interactive than lectures and proctored written examinations.

Historically, the emphasis of NRP has been on assimilation of content knowledge and demonstration of the technical skills necessary for neonatal resuscitation. Yet, content knowledge and technical skills alone are insufficient for the delivery of optimal care while working as a team under intense time pressure. Behavioral skills, such as effective communication, teamwork, and leadership, also are critically important during crises such as resuscitation of the newborn, yet little attention has been paid to training methodologies that facilitate acquisition of such skills (Table 3). The Joint Commission published a *Sentinel Event Alert* in 2004 that found ineffective communication to play a role in almost 75% of the cases of neonatal mortality or severe neonatal morbidity reported to that agency. (8) It subsequently recommended that all health-care organizations responsible for delivering newborns establish a system of training that incorporates behavioral skills such as teamwork and effective communication and regularly conduct clinical drills followed by constructive debriefings. The NRP has begun to address the importance of behavioral skills and other elements of crew resource management strategy (first developed by the commercial aviation industry in an effort to improve safety) by incorporating some of these concepts into the learning objectives of the NRP. (9)(10)(11)

All of these developments point to a new emphasis on learning (and the adult learner) rather than teaching (and the teacher). Realization that not everything that is taught necessarily is learned is ending the days of "death by PowerPoint" in which instructors unfamiliar with the material simply read what is on the slides and move on to the next

Table 3. Key Behavioral Skills

1) Know your environment.
2) Anticipate and plan.
3) Assume the leadership role.
4) Communicate effectively.
5) Delegate workload optimally.
6) Allocate attention wisely.
7) Use all available information.
8) Use all available resources.
9) Call for help when needed.
10) Maintain professional behavior.

exercise. An appreciation for the tenets of adult learning is producing more interactive, intellectually stimulating environments in which the instructor functions to facilitate rather than dominate the learning process. (12)

Keeping instructors informed of recent developments is a mandatory component of the NRP. To facilitate communication with its 27,000 instructors* the NRP publishes a semiannual *NRP Instructor Update* that is downloadable from the NRP's website. (13) This is complemented by the opportunity to interact with NRP Steering Committee members at the NRP Current Issues Seminar held annually immediately prior to the AAP's National Conference and Exhibition. Each seminar is developed around a central theme deemed timely for instructors, and summaries of recent basic science and clinical medicine topics pertinent to neonatal resuscitation are presented. Breakout sessions allow instructors to focus on topics of special interest. All of the presentations (in PDF) are available on the NRP website for downloading.

Another novel and very successful aspect of the NRP is the NRP Grant Program. (14) Since its initiation in 1994, it has funded more than 35 studies† conducted by investigators from the United States and other countries. Both established and new ("Young Investigator") researchers are encouraged to apply. This mechanism has proven very effective for stimulating research in areas deemed to be of high priority to the community of clinicians and investigators interested in resuscitation of the newborn.

New Challenges

Despite tremendous efforts to generate evidence-based clinical guidelines, gaps remain in knowledge of the physiology and treatment of the patient in need of resuscitation. The Pediatric Advanced Life Support (PALS) program of the AHA provides training in advanced cardiac life support for children. It, too, has gained wide acceptance in the United States as the standard for pediatric (non-neonatal) resuscitation. The NRP recommends a compression-to-breath ratio of 3 compressions to 1 breath for all newborns (in the presence of single or multiple rescuers), but the PALS program recommends a ratio of 30:2 for all patients, except newborns, when a single rescuer is present. (15)(16)(17) Thus, the questions arise: How does one define what constitutes a newborn, and when should health-care professionals follow NRP guidelines and when should they follow PALS guidelines? It is likely that the degree of granularity of the supporting data never will be sufficient to produce a precise answer (especially given the difficulty in conducting prospective, randomized, controlled clinical trials in neonatal and pediatric resuscitation), and anyone wishing for an answer that has an absolute cutoff (involving both gestational and chronologic ages) is likely to be disappointed. Similar uncertainties exist regarding

*2011 statistics: 28,000 instructors
†The NRP Grant Program has funded more than 55 studies

the relative utility of endotracheal intubation versus the laryngeal mask airway and emergency umbilical venous cannulation versus intraosseous access. However, consensus may be possible to achieve, if based only on rational conjecture, as to how to proceed. For example, it makes sense to consider not just the patient's gestational and chronologic ages, but also the underlying pathophysiology when deciding what resuscitation guidelines to follow in particular clinical situations. This means that health-care professionals caring for growing preterm infants, sick term infants undergoing prolonged hospitalization, and patients in the first postnatal weeks presenting in extremis to emergency departments and clinics require accurate diagnostic skills and familiarity with a range of potential therapies. This is likely to be an active area of basic science and clinical investigation in the years to come. In the meantime, health-care professionals need to exercise their best judgment when faced with situations for which clear clinical guidelines do not exist.

Historically, trainees and instructors alike have expected some percentage of face-to-face time during the training program to be dedicated to didactic instruction for content knowledge to be "passed" from instructor to trainee. This expectation is not in line with adult education theory that emphasizes active participation by trainees. Despite efforts by the NRP Steering Committee to recommend limiting the time spent in passive exercises such as lecture, data presented at the 2007 NRP Seminar by Gary Weiner, MD, confirm that many instructors continue to devote an inordinate amount of time to lecturing. (18) Results of a national survey of NRP instructors indicate that most spend the greatest percentage of time in a NRP provider course using slides to lecture on the content information *already included* in the NRP provider manual. This same group of instructors, when asked to rate the effectiveness of various learning methodologies, indicated that they felt lectures were relatively *ineffective*. To create a more interactive and productive learning experience, the responsibility for acquisition of content knowledge must shift from the instructor to the trainee, and time spent in lecture (reviewing material that theoretically already should have been mastered by trainees) will need to be de-emphasized further or eliminated entirely.

Successful completion of NRP provider training requires achieving the minimum passing score on a multiple-choice written examination of content knowledge and demonstration of pertinent technical or procedural skills on task trainers while being observed by an instructor. The text on the NRP provider card given to those completing the program states that the holder of the card "has successfully completed the national cognitive and skills evaluations indicated on the reverse side in accordance with the curriculum of the American Academy of Pediatrics/American Heart Association Neonatal Resuscitation

Program." The *Textbook of Neonatal Resuscitation* states, "Completion of the program does not imply that an individual has the competence to perform neonatal resuscitation. Each hospital is responsible for determining the level of competence and qualifications required for someone to assume clinical responsibility for neonatal resuscitation." (19) Nowhere does material issued by the NRP claim that an individual who has successfully completed the program is competent to resuscitate real newborns at the time of delivery. Despite the cautionary stance taken by the NRP and the AAP, it is common to hear or see the words "certified in NRP" or "NRP-certified" used in reference to successful completion of the NRP by individuals outside of the NRP Steering Committee and its staff and liaisons. Although no one argues that participation in a well-run NRP training session is harmful, certainly there is potential harm in interpreting possession of a course completion card as indicative of competence in the real delivery room. The NRP never was intended to be used as a measure of the competence of health-care professionals (especially those already experienced in neonatal resuscitation); rather, it was developed to facilitate acquisition of the elemental content knowledge and technical skills necessary to resuscitate a newborn. In the absence of data indicating that professionals experiencing the NRP perform at a higher level when caring for real patients when compared with non-NRP-trained individuals (and also that the patients cared for by such professionals have better outcomes), the relationship between successful completion of the NRP and trainee competence remains hypothetical. Better delineation of this relationship requires the development of more realistic training scenarios and reliable performance metrics.

Many hospitals in the United States have policies mandating successful completion of the NRP and possession of an active NRP provider card as a condition for employment for any health-care professional bearing responsibility for the direct care of newborns. This is certainly laudable, but creates a paradox: To remain in compliance with their own policies and facilitate participation by what may be hundreds of staff in NRP on a biennial basis, hospitals often must limit severely the time allotted for training so that all staff may take (and pass) the written test and demonstrate technical skills to an instructor. This focus on compliance rather than achievement of learning objectives by trainees is misplaced and diminishes the value of the training.

Evolution

The NRP will continue to evolve, both in content and in process, to meet the needs of the professionals looking to it for support. Development of a career-long learning program in neonatal resuscitation that is relevant to professionals from multiple disciplines at all levels of experience and is embedded with robust learning opportunities and valid performance metrics is the focus of the NRP. Accomplishing this requires a change in the very culture of healthcare education and training. Elements of this culture change necessarily include:

- Extending evidence-based practice to education and training practices and adopting strategies that follow from adult learning theory.

- Transitioning the role of teacher to that of a facilitator of learning and empowering the learner to take control of his or her own education.

- Moving from a model of sporadic or intermittent "bolus" training to one that facilitates learning on a continuous basis throughout a career.

- Embracing high-fidelity, high-stakes simulation-based training as the standard in preparation for and assessment of performance in the real environment.

- Encouraging development of challenging training experiences and expecting and accepting failure during these experiences so trainees may learn from their mistakes.

- Focusing on staff competency rather than regulatory compliance.

Reviewing available evidence and reaching international consensus under the auspices of ILCOR continues to be an effective method of generating guidelines for clinical care, and this methodology soon will be extended to guidelines for education and training. It is anticipated that education and training guidelines addressing the optimal methods for facilitation and assessment of learning will be published in 2010 alongside clinical guidelines as part of the ILCOR process.

The stage is being set for a major shift in learning methodology within the NRP. This shift alters the role of an instructor from someone who *imparts* knowledge and skill *to* the trainees to one who *facilitates* acquisition of such knowledge and skills *by* the trainees. Such a shift demands that trainees play an active role in assuming responsibility for their progress and that instructors cede control of the learning process to the trainees. The Instructor Development Task Force began meeting in early 2007 to plan how to prepare NRP instructors for this major shift and create the learning materials that will be required to support instructors in their new role.

Participation in NRP currently is recommended on a biennial basis as a single isolated training experience. Renewal of NRP provider status (commonly and incorrectly referred to as "recertification") typically is a single experience consisting of several hours of training that involves the NRP written examination, technical skills stations, and a

"Megacode," in which trainees are required to integrate all of their knowledge and skills. The NRP Steering Committee recognizes that even though a single training experience once every 2 years facilitates compliance with institutional policies, it often is not consistent with achieving optimal educational outcomes. Thus, the NRP is poised to transition to a career-long learning model in which trainees are required to review different aspects of neonatal resuscitation regularly using an assortment of learning methodologies. This requires development of new learning materials, many of which will be accessible online from anywhere in the world where internet access is available. Such availability will allow rapid updating of content to reflect new evidence, embedding many more visual and auditory cues into training materials to stimulate learning, and creating a large database of challenging interactive case-based learning modules, replete with references, that will prove valuable to even the most experienced of delivery room professionals.

Simulation-based training, where trainees are immersed in highly realistic re-creations of actual real-life clinical events, will play a major role in the evolution of NRP. This type of training has been used successfully for decades in a number of other industries where the risk to human life is high. Although relatively new to the health-care field in general, work has been ongoing in simulation-based training in neonatal resuscitation at the Center for Advanced Pediatric & Perinatal Education at Packard Children's Hospital at Stanford for more than 10 years, and this effort and others have led to a number of methodologic and technologic innovations that will transform training in neonatal resuscitation radically. (20)(21) Such hands-on, practical training can be conducted either in the real clinical environment or physical space equipped to replicate the real environment with a high level of fidelity.

Mastery of the technical skills required for successful resuscitation of the newborn requires not only an understanding of when those skills should be used but also the ability to interpret visual, auditory, and tactile cues to perform the appropriate manual tasks in the correct sequence. Although technical skills may improve with increasing clinical activity in the real delivery room caring for real patients, it is also possible (and preferable) to acquire and maintain such skills on suitable models (human patient simulators). Such models need to possess a level of fidelity similar enough to a real human newborn that the important cues are presented accurately to the trainee, allowing achievement of learning objectives. To date, most human neonatal models have had a low level of anatomic fidelity and little or no ability to represent the physiologic alterations intrinsic to the neonate in distress. To stimulate interest in development of a realistic human neonatal patient simulator, a list of characteristics was drawn up and vetted by the NRP Steering Committee and published online in 2005 as a request for proposals (RFP) to industry. This was a seminal moment in patient simulator history, marking the first time that development of a highly realistic patient simulator was driven by the learning objectives put forth by a professional body rather than by the internal marketing imperatives of industry. This RFP now functions as an open invitation to industry that should guide initiatives in this field for years to come and provide NRP trainees and instructors with tools to facilitate the acquisition and refinement of the cognitive, technical, and behavioral skills necessary for successful resuscitation of the newborn.

Achieving high scores on examinations of knowledge and skill long has been expected of health-care professionals. Indeed, successful completion of the NRP requires achieving a minimum passing score on a multiple-choice written examination and successfully performing various technical skills, such as bag-mask ventilation and chest compressions, while under the watchful gaze of an instructor. Failure, when it occurs, is seen uniformly as a negative experience and results in embarrassment at best and denigration and denial of a NRP provider card at worst. Thus, trainees often are guided by instructors, not being allowed to deviate in the slightest from the path deemed most appropriate by the instructors, that they may "learn." Yet how does learning occur? It may be argued that we learn best from our mistakes. As human beings, we often make mistakes, especially when operating in high-stakes situations under intense time pressure. If those mistakes occur when caring for patients, they may carry lifelong consequences for those patients. In episode 6, Mare Tranquilitatis, of the HBO television miniseries "From the Earth to the Moon," Neil Armstrong (played by actor Tony Goldwyn) and crewmate Buzz Aldrin (actor Bryan Cranston) prepare to land on the moon for the first time in human history. This was obviously a high-stakes endeavor because failure not only would have engendered national embarrassment at missing John Kennedy's vow to place a man on the moon by 1970 but also could have cost the astronauts their lives. During one particularly challenging training exercise in the lunar module simulator, the astronauts failed to abort the landing and crashed the simulator into the artificial moon's surface. During the debriefing that follows, it is obvious that egos were bruised and anger bubbles to the surface. Despite all of this, it is during a quiet moment after the simulator session and debriefing that Neil Armstrong turns to Buzz Aldrin and states simply, "Sims (simulations) are for learning." The training model used in aerospace is radically different from that historically used in health care. The underlying assumption in aerospace is that things WILL go wrong and crews must know how to handle every contingency. Thus, those responsible for training astronauts design programs that encompass every possible failure so the crews have the opportunity to practice solving particular problems prior to encountering them in actual spaceflight. The expectation is that failure will occur during training and that the professionals undergoing such training will learn from their failures and not repeat them during future training missions or actual spaceflight. Compare this to training in health care where success, not failure, is the focus. By not pushing trainees to fail in difficult training scenarios, they may leave training with a false sense of confidence and are set up to fail when working in the real clinical environment.

Summary

The NRP has set the standard for training in neonatal resuscitation for more than 2 decades. Part of this success is attributable to its ability to adapt to the ever-changing needs of its instructors and trainees. The next decade will bring even more substantial methodologic and technologic innovations as the NRP becomes more learner-focused and learner friendly and embraces methodologies such as simulation and technologies such as online libraries of interactive case-based scenarios. This continuing evolution of NRP should make it even more useful to the practicing neonatologist as a source of continuing medical education and career-long learning.

ACKNOWLEDGMENTS.

The author acknowledges the kind contribution of the following individuals to the material included in this work: John Kattwinkel, MD, Bill Keenan, MD, Susan Niermeyer, MD, George Peckham, MD, Wendy Simon, MA.

References

1. Summary notes. Goals. Resuscitation of the Newborn Task Force. September 25–26, 1980. Courtesy of George J Peckham, MD

2. Keenan named resuscitation giant. *NRP Instructor Update*. 2005;14(1):2. Available at: http:www.aap.org/nrp/newsletter/2005_springsummer_iu.pdf

3. Chamberlain D. The International Liaison Committee on Resuscitation (ILCOR)-past and present. Compiled by the founding members of the International Liaison Committee on Resuscitation. *Resuscitation*. 2005;67:157–161

4. *Your Guide to the 2005 International CoSTR Conference*. Dallas, Tex: American Heart Association; 2005. Available at: http://www.c2005.org/presenter. jhtml?identifier_3022536

5. *C2005 Evidence Evaluation Worksheets: International Liaison Committee on Resuscitation 2005 Consensus on ECC & CPR Science and Treatment Recommendations*. Dallas, Tex: American Heart Association; 2005. Available at: http://www.c2005.org/presenter. html?identifier_3026177

6. From the 2005 International Consensus Conference on Cardiopulmonary Resuscitation and Emergency Cardiovascular Care Science With Treatment Recommendations, hosted by the American Heart Association in Dallas, Texas, January 23–30, 2005. Section 1. Part 7: Neonatal resuscitation. *Circulation*. 2005;112(suppl 1):III-91–III-99. Available at: http://circ. ahajournals.org/cgi/content/full/112/22_suppl/III-91

7. Kattwinkel J, ed. *Textbook of Neonatal Resuscitation*. 5th ed. Elk Grove Village, Ill and Dallas, Tex: American Academy of Pediatrics and American Heart Association; 2006

8. The Joint Commission. Preventing infant death and injury during delivery. *Sentinel Event Alert*. 2004;30. Available at: http://www.jointcommission.org/SentinelEvents/ SentinelEventAlert/sea_30.htm

9. Helmreich RL, Wilhelm JA, Gregorich SE, Chidester TR. Preliminary results from the evaluation of cockpit resource management training: performance ratings of flightcrews. *Aviat Space Environ Med*. 1990;61:576–579

10. Helmreich RL, Chidester TR, Foushee HC, Gregorich S, Wilhelm JA. How effective is cockpit resource management training? Exploring issues in evaluating the impact of programs to enhance crew coordination. *Flight Saf Dig*. 1990;9:1–17

11. Zaichkin J, ed. Optional activities. In: *Instructor's Manual for Neonatal Resuscitation*. 4th ed. Elk Grove Village, Ill, Dallas, Tex: American Academy of Pediatrics and American Heart Association; 2006:chapt 8

12. Zaichkin J, ed. Educational foundations of the Neonatal Resuscitation Program. In: *Instructor's Manual for Neonatal Resuscitation*. 4th ed. Elk Grove Village, Ill, Dallas, Tex: American Academy of Pediatrics and American Heart Association. 2006: chapt 1

13. Neonatal Resuscitation Program Web site. Available at: http://www.aap.org/nrp/

14. *2008 Sponsored Research Grant Program and Young Investigator Award Application and Guidelines*. Available at: http://www.aap.org/nrp/science/science_grant.html

15. 2005 American Heart Association Guidelines for Cardiopulmonary Resuscitation and Emergency Cardiovascular Care. Part 13: Neonatal resuscitation guidelines. *Circulation*. 2005;112:IV-188–IV-195

16. 2005 American Heart Association Guidelines for Cardiopulmonary Resuscitation and Emergency Cardiovascular Care. Part 1: Introduction. *Circulation*. 2005;112:IV-1–IV-5

17. 2005 American Heart Association Guidelines for Cardiopulmonary Resuscitation and Emergency Cardiovascular Care. Part 11: Pediatric basic life support. *Circulation*. 2005;112:IV-156–IV-166

18. Weiner G. *NRP 2007: What It Is and Isn't, What Works and Doesn't*. Presented at American Academy of Pediatrics National Conference and Exhibition. Available at:http://www. aap.org/nrp/pdf/NRPToday. pdf

19. Kattwinkel J, ed. Neonatal Resuscitation Program provider course overview. In: *Textbook of Neonatal Resuscitation*. 5th ed. Elk Grove Village, Ill, and Dallas, Tex: American Academy of Pediatrics and American Heart Association; 2006:ix

20. Halamek LP, Kaegi DM, Gaba DM, et al. Time for a new paradigm in pediatric medical education: teaching neonatal resuscitation in a simulated delivery room environment. *Pediatrics*. 2000;106:e45. Available at: http://www.pediatrics.org/cgi/content/full/106/4/e45

21. *A New Vision for Pediatrics and Perinatal Education*. Palo Alto, Calif: Center for Advanced Pediatric & Perinatal Education. Available at: http://www.cape.lpch.org

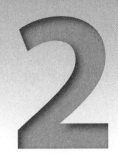

Core Elements and Course Requirements

The Neonatal Resuscitation Program™ (NRP™) now uses a different education model than what learners and instructors have experienced in the past. The NRP course format now requires learners to study the material from the *Textbook of Neonatal Resuscitation, 6th Edition*, and take an online examination *before* attending their NRP course. Learners attend an interactive course that includes little or no lecture about textbook content, uses course time for skills stations and supervised practice, and uses simulation and debriefing as an important part of the learning experience.

This chapter will help you understand how NRP education materials are developed and the changes in education methodology, and includes information needed to create the ideal NRP Provider Course curriculum. The "how-to" information for each element, such as administering the online examination, setting up Performance Skills Stations, and conducting simulation and debriefing, can be found in its own chapter.

In Chapter 2 you will learn about

- **How NRP education materials are developed**
- **Why the NRP course format changed**
- **The pathway to NRP provider status**
- **Core elements and course requirements of the NRP Provider Course**

"Instructor Self-assessment" for Chapter 2 begins on page 191.

After studying this chapter, complete the Chapter 2 questions, using the answer sheets that begin on page 188. Your regional trainer may ask you to bring the answer sheets to your NRP Instructor Course.

Where do NRP materials come from?

Revised NRP materials result from the work of the International Liaison Committee on Resuscitation (ILCOR), a multinational group that provides a coordinated forum for researching, reporting, and developing international resuscitation guidelines supported by scientific data. Every 5 years, ILCOR coordinates the research, debates the science, and determines new international resuscitation treatment recommendations. (See the diagram on page 17.)

In 2007, the American Academy of Pediatrics/American Heart Association NRP Steering Committee again joined forces with 8 internationally based groups to spearhead the ILCOR Neonatal Delegation.

- Australian Resuscitation Council (ARC)

- Council of Latin America for Resuscitation (CLAR)

- European Resuscitation Council (ERC)

- Heart and Stroke Foundation of Canada (HSFC)/Canadian Pediatric Society (CPS)

- Pediatric Society/Resuscitation Council of Asia (RCA)

- New Zealand Resuscitation Council (NZRC)

- Resuscitation Council of South Africa (RCSA)

- World Health Organization (WHO)

- American Academy of Pediatrics/American Heart Association NRP Steering Committee

The International Liaison Committee on Resuscitation identifies controversial issues regarding resuscitation. Delegates are assigned questions and develop worksheets based on the data gathered on their particular questions.

The ILCOR Neonatal Delegation worked on numerous worksheets. Questions for research and debate included the following:

- For newborns requiring resuscitation, is any adjunct measure (eg, carbon dioxide [CO_2] detection, pulse oximeter) as effective as the usual clinical findings (eg, heart rate, chest movement) in improving outcome?

- In newborns receiving chest compressions, do other ratios (5:1, 15:2) versus a 3:1 improve outcomes?

- In depressed newborns with clear amniotic fluid, does suctioning of the mouth and nose versus none improve outcome?

How Neonatal Resuscitation Guidelines and NRP Materials Are Developed

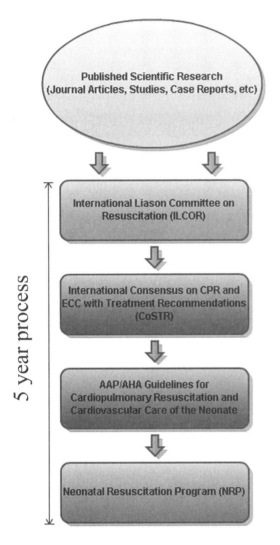

ILCOR includes eight international resuscitation councils: the American Heart Association (AHA), European Resuscitation Council (ERC), Heart and Stroke Foundation of Canada (HSFC), Resuscitation Council of Asia (RCA), Resuscitation Council of Southern Africa (RCSA), the Australia and New Zealand Council on Resuscitation (ANZCOR), and the InterAmerican Heart Foundation (IAHF).

Hundreds of volunteer experts from around the world review and evaluate the peer-reviewed literature, and then develop a summary of knowledge for each resuscitation topic. This summary is reviewed, debated, and the level of evidence rated and classified. The summary is posted online for public comment. Finally, based upon the consensus of the assembled international experts, treatment recommendations are generated. This document, known as CoSTR, is the *international* consensus on resuscitation science for newborns, children, and adults.

Each resuscitation council that makes up ILCOR develops resuscitation guidelines based upon the CoSTR that are applicable to their country/practice. AAP/AHA resuscitation guidelines for newborns are published in the journals *Resuscitation*, *Circulation*, & *Pediatrics*.

The Neonatal Resuscitation Program Steering Committee develops educational materials based upon the AHA/AAP Guidelines.

- When resuscitating or stabilizing newborns at birth, is there an oxygen administration strategy that is superior to any other in improving outcome?

- In preterm newborns in the delivery room under radiant heaters, what are the preferred methods of decreasing heat loss (room temperature, wrapping, warming mattresses, etc) compared to newborns receiving standard traditional management to achieve optimal temperatures, and does a combination of treatments cause hyperthermia?

- In newborns at the limits of viability or anomalies associated with lethal outcomes, does the noninitiation versus initiation of resuscitation result in an outcome that is ethically justified?

- In depressed newborns requiring positive-pressure ventilation (PPV), does the administration of longer inspiratory times, higher inflation pressures, or the use of positive end-expiratory pressure (PEEP), as compared to standard management, improve outcome?

- For health care professionals, do simulation-based learning methodologies, when compared to traditional (lectures) training, improve the acquisition of content knowledge, technical skills, and behavioral skills required for effective and safe resuscitation?

These many worksheets resulted in evidence classified by the strength of the study design, and a recommendation class based on the strength of the evidence. At a series of meetings held around the world, the worksheets and proposed revised guidelines were discussed and debated. After hundreds of hours researching, analyzing, and discussing scientific data related to neonatal resuscitation, the ILCOR team helped determine new international resuscitation treatment recommendations, known as the Consensus on Science and Treatment Recommendations (CoSTR).

Each resuscitation council then developed resuscitation guidelines for its own region of the world, based on the scientific principles in the CoSTR document. The neonatal portion of the US Treatment Guidelines was published in the journals *Circulation, Resuscitation*, and *Pediatrics* in October 2010, and is reprinted in the back of the *Textbook of Neonatal Resuscitation, 6th Edition.*

The NRP Steering Committee translated these most recent guidelines into the *Textbook of Neonatal Resuscitation, 6th Edition,* and the accompanying education materials that support the efforts of NRP instructors and providers.

⌐**www**

To learn more about the development of new guideline recommendations, go to **www.aap.org/nrp** and click on "Science".

Why did the NRP Steering Committee change the education methodology and NRP course format?

The NRP has been a very successful program and we certainly are hesitant to make any significant changes without careful consideration. We believe that the program's future success and the lives of newborns touched by its participants are best served by allowing instructors to spend as much time as possible working hands-on with participants by using self-directed education for the cognitive portion of the course.

The previously acceptable method for conducting an NRP course often involved a slide and lecture format. Courses varied in length from 8 to 24 hours for a Provider Course to 4 to 8 hours for a Renewal Course. This format worked well for many years. However, as the program continued in this format and learners attended numerous Renewal Courses, many learners would arrive at the course with the *Textbook of Neonatal Resuscitation* still in its plastic wrapper. Learners knew they could depend on the instructor to "spoon feed" them the contents of the textbook over the course of many hours. In this way, passive learners would retain enough information to pass the written test. The Megacode performance (the demonstration of resuscitation skills in correct sequence and with proper technique) was often coached by the instructor to ensure that learners could "pass" the NRP course and attain provider status.

This methodology certainly achieved the goal of complying with the American Academy of Pediatrics (AAP) recommendation that learners "pass" an NRP course every 2 years. Instructors are sometimes pushed to pass a great number of health care professionals who are required to maintain NRP provider status as a condition of employment. Courses usually are conducted in the fastest, most cost-effective way possible, and it is to the instructor's advantage to pass every participant. However, this focus on compliance often diminishes the value and purpose of NRP training.

Although the program is based around adult learning principles and was designed to meet multiple learning styles, data obtained from a national survey of instructors indicated that the largest percentage of instructor time is spent giving didactic lectures and administering the written evaluations. The NRP Steering Committee believes that this is not the best use of our instructors' expertise. Our goal is to have the majority of instructor-participant interaction focused on hands-on learning, immersive simulations, and constructive debriefings. To achieve this goal, we believe that most participants should complete the

> The NRP education methodology changes with the 6th Edition materials. Instructors no longer will give lectures or administer the written examination. The majority of instructor-participant interaction is now focused on hands-on learning, immersive simulations, and constructive debriefings.

cognitive components at their own pace, using self-directed educational materials, such as the *Textbook of Neonatal Resuscitation, 6th Edition,* and the accompanying DVD.

The shift to making the instructor less of a "teacher" and more of a "learning facilitator" means that the learner must now take responsibility for his or her own learning. The course participant studies the textbook and learns the content knowledge prior to attending an interactive course that involves hands-on skills practice and simulation-based training and debriefing, and little or no lecture about material that he or she should have already learned through self-study and online examination. This methodology allows the instructor to tailor the Provider Course to meet the learning needs of the participants.

> **Every learner takes an NRP Provider Course. There is no longer an NRP Renewal Course. The NRP instructor tailors the core elements of each course to suit the learning objectives of the trainees.**

The other reason for the change involves a shift from the philosophy that passing scores indicate adequately prepared learners. In our previous model of NRP training, the instructor imparts knowledge "to" the learner through slides and lecture, expects a passing score on the written examination, ensures that all but the most incompetent learners get through the Megacode performance (which may involve extensive coaching and teaching during the Megacode), and "passes" the learner. This may be a major disservice to the learner, who leaves the NRP course with a false sense of security about the adequacy of his or her skills and ability to manage complications during an actual resuscitation. Passing scores do not always mean that learners have the necessary skills to perform well under actual circumstances.

Health care training has always focused on success, and failure results in embarrassment and poor morale. Simulation-based training changes this perspective, and advocates believe that the best learning often comes from making an error. As a result of this philosophy, the NRP is shifting part of the course curriculum to simulation training, where learners are allowed to make mistakes and learn from them in a safe and supportive training environment, instead of during actual patient care.

For all of these reasons, the NRP is moving to a more self-directed learning model, which allows the learner to spend course time engaged in hands-on, interactive learning. Course elements can be tailored to meet the learning needs of the participants. We believe that the objectives and educational goals that form the foundation of the NRP will be best served for the future by moving to this format.

The Learning Path to NRP Provider Status
Learner(s) and instructor(s) agree on the need for a Provider Course.
Date and time of the NRP Provider Course is determined.

Instructor responsibilities

Instructor uses institutional process to determine which learners plan to take the scheduled course.

Instructor plans the course based on the number of learners and the anticipated learning objectives.

Instructor may assess learning needs by requesting an Experience Survey from each registrant.

Instructor informs learners about their responsibilities, how to prepare for the course, and requirements for successful completion.

Instructor is available to learners for assistance, if necessary.

Instructor administers the course on the scheduled date, ensuring that supplies, equipment, and staff are available.

Instructor completes administrative duties as necessary after the course.

Learner responsibilities

Learner self-studies the *Textbook of Neonatal Resuscitation, 6th Edition.*

Learner may practice hands-on skills, if needed prior to the course.

Learner may access instructor for assistance, if needed.

Learner takes and passes the NRP online examination prior to the course.

Learner takes the scheduled NRP Provider Course.

Learner should maintain and improve skills by participating in unit activities, such as mock codes.

Learner renews their NRP provider status every 2 years at a Provider Course.

What are the core elements of the Neonatal Resuscitation Program Provider Course?

The NRP curriculum has 3 primary components:

1. Knowledge (such as knowing the correct dose of epinephrine)
2. Skills (such as knowing how to administer PPV)
3. Teamwork and communication (making it all work)

The NRP curriculum consists of core elements in each of these 3 components. The NRP core elements include both learning activities and evaluation components. At a minimum, every participant in an NRP Provider Course must complete a knowledge evaluation (online examination), skills evaluation (Integrated Skills Station), and simulation-debriefing experience. Based on the learners' needs, instructors may customize their course by selecting additional core elements and using a variety of teaching methodologies.

Knowledge

Learning Activity: Textbook and/or DVD Self-study
The cognitive portion of the NRP curriculum includes the knowledge base that providers must have to understand neonatal risk factors, physiology, anatomy, and the pharmacology of resuscitation. This material is covered in the *Textbook of Neonatal Resuscitation, 6th Edition,* and the accompanying textbook DVD. Students are expected to acquire this cognitive material by self-study prior to arrival at your course.

> Instructors no longer use slides and lecture during an NRP course. Instead, instructors are encouraged to use this time for hands-on, interactive learning.

> A basic NRP Provider Course must include *at least* Lessons 1 through 4 *and* Lesson 9.

Learners can study every lesson and may be encouraged to expand their knowledge in this way. Hospitals may choose to have their participants study only a subset of lessons based upon their job responsibilities and scope of practice. A basic NRP Provider Course must include *at least* Lessons 1 through 4 *and* Lesson 9.

Students must have access to a textbook and textbook DVD before their course to allow time for self-study. Ideally, students should have a textbook about 1 month before the course date. The time learners need for self-study varies according to their learning level and experience. New learners require an average of 7 to 8 hours for study, with the lessons on PPV (Lesson 3) and medications (Lesson 6) requiring the most time. Experienced NRP learners average about 3 hours for study.

Knowledge Evaluation: NRP Online Examination (Required)
Successful completion of the online written examination is required *before* participants attend the classroom portion of the NRP course. Participants will be prompted to print an online examination verification that they will bring to their class and present to the instructor. Learners must attend the classroom portion of their NRP course within 30 days of completing the online examination. A hard-copy test format is no longer available. There is a fee for the online testing. See Chapter 4 for detailed information about using the online examination.

Hands-on Skills

Successful completion of the online NRP written examination is required *before* attending the classroom portion of the NRP course.

Learning Activity: Self-directed Skills Practice

Participants may acquire or refine their resuscitation skills prior to attending their NRP course using self-directed practice. Both new and experienced providers can use the *Simply NRP* self-directed teaching kit to learn or review the basic resuscitation skills described in Lessons 1 through 4 of the *Textbook of Neonatal Resuscitation, 6th Edition* (equipment check, initial steps, PPV, and chest compressions). An inflatable neonatal manikin, instructional DVD, and all the equipment required to learn and practice these skills are included in the kit. The *Simply NRP* DVD uses a "watch as you practice" method with an on-screen instructor and assistant demonstrating each skill followed by an opportunity for the learner to practice with the instructor using his or her own manikin. The *Simply NRP* kit allows learners the flexibility to use materials when it is most convenient, control the pace of the instruction, repeat portions of the instructions if necessary, and practice skills as often as necessary outside of the hospital in a private setting free from scrutiny by their colleagues.

Instructors also may set up self-directed practice stations in an accessible area, such as in a conference room or on an available radiant warmer, for more experienced providers to practice their skills prior to attending their scheduled course. In particular, providers may benefit from practicing face-mask placement, umbilical venous catheter preparation, and filling epinephrine syringes. Practice stations should be set up approximately 1 to 2 weeks prior to the scheduled class time and must be accessible to staff members on all shifts. Allowing participants an opportunity to practice infrequently used skills prior to their course may decrease performance anxiety and identify areas requiring more guided instruction.

Learning Activity: Performance Skills Stations

The classroom portion of most NRP Provider Courses will begin with Performance Skills Stations to teach or review hands-on resuscitation skills. This is an opportunity for instructors to demonstrate the proper technique and timing of the skills and for learners to receive guided one-on-one instruction. Instructors determine which, if any, stations need to be included in their course based upon an assessment of their learners' needs. Most learners benefit from instructor-guided review and practice. Experienced providers may only require skills stations for new (eg, laryngeal mask airway) or infrequently used (eg, medication administration) skills. If the instructor determines that structured review is unnecessary based on the learner's expertise, individual Performance Skills Stations are not required.

Ideally, Performance Skills Stations should be placed in an area that closely simulates a clinical setting. Instructors may use the scenario-based format described in the Performance Checklists (Lessons 1 through 6) to help learners practice more than one intervention in proper sequence. The Performance Skills Stations should be interactive, with instructors asking learners questions about the indications for each intervention, how to evaluate its efficacy, when to discontinue, and the anticipated next steps. This practice continues until the instructor and learner agree that the learner can perform the skill correctly and smoothly and without coaching within the context of a short clinical scenario. Each scenario of a Performance Skills Station should build on the skills practiced in the scenarios before it, beginning with the Equipment Check and ending with the skill that is the focus of the Performance Skills Station. Each participant participates in the assessment of the performance by answering Reflective Questions. This style of analyzing the performance prepares the instructor and the learner for the Simulation and Debriefing component of the course.

Learners can study every lesson and may be encouraged to expand their knowledge in this way. Hospitals may choose to have their participants study only a subset of lessons based upon their job responsibilities and scope of practice. A basic NRP Provider Course must include the hands-on skills described in Lessons 1 through 4 and the ethics information in Lesson 9. If learners study additional lessons and procedures, such as intubation or umbilical line placement, they may obtain course credit for these components; however, NRP course credit does NOT certify the learner to perform these procedures in the birth setting. Completion of a lesson, or demonstration of a procedure in an NRP course, does NOT indicate competence or authorization to perform that procedure in a clinical setting. Professional governing bodies, regulatory agencies, and institutional job descriptions define an individual's scope of practice. Although participants may study all of the procedures in the NRP course, they must remain within their scope of professional practice during patient care. This is a critical distinction that instructors must emphasize.

> Learners may practice any skill in the NRP course. Neonatal Resuscitation Program course completion does **NOT** certify the learner to perform procedures within the hospital or indicate clinical competence.

Skills Evaluation: Integrated Skills Station (Required)
The final Performance Skills Station is called the Integrated Skills Station, and it is a required element for all Provider Courses. The Integrated Skills Station is an opportunity for each provider to

demonstrate the steps in the NRP flow diagram using the proper sequence, timing, and technique. This is an individual evaluation intended to ensure that all learners understand the "what, when, and how" of the resuscitation skills. Unlike the other Performance Skills Stations, the instructor does not coach the learner or interrupt the demonstration. Depending upon the skills included in each course, instructors may choose to evaluate the participant's skills using a single comprehensive clinical scenario or present several shorter clinical scenarios. Participants should be given an opportunity to demonstrate the skills from each lesson included in their course. The Integrated Skills Station Performance Checklists for both the Basic (Lessons 1 through 4) and Advanced (Lessons 1 through 6) performances are included in Appendix E, and in the *Textbook of Neonatal Resuscitation, 6th Edition.*

If an instructor determines that the participant has arrived at the course fully prepared from self-study or previous experience, the learner may begin with the Integrated Skills Station. If weaknesses are identified, additional practice at a Performance Skills Station may be required.

If the provider makes significant mistakes in the sequence, timing, or technique of the individual skills, he or she should return to the appropriate Performance Skills Station for additional practice before moving to the Simulation and Debriefing component of the NRP course. While technical skills can be refined during the simulation component, significant deficiencies in skills interfere with the intended focus on teamwork and communication.

> The Integrated Skills Station is an individual assessment of hands-on skills and is a required component of every NRP Provider Course. The Integrated Skills Station should be completed before proceeding to the Simulation and Debriefing component.

Teamwork

Learning Activity: Simulation (Required)

Simulation is an education methodology that uses visual, auditory, and tactile cues to replicate the essential components of a real situation. By simulating an actual resuscitation experience, learners can work through high-risk situations in a safe environment and then reflect on the experience and critically evaluate their actions. Unlike the Performance Skills Stations that focus on individual performance and correct technique, simulation activities focus on how individuals work together as a team. Rather than trying to achieve a "perfect" performance, teams are challenged with progressively difficult scenarios to identify weaknesses and learn from them. Simulation is most valuable when the learners are able to "suspend disbelief" and become fully immersed in the clinical scenario. Simulation training, and the debriefing that follows, does not require expensive supplies and equipment. It does require instructors to dedicate additional time to creating realistic learning environments and to learn the skills necessary to evaluate teamwork and communication. Simulation and debriefing adds a new dimension to your NRP course that allows learners to take responsibility for much of their own learning.

The scenario used during simulation training is based on the learning objectives of the NRP trainees. Simulation training depends on good methodology, not technology; therefore, expensive simulators and equipment are not necessary. The NRP instructor usually can work with manikins and equipment already present for NRP training, and add simple visual cues such as blood and meconium (made from common household items). It is helpful if the simulation can be videotaped, using basic video-recording equipment, for the subsequent debriefing.

> Simulation focuses on developing effective teamwork and communication. It is meant to replicate the way that health care professionals actually practice in real clinical situations. Simulation is an essential element of an NRP Provider Course.

Teamwork Evaluation: Debriefing (Required)

Many NRP instructors are accustomed to the "score sheet" method of evaluation that focuses on what interventions should have occurred during a scenario, giving direct feedback to individuals on what is needed for improvement, and determining if individuals "pass" or "fail." In contrast, debriefing is the evaluation method used during the simulation component of the NRP Provider Course. Debriefing usually does not require critique or feedback from the instructor to the learners. Instead, the instructor guides a participant-directed discussion by asking questions and leading the learners on a path of reflection and self-discovery. Participants discuss what occurred during the simulation, what worked well, and what did not work well. Ultimately, participants themselves identify how to improve their team's performance. If significant weaknesses are identified, the team can return to the simulation environment and repeat the clinical scenario, employing the strategies identified in their debriefing. Although the simulation itself is engaging and educational, the most important learning occurs during debriefing. The focus of the debriefing should be on teamwork and communication, not on individual technical skills. By the time providers have proceeded to the Simulation and Debriefing component of the course, they should have firmly established skills.

Facilitating an effective debriefing is a new skill for most NRP instructors. The *NRP Instructor DVD: An Interactive Tool for Facilitation of Simulation-based Learning* is a self-directed learning activity that is intended to help NRP instructors become familiar with simulation and debriefing. It is *required* learning for every NRP instructor. (See Chapter 9 for more information about NRP instructor requirements.)

> Debriefing focuses on teamwork and communication. The instructor guides the discussion with open questions and allows reflection and self-discovery.

Instructor Q & A

How can I learn more and stay informed about NRP?

There are many resources for NRP instructors. Following are 2 of the most important resources:

- *NRP Instructor DVD: An Interactive Tool for Facilitation of Simulation-based Learning*

  To facilitate the transition to a simulation-based training methodology, a comprehensive, interactive DVD with video-based depiction of the technology, skills, techniques, and attitudes for effective scenario development and debriefing has been created. This new tool will familiarize instructors with simulation and guide them in how to incorporate this innovative methodology into NRP courses. Each current and future NRP instructor will be required to purchase his or her own DVD, which will offer continuing education credit in accordance with state policies and regulations.

- **American Academy of Pediatrics Neonatal Resuscitation Program Web site**

  http://www.aap.org/nrp/nrpmain.html   ⌨www

  The NRP home page is where instructors log in to submit NRP Course Rosters. However, the NRP home page is also an excellent resource for staying informed. Find out what is new with the NRP, peruse the instructor and provider resources, learn more about online testing, and find tools to help you create quality NRP courses. The *NRP Instructor Update* newsletter is also found online and is your most efficient means of staying up-to-date with the NRP.

I'm really worried that my NRP students will have trouble understanding the material and passing the online test without my lecture and slides.

Neonatal Resuscitation Program learners who work in a professional capacity in a health care setting are more than capable of reading and understanding the *Textbook of Neonatal Resuscitation, 6th Edition*, which follows the same format that has earned the textbook critical acclaim for its simplicity and ease of use for many years. If learners prefer, they can use the DVD that accompanies each textbook and study that way instead of reading the textbook. Many learners enjoy the interactive components of the DVD more than reading the textbook.

Many instructors voluntarily implemented the self-study and online examination requirement a few years ago and, thus far, have received positive feedback from learners. In fact, most participants appreciate being able to self-study and take the online examination at their convenience instead of sitting through a lengthy class that includes lectures and waiting for fellow students to finish their hard-copy examinations.

Does the NRP forbid me from reviewing material with learners prior to the online examination and Provider Course?

Nothing in the revised NRP education methodology forbids an instructor from assisting students during the self-study period of the course. An NRP instructor should be available to students to answer questions or clarify information as needed. You also may encourage small groups of learners to prepare for their NRP course by studying together. The instructor may lead self-study groups if desired. However, the instructor who leads the self-study group by lecturing about every lesson in the textbook to a passive group of learners is doing the learners a disservice. Instead, the instructor should encourage the students take an active role in the learning (eg, by assigning each lesson to a learner and asking that learner to lead a discussion about the Key Points of the lesson). Most importantly, the group-study students should use the opportunity to practice hands-on technical skills, using the actual equipment in an unoccupied newborn resuscitation area or in your NRP skills area, or by using the *Simply NRP* equipment and DVD for practicing skills in Lessons 1 through 4.

I enjoyed lecturing and showing the slides. I do not want to learn how to create scenarios and lead debriefings. I'm considering letting my instructor status expire.

The NRP Steering Committee realizes that not every instructor will want to learn new skills and responsibilities. It is acceptable to allow your NRP hospital-based instructor or regional trainer status to become inactive if you feel that the changes do not fit your teaching style, abilities, or interests. As a learner in an NRP Provider Course, your previous experience as an instructor will give you renewed appreciation for what you expect and value from your Provider Course. The NRP appreciates your commitment to the NRP and your continued support of the program.

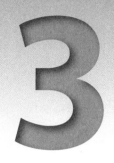

Course Planning: Who Learns What, and How?

The Neonatal Resuscitation Program™ (NRP™) instructor is responsible for knowing who benefits from an NRP course, how to plan the course, and requirements for successful completion. This chapter helps the NRP instructor understand how to incorporate the core elements of the NRP into courses that best meet the needs of the learners.

In Chapter 3 you will learn about

- Who should take an NRP Provider Course

- Requirements for completion of an NRP Provider Course

- Core elements of the course and strategies learners may use to prepare

- Sample agendas for a Provider Course developed to meet learners' needs

- Basic information about course continuing education credit

- A sample timeline for planning an NRP course

- Teaching NRP outside the United States: Things to Know

"Instructor Self-assessment" for Chapter 3 begins on page 192.

After studying this chapter, complete the Chapter 3 questions, using the answer sheets that begin on page 188. Your regional trainer may ask you to bring the answer sheets to your NRP Instructor Course.

> The NRP Provider Course is designed for health care professionals involved in any aspect of neonatal resuscitation. The NRP also may be useful to prehospital professionals and other in-hospital professionals who desire in-depth training specific to neonatal resuscitation.

How do I identify or justify the need for an NRP course?

The NRP is designed primarily for those who participate in neonatal resuscitation in the delivery room and newborn nursery. Neonatal Resuscitation Program courses are offered in community hospitals by hospital-based instructors or are provided as a service to community hospitals and providers by regional trainers and hospital-based instructors, usually based at regional medical centers.

In many institutions, the NRP is conducted to

- Improve the quality of neonatal resuscitation.

- Meet performance expectations or attain hospital privileges or credentialing for staff who attend births or care for newborns.

- Serve as a quality management strategy to improve the process and outcome of neonatal resuscitation.

- Meet regulatory agency requirements for evidence of an education program that supports competency-based practice.

Although Advanced Pediatric Life Support (APLS) and Pediatric Education for Prehospital Professionals (PEPP) courses are appropriate for those who participate in resuscitation outside the delivery room, the NRP also may be useful to prehospital professionals and other in-hospital professionals who desire in-depth training specific to neonatal resuscitation.

Who takes an NRP Provider Course?

The NRP Provider Course is designed for health care professionals involved in any aspect of neonatal resuscitation. This includes physicians, nurses, advanced practice nurses, nurse midwives, licensed midwives, respiratory care practitioners, and other health care professionals who provide direct care during neonatal resuscitation.

Neonatal Resuscitation Program instructors sometimes receive requests from students in a health care profession who want to take an NRP course to better prepare them for clinical rotations. This is up to the instructor's judgment; however, the NRP is of little benefit to those students in health care professions who have no delivery room experience or have not seen the birth of a healthy term newborn. Basic knowledge and experience in what is clinically normal is beneficial before learning about neonatal resuscitation.

Sometimes I am asked to teach an NRP course for those who attend births outside the hospital setting, such as paramedics. How can I modify the NRP to meet their needs?

Fortunately, birth is a natural process, and most babies require few interventions from birth attendants. When complications are unexpected or unavoidable outside the hospital setting, health care providers should have the knowledge and abilities to perform basic lifesaving procedures for the newborn.

Basic resuscitation of the newborn is the same in any setting. Prehospital professionals, or anyone whose job responsibilities might include neonatal resuscitation outside the hospital setting, should have the equipment and skills necessary to provide initial steps of resuscitation and mask ventilation, and perform chest compressions (*Textbook of Neonatal Resuscitation, 6th Edition*, Lessons 1 through 4). Paramedics and other prehospital professionals may have endotracheal intubation, laryngeal mask airway placement, and medication administration within their scope of practice (Lessons 5 and 6). Lesson 7 covers topics appropriate to newborn resuscitation outside the delivery room setting. Remember that, to obtain NRP provider status, the participants of the course must successfully complete at least Lessons 1 through 4 *and* Lesson 9.

Plan some extra time during your course to ensure that these providers have an opportunity to discuss modifications and equipment alternatives for their setting. For example, Lesson 7 covers resuscitation outside the hospital setting, and participants may appreciate extra time to discuss strategies to meet their unique challenges.

The Experience Survey may be helpful as a pre-course planning tool. (See pages 32 and 214.) In addition, talk with the person who identified the need for an NRP course and find out what skills are appropriate and what equipment is available to meet the learning needs of these participants. If you provide NRP courses often for prehospital professionals, you may wish to tailor the survey so that it reflects the specific learning objectives and job responsibilities of the learners in your community.

Experience Survey

Complete and submit to instructor prior to course.

Name _____

E-mail address _____

Contact number _____

Institution _____

Credentials:

MD _____   RN _____   LPN _____   Respiratory Therapist _____

Advanced practice RN (specify type: CRNP, NNP, PNP, CNM, etc) _____

Prehospital professional (specify) _____

Other (specify) _____

Current position

MD: Obstetrics/Gynecology _____   Neonatology _____   General Pediatrics _____

Family Medicine _____   Emergency Medicine _____   Anesthesiology _____

Other (specify) _____

RN/LPN: Labor and Delivery _____   Newborn Nursery _____

Special Care Nursery/NICU _____

Nursing Education _____   Operating Room _____   Emergency Department _____

Other (specify) _____

Other health care professional (specify) _____

Is this your first NRP course? Yes _____   No _____

What is your role at a newborn resuscitation?

_____ I have primary responsibility for all aspects of resuscitation, including airway management, umbilical line placement, and administration of medications.

_____ I have primary responsibility for providing initial steps, positive-pressure ventilation (PPV), and chest compressions until help arrives.

_____ I have primary responsibility for providing initial steps, and PPV, assisting with airway management, drawing up and administering medications, and assisting with umbilical line placement.

_____ I have a different role than any described above. My role is: _____

In the past 6 months, how many times have you participated in the resuscitation of a newborn?

None _____ 1-4 _____ 5-9 _____ 10-20 _____ More than 20 _____

During those resuscitations, how many times have you performed the following:

Initial steps _____ Bag-and-mask ventilation _____ Ventilation with T-piece resuscitator _____

Chest compressions _____ Endotracheal intubation _____ Laryngeal mask airway _____

Preparation and/or administration of epinephrine _____

Preparation and/or insertion of emergency umbilical venous catheter _____

In the next 6 months, how many times do you anticipate participating in newborn resuscitation?

None _____ 1-4 _____ 5-9 _____ 10-20 _____ More than 20 _____

What specific goals do you have for the course?

Improve team communication _____

Participate in simulation-based training _____

Improve skills performance:

Ventilation with bag and mask _____ Ventilation with T-piece resuscitator _____

Chest compressions _____

Endotracheal intubation (assist or perform) _____

Laryngeal mask airway placement _____

Epinephrine and volume administration _____

Emergency umbilical venous catheter placement (assist or perform) _____

Other personal objective for attending this course: _____

Have you participated in simulated neonatal resuscitations, mock codes, or similar exercises in the past 2 years?

Yes _____ No _____

Please add any other comments you think would help the instructor in meeting your educational goals:

_____
_____
_____
_____

I occasionally have a request from a social worker, physical therapist, chaplain, or other member of the health care team to attend an NRP course to find out more about neonatal resuscitation. Is this allowed?
With the permission of the instructor and at the discretion of the local institution, persons who do not provide direct medical care but who have a professional interest in NRP may be permitted to observe or "participate" in a course. The instructor should consider the number of outside observers or participants requesting a place in a class and whether including them is a wise use of instructor time and resources. The member of the health care team who is interested in attending an NRP course may meet his or her objectives with options other than actually attending a class, such as reading the textbook or viewing the accompanying DVD. If the requestor is interested in simulation and debriefing, viewing the *NRP Instructor DVD: An Interactive Tool for Facilitation of Simulation-based Learning* may meet this person's needs.

If the person still wishes to take part in an NRP course, the instructor should clearly communicate to the participant that

- The instructor's priority is meeting the needs of NRP course participants.

- The purpose of observing or participating in the course is for educational enrichment only.

- Course Completion Cards are not issued to affiliated health care team members who only observe the course.

This person also may be useful as a simulation participant, playing his or her professional role during simulation. Adding a social worker, chaplain, or other health care professional who may be present in the scenario adds realism to the exercise; however, this person should be aware of the learning objectives and help ensure that the scenario stays focused on the stated objectives.

Who takes which lessons?
Staff members who provide care for antepartum patients and/or healthy newborns may wonder how the NRP applies to their job responsibilities. Neonatal resuscitation skills are essential for these staff members because a newborn may unexpectedly require resuscitation outside the delivery setting, or these staff members may be called upon to assist with resuscitation. If these staff members have trouble relating to delivery room scenarios, see page 111 for additional scenarios that may be more applicable and relevant to them.

Not everyone who takes an NRP course is required to study material from all 9 lessons in the *Textbook of Neonatal Resuscitation*, 6th Edition. Depending on job responsibilities, learners may choose to take the comprehensive course (Lessons 1 through 9) or Lessons 1 through 4 and 9, which is the minimum requirement for completion of the Provider Course.

Administrative and clinical leaders at each hospital determine which additional lessons are required for staff at their institution. It is recommended that persons responsible for performing a complete resuscitation (or providing direct assistance) should complete all 9 lessons.

Each hospital must determine what NRP lessons are required for the staff at their institution; however, learners can participate in any lesson and may be encouraged to expand their knowledge in this way. If learners take lessons and demonstrate procedures, such as intubation or umbilical line placement, but do not perform these procedures as part of their professional responsibility, they still may get credit for completing those components of the course. Remember that **NRP courses do not certify the learner to perform any resuscitation technique,** and course participants should not exceed their scope of practice defined by their professional governing body and institutional job descriptions.

Instructors also may teach or request that learners read sections or Key Points from lessons that are optional for participants, but choose not to formally evaluate learners on the material. This way, learners are exposed to information that expands their knowledge base, but reduces anxiety about "being tested" beyond their required skills.

Why does everyone take Lesson 9?

Lesson 9 (Ethics and Care at the End of Life) in the textbook was written in response to many requests from NRP providers and instructors for more information and guidelines on this topic. The NRP Steering Committee believes that ethics should be integrated into all decision making before, during, and, potentially, after resuscitation. Because ethical issues cannot be separated from neonatal resuscitation, the NRP requires that participants learn the information and factor guidelines for ethical decision making into their practice.

Does everyone need to know all the steps of the NRP flow diagram?

Learners who do not have job responsibilities beyond positive-pressure ventilation (PPV) and chest compressions (Lessons 1 through 4) are still required to know the steps and decision points of the entire resuscitation flow diagram. (See page xi.) These learners often are called upon to assist at a resuscitation, and may be asked to prepare equipment or serve as the recorder to document events. It is imperative that these learners know what is happening at the moment, what is likely to happen next, and what is important to document on the resuscitation record.

Can a hospital require an NRP Provider Course for health care professionals and those wishing to retain hospital privileges more often than the American Academy of Pediatrics (AAP) requirement of every 2 years?

Yes, a hospital can set its own requirements for maintenance of provider status within the institution. For example, some hospitals have

> Neonatal Resuscitation Program providers are not "certified" or authorized to perform resuscitation procedures.

written their policy to indicate that providers of neonatal resuscitation must complete an annual NRP Provider Course to improve retention of the material. These Course Rosters should be completed and sent to the AAP; however, participants need only appear on a Course Roster every 2 years to maintain NRP provider status from the AAP. No matter what the institutional policy states, providers who successfully complete a minimum of Lessons 1 through 4 *and* Lesson 9 are entitled to NRP provider status by the AAP. Consequences of failing to abide by the institutional policy for required training are determined by the institution.

The Provider Course Agenda

I understand that the NRP allows for a great degree of flexibility in planning the course agenda. What are my options?
Instructors should plan NRP courses in a way that best meets the needs of the learners. Instructors can be creative when planning their curriculum and course agenda. The goal is to provide an interactive environment that challenges and stimulates adult learners. While ensuring that the core components are included, instructors should tailor the curriculum of each course to meet their learners' objectives.

Neonatal Resuscitation Program courses are not of any prescribed length because the length of the course is dependent on the number of learning objectives and the skill level of the learners.

> Successful completion of the NRP Provider Course requires that the learner pass the online NRP examination, successfully complete the Integrated Skills Station, and participate in the Simulation and Debriefing component of the course.

What is the suggested instructor:learner ratio for an NRP Provider Course?
Most NRP Provider Courses require 1 instructor for every 3 or 4 learners.

What are the core elements of an NRP course?
Learning Activity: Textbook and/or DVD Self-Study
Regardless of the pre-course study format used, the participant is responsible for learning the program content by studying the *Textbook of Neonatal Resuscitation, 6th Edition* (either in print or on DVD). This is in contrast to many resuscitation programs in which the content is provided through lectures, with the textbook serving mainly for reference or review. Participants must be made aware of their responsibility to study the material thoroughly prior to the course offering and pass the online examination prior to the NRP Provider Course.

Students may self-study in various ways prior to taking the online examination.

- Study independently, without interacting with others. In this way, learners who are already practiced and experienced in neonatal resuscitation do not need to spend long hours reviewing material already familiar to them.

- Study in groups, and reinforce textbook material by discussing what they read in the textbook or studied on the DVD. This is especially valuable for participants who have difficulty reading, or for whom English is a second language. Be aware that group study does not entail an instructor lecturing to a group of passive learners. Neonatal Resuscitation Program learners are responsible for reading the textbook or viewing the textbook DVD. The instructor may be present, if necessary, to answer questions or facilitate group discussion.

Learning Activity: Self-directed Skills Practice

It is possible for a learner to practice hands-on resuscitation skills independently. The learner may use the *Simply NRP* kit (for Lessons 1 through 4) or practice skills with actual resuscitation equipment while watching the Resuscitation Skills videos on the textbook DVD. However, after the Equipment Check and Initial Steps, a team approach to resuscitation necessitates 1 or 2 other learners for the most useful practice session.

Practicing technical skills in groups gives learners the opportunity to practice resuscitation skills as a team. If needed, an instructor can designate supervised practice time with participants and individualize the practice activities to meet specific needs. This may be beneficial for inexperienced participants and for those participants who learn more slowly than others.

Determine how to set up your practice site and keep it in good order. Devise a process for periodically checking equipment availability and repair. Your NRP practice site may include a DVD player and access to a computer with a DVD drive and Internet access for obtaining NRP learning resources.

Examples of practice facilities include the following (see chapter 5 for photos and more information about setting up practice stations):

- A box or bag of resuscitation supplies that learners take to a radiant warmer that is not currently in use for patient care

- An overbed table or cart stocked with essential resuscitation supplies that is stored in a unit closet and pulled out for practice

- A surplus radiant warmer stocked with essential resuscitation supplies that is stored on the unit and accessible to any learner

- A radiant warmer or table with essential resuscitation supplies in a unit classroom accessible by checking out a key from a designated person

- A room with a table and an appropriate device to use a *Simply NRP* kit. The kit contains an instructional DVD, an inflatable baby manikin, and actual supplies needed for practicing textbook Lessons 1 through 4.

Evaluation Activity: Online examination prior to the NRP course
As described previously, the minimum requirement for an NRP Provider Course is Lessons 1 through 4 and Lesson 9. The online examination is required of all NRP learners prior to the NRP course, but no sooner than 30 days prior to the course. Learn more about the online examination in Chapter 4.

Learning Activity: Performance Skills Stations
The Performance Skills Stations at your NRP course give your learners the opportunity to

- Work with an NRP instructor who will review indications for why and when to use the intervention, and answer questions related to the intervention (cognitive component).

- Practice or review how to perform the intervention with the assistance of an NRP instructor (technical component). When the learner and instructor agree that the learner can perform the intervention smoothly and without assistance, the learner incorporates the intervention into a clinical scenario. Each Performance Checklist scenario builds on the scenario that precedes it. The scenario always begins with the Equipment Check and includes all skills up to and including the skill that is your focus of the Performance Checklist. This repetition prepares the learner for the Integrated Skills Station and simulation training.

Although most learners benefit from instructor-guided review and practice, Performance Skills Stations are not required of all learners in every NRP Provider Course. If the instructor has supervised pre-course practice sessions and has already evaluated the learners' abilities to perform the skills, Performance Skills Stations would be unnecessary at the NRP Provider Course. If the instructor knows the learners well (eg, works with the learners performing frequent complex resuscitations) and is assured that the learners have the expertise to perform NRP technical skills, the instructor may omit Performance Skills Stations at the Provider Course. Perhaps the instructor has assessed the learners' needs and determines that Performance Skills Stations are required only for new skills (such as laryngeal mask airway placement) or infrequently used skills (such as medication administration). If it becomes apparent during the Integrated Skills Station that the learner has gaps in knowledge or technical skills, the learner may need to review, practice, and be evaluated at the appropriate Performance Skills Station.

See Table 3-1 for examples of how the instructor might determine which components to include in a course to best meet the learning objectives of the participants.

Evaluation Activity: Integrated Skills Station
The Integrated Skills Station is required of all learners. The Integrated Skills Station is a performance station that evaluates the learner's ability to integrate the what, when, and how of the resuscitation interventions appropriate to their NRP learning objectives. If the instructor determines that the learner has arrived at the NRP Provider Course fully prepared and not needing any of the Performance Skills Stations for review or practice, the NRP Provider Course may begin with the Integrated Skills Station.

The instructor may evaluate the learner by using one comprehensive scenario or a series of several shorter clinical scenarios. The instructor does not interrupt, coach, or assist the learner during the scenario.

Table 3-1. Tailoring the Neonatal Resuscitation Program Provider Course to Meet Learner Needs: Examples of Who Needs What

Who Are Your Learners?	Which Textbook Lessons ?	Which Activities?
Four newly hired nursery RNs who do not attend births; neonatal intensive care unit (NICU) team attends neonatal emergencies	Lessons 1-4 and Lesson 9	Performance Skills Stations for Lessons 1-4; Integrated Skills Station; Simulation and Debriefing (newborn nursery scenarios)
Level II nursery RNs and MDs, most of whom have worked together >10 years; resuscitate high-risk newborns about 12 times/year	Lessons 1 through 9	All Performance Skills Stations; Integrated Skills Station; Simulation and Debriefing (low- and high-risk birth; focus on teamwork and communication)
20 first-year pediatric residents with no delivery room experience who will attend all births	Lessons 1 through 9	All Performance Skills Stations; Integrated Skills Station; Simulation and Debriefing (healthy baby and at-risk birth scenarios)
Six busy community physicians, frequently attend births on-call for Level II nurseries; recently resuscitated baby with difficult airway; want to improve teamwork and communication	Lessons 1 through 9 (Encourage multidisciplinary participation in course.)	Allow physicians to choose which Performance Skills Stations to review and practice; focus on airway management skills; Integrated Skills Station; Simulation and Debriefing (include difficult airway scenario and focus on teamwork and communication)
Pediatric RN reviewed skills with *Simply NRP* kit at home; does not attend births; cares for newborns readmitted to pediatric unit	Lessons 1-4 and 9	RN chooses to skip Performance Skills Stations; goes directly to Integrated Skills Station; Simulation and Debriefing (includes pediatric unit scenarios)
Neonatal Nurse Practitioners, Transport Team RNs and RTs from regional medical center NICU	Lessons 1-9	Allow participants to choose needed Performance Skills Stations; Integrated Skills Station; Simulation and Debriefing (delivery room and high-risk neonatal transport scenarios)

Those learners studying Lessons 1 through 4 and Lesson 9 are assessed using the Basic Integrated Skills Station Performance Checklist, and those doing the comprehensive NRP course are assessed using the Advanced Integrated Skills Station Performance Checklist (Appendix E). For major deficiencies in knowledge, or if the trainee requires extensive coaching or assistance from team members, the learner is directed to the appropriate Performance Skills Stations for additional review and practice. The Integrated Skills Station should be successfully completed by every learner before proceeding to the Simulation and Debriefing component of the course.

Detailed information about how to administer the Integrated Skills Station is in Chapter 6.

Learning Activity: Simulation and Debriefing
Simulation and debriefing add a new dimension to NRP learning. By replicating the most important visual, auditory, and tactile cues into the resuscitation setting, learners can "suspend their disbelief" and immerse themselves into a realistic neonatal resuscitation experience. Simulation demands that the instructor base the clinical scenario on learning objectives and allow learners to take their own path through the resuscitation, based on the team's evaluation of their interventions and the perceived responses of the "patient." Simulation differs from the Integrated Skills Station in that resuscitation interventions are not prescribed for the purposes of student evaluation (eg, chest compressions may not be indicated). Although technical skills are an important component of resuscitation, the focus of simulation and debriefing is communication and teamwork.

Debriefing is a team discussion facilitated by the NRP instructor that enables the team to self-discover what worked well during the resuscitation, what did not work well, and what should be done differently the next time. The bulk of the learning occurs during debriefing, not during the scenario. Therefore, sufficient time should be allowed for debriefing.

How can I document each NRP course participant's progress through the NRP course?
Consider using the Individual Recording Sheet (pages 41 and 245). Tailor the document to fit the components of your NRP Provider Course. For example, your course participants may not need to review and practice at each Performance Skills Station. The document should be useful to the instructor for documenting information about each learner and what was accomplished at the course.

To document all participants' learning experiences on one form, consider using the Master Recording Sheet (pages 42 and 246). Unlike the AAP Course Roster (pages 175 and 176), the Master Recording Sheet documents each component of every learner's experience.

Neonatal Resuscitation Program™ Provider Course Individual Recording Sheet: Sample
(hospital name)

RETURN THIS SHEET TO ANY INSTRUCTOR AT THE END OF THE COURSE

Provider Course Date: _____

Name: _____

Credentials: RN MSN NNP RT MD DO PA Other _____

Mailing Address: (your NRP™ Provider Card will be *mailed in an envelope* to you at this address, if necessary) _____

Phone or e-mail: _____ Hospital: _____

_____ Online examination verification received

_____ **Lessons 1-9** _____ **Lessons 1-4 and Lesson 9** _____ **Lessons 1-4, 9 and** _____

Performance Skills Stations

Instructor Initials

_____ Equipment Check

_____ Initial Steps

_____ Positive-Pressure Ventilation

_____ Chest Compressions

_____ Intubation (perform or assist)

_____ Laryngeal Mask Airway

_____ Draw up epinephrine

_____ Administer epinephrine via endotracheal tube

_____ Administer epinephrine via emergency umbilical venous catheter (UVC)

_____ Prepare emergency UVC for placement

_____ Place or assist with placement of emergency UVC

_____ **Integrated Skills Station** _____ **Basic** _____ **Advanced**

_____ **Simulation and Debriefing**

INSTRUCTOR INITIALS/SIGNATURES

_____ _____ _____ _____

_____ _____ _____ _____

Instructor Reminder: Participant must pass all components of the course within 1 month of beginning the NRP online examination.

_____ Participant's name recorded on AAP Course Roster

_____ Instructors' names recorded on AAP Course Roster

Master Recording Sheet

American Academy of Pediatrics/American Heart Association Neonatal Resuscitation Program™ Provider Course

Date of course _____   Course location _____

Lead instructor _____   Asst. instructor _____

Asst. instructor _____   Asst. instructor _____

Continuing education credit awarded _____   _____   _____

Place a check in the appropriate box of each completed course component.

Student Name	Online examination verification received	Lessons 1-4 and Lesson 9	Lessons 1 through 9	Lessons 1-4, 9 and (additional) _____	Performance Skills Stations Lessons 1-4, 5, 6	Integrated Skills Station BASIC or ADVANCED	Simulation and Debriefing	Date completed (if different than course date)

How do I organize the NRP for my unit?

Every hospital unit must determine how best to organize the NRP so that all health care professionals maintain NRP status by attending an NRP Provider Course every 2 years. With self-study and online examination prior to the NRP course, instructors no longer need to plan lecture or examination time into the agenda. However, simulation and debriefing do take time that, according to learners who have experienced skilled simulation and debriefing, is "unlike any other learning experience and well worth the time spent."

Some units have large numbers of providers to train. When possible, it is preferable to break the courses into small groups of learners. The focus should be on learning, not throughput. Neonatal Resuscitation Program learning experiences are about quality, not quantity.

How does my NRP course agenda look?

The NRP course agenda varies, depending on the number of learners in your course and how much time each individual requires to complete the course, the number of instructors available, and your available resources, such as classroom space and quantity of NRP supplies and equipment, including newborn manikins.

Assumptions:

- Course time does not include setup or cleanup time, administrative time for sending out course notices, time for documenting attendance, or time for completing the online roster.

- These sample course agendas are 4 hours in length and use 1 instructor for every 3 to 4 learners who have self-studied the text and passed the online examination prior to the course. This allows learners to participate in a team of 3 to 4 learners at a completely equipped station used for all course components. Learners are involved in activities at all times, instead of waiting for a turn with an instructor.

- Your learners may require more or less course time.

May I teach an NRP Provider Course for only one person?

A single-person course is possible, but is inconvenient to arrange and an inefficient use of the instructor's time and resources. The solo learner must recruit at least 2 colleagues who are capable of acting as part of a competent resuscitation team as the learner is evaluated at the Integrated Skills Station. In addition, these colleagues must participate in the scenarios that meet the requirement for the simulation and debriefing components of the course. Although these team members may benefit from practicing neonatal resuscitation with the learner, they add to the staff resources necessary to achieve one person's NRP provider status. It is more efficient to arrange designated course times and dates for groups of learners who can attend the course together and perform resuscitation as a team.

Sample NRP Course Agenda #1

Learners: Community Hospital Physicians, Special Care Nursery RNs, and Labor and Delivery RNs

Time	Activity	Notes
8:00-8:15 am	Introductions, paperwork.	Ensure that all learners have online examination verification. Orient learners to written materials, such as confidentiality agreement.
8:15-8:20 am	What NRP is, what it is not.	The NRP is not a certification course. Learners may practice all skills, but must stay within the designated scope of practice during actual resuscitation. Learners renew provider status every 2 years.
8:20-8:30 am	How the day works.	Course requirements: What do learners need to do? This may vary depending on learners' needs. See Table 3-1 for examples. (See sample script on pages 86-87.)
8:30-8:45 am	"What's the Baby Doing Now?"	Orientation to breathing, heart rate, oximetry. Allow learners to see, hear, and touch manikin and methods of physiologic feedback, such as metronome. Orient to supplies and equipment.
8:45-8:55 am	Demonstrate simulation and debriefing using short scenario.	Allow learners to see how learners prepare for resuscitation, talk through actions as they perform them (no pretending), receive physiologic feedback from the manikin, and observe instructor/learner roles during debriefing.
8:55-9:00 am	Divide into teams based on learning needs.	Each team of 3 or 4 learners is assigned an instructor who is aware of the group's learning objectives.
9:00-11:50 am Instructor manages time for each component based on learners' needs	Each instructor has a complete resuscitation setup and manikin, and takes the team of 3 or 4 learners through Performance Skills Stations in place. Rotate to Laryngeal Mask Airway Performance Skills Station. Rotate to Medication Performance Skills Station.	Each team progresses at its own pace. In this course, the Laryngeal Mask Airway and Medication Performance Skills Stations are separate stations so that each learner can have a setup and practice/review the procedure simultaneously. If each team has one setup for laryngeal mask airway placement and one setup for umbilical venous catheter line placement and medications, learners must practice one person at a time.
	Integrated Skills Stations in progress.	The NRP instructor decides when each learner is ready for the Integrated Skills Station.
	Simulation and Debriefing in progress.	The NRP instructor may conduct Simulation and Debriefing at the same station where practice and learning occurred, or at a different station with additional instructor assistance.
11:50 am-12:00 noon	Evaluation and adjournment.	Learners turn in their Individual Recording Sheet, online examination verification, and course evaluation.

Sample NRP Course Agenda #2

Learners: Neonatal nurse practitioners, neonatal intensive care unit (NICU) RNs, and respiratory therapists who are the Delivery Room Resuscitation Team in a Busy Level III setting. *Prior to the course, instructors and the NICU Resuscitation Team collaborated on what to include at a "Delivery Room Management of the ELBW Infant" Performance Skills Station (based on the Resuscitation Skills Video of the same name in the textbook DVD) to meet this team's learning needs.*

Time	Activity	Notes
8:00-8:15 am	Introductions, paperwork.	Ensure that all learners have online examination verification. Orient learners to written materials such as confidentiality agreement.
8:15-8:20 am	What NRP is, what it is not.	The NRP is not a certification course. Learners may practice all skills but must stay within designated scope of practice during actual resuscitation. Learners renew provider status every 2 years.
8:20-8:30 am	How the day works.	Course requirements: What do learners need to do? (NRP instructors assessed the group's needs and selected specific Performance Skills Stations.)
8:30-8:45 am	"What's the Baby Doing Now?"	Orientation to breathing, heart rate, oximetry. Allow learners to see, hear, and touch manikin and methods of physiologic feedback, such as metronome. Orient to supplies and equipment.
8:45-8:55 am	Demonstrate simulation and debriefing using short scenario.	Allow learners to see how learners prepare for resuscitation, talk through actions as they perform them (no pretending), receive physiologic feedback from the manikin, and observe instructor/learner roles during debriefing.
8:55-9:00 am	Divide into teams composed of typical resuscitation team (NNP, 2 RNs, RT for this course).	Each team of 3 or 4 learners is assigned an instructor who is aware of the group's learning objectives.
9:00-10:00 am	Four teams rotate to 4 stations. (Instructors added Station 4 to this course based on learners' needs and followed recommendations in the *NRP Instructor DVD* Resuscitation Skills videos of the same title.)	Station 1: Intubation Performance Skills Station (including meconium management) Station 2: Medication Performance Skills Station Station 3: Laryngeal Mask Airway Performance Skills Station Station 4: The ELBW: Aspects of Delivery Room Management (additional station created by NRP instructors)
10:00-10:30 am	Integrated Skills Stations in Progress.	The NRP instructor decides when each learner is ready for the Integrated Skills Station.
10:30-11:50 am	Simulation and Debriefing in Progress.	The NRP instructor may conduct Simulation and Debriefing at the same station where practice and learning occurred, or at a different station with additional instructor assistance.
11:50-12:00 noon	Evaluation and adjournment.	Learners turn in their Individual Recording Sheet, online examination verification, and course evaluation.

Sample Timeline for Neonatal Resuscitation Program Course Preparation*

Choose the tasks applicable to your course.

Setting a date for a course
- ❑ Determine need for course and what type of course (Provider, Hospital-based Instructor, or Regional Trainer Course).
- ❑ Determine need to jointly sponsor or desire to cosponsor with another institution or organization.
- ❑ Select potential participants.
- ❑ Determine date(s) of course.
- ❑ Research continuing education application(s).
  - — Submission deadlines vary from 6 weeks to 12 months prior to offering.

Three to 12 months before the course
- ❑ Prepare mailing list.
- ❑ Arrange and reserve space for practice, if necessary.
- ❑ Select course location.
- ❑ Choose faculty and verify instructor status.
- ❑ Have faculty planning meeting.
- ❑ Notify person who is responsible for staffing/scheduling of the course date to facilitate course attendance.
- ❑ Determine how learners will access the online examination.
- ❑ Prepare budget.
- ❑ Prepare course flyer or announcement.
- ❑ Submit continuing education application(s), if not already done.

Six to 8 weeks before the course
- ❑ Advertise course and mail flyer to participants outside your institution.
- ❑ Order textbooks for participants if you supply them.
- ❑ Order additional Neonatal Resuscitation Program (NRP) supplies if needed.

Four to 6 weeks before the course
- ❑ Begin registration list of participants' names, addresses, and phone numbers.
- ❑ Distribute textbooks (if applicable to your course procedure) with instructions to read and study the textbook and/or accompanying DVD and pass the online examination prior to course.
- ❑ Send confirmation letter and attachments (map, study aids, Experience Survey) as registrations are received.
- ❑ Arrange for food and beverages, if applicable.
- ❑ Order additional course supplies.
- ❑ Inventory equipment and make arrangements to borrow supplies, if necessary.
- ❑ Plan time for faculty planning meeting; plan site visit if teaching at an unfamiliar institution.
- ❑ Arrange opportunity for practice periods, if necessary for your course.

Two weeks before the course
- ❑ Write or request checks for honoraria and other expenses due, if applicable.
- ❑ Review responses to Experience Survey for NRP Provider Course.
- ❑ Prepare written handouts.
- ❑ Prepare administrative handouts and directional signs.
- ❑ Have faculty planning meeting periods, if necessary for your course.
- ❑ Continue opportunities for learners to practice, if necessary for your course.
- ❑ Confirm course date(s) and expectations of instructors.
- ❑ Remind participants of the requirement to study the material and pass the online examination before the course.

One week before the course
- ❑ Collate written handouts for learners.
- ❑ Organize resuscitation supplies to take to classroom.
- ❑ Confirm room reservation, catering arrangements, and audiovisual equipment.

Day of the course
- ❑ Arrive early.
- ❑ Post directional signs.
- ❑ Check classroom and, if necessary, refreshment setup.
- ❑ Set up Performance Skills Stations, Integrated Skills Stations, and area for simulation and debriefing.
- ❑ Test audiovisual equipment.
- ❑ Ensure that you have or can access instructor information for the Course Roster (full name and instructor ID number).

After the course
- ❑ Clean up, restock, and reorganize NRP equipment. Replace and repair equipment, if necessary.
- ❑ Return borrowed equipment.
- ❑ Complete American Academy of Pediatrics (AAP) Course Roster electronically at www.aap.org/nrp, make a copy for your file, and submit to the AAP.
- ❑ Summarize evaluations and distribute to faculty and continuing education provider, if applicable.
- ❑ Make personal notes of what worked well and what to do differently next time.
- ❑ Notify students' supervisors of students' attendance, if necessary.
- ❑ Make copies for your file, then send continuing education forms, evaluation summary, and budget to appropriate parties.
- ❑ Send thank-you notes as appropriate.
- ❑ Complete and distribute NRP Course Completion Cards when received from the AAP.

*Each of these steps is described in detail in Appendix C. The timeline is created for use in planning a comprehensive NRP Provider Course for community participants. Choose the steps most applicable to your planning needs and make your own course-planning timeline.

Continuing Education Credits

Do course participants automatically receive continuing education credits for attending an NRP course?

Although the AAP and the American Heart Association (AHA) developed the course materials, they **grant continuing education credits only for the online examination portion of NRP courses and for the *NRP Instructor DVD: An Interactive Tool for Facilitation of Simulation-based Learning*.**

There are several reasons for this. The organization jointly sponsoring the activity must be involved in all stages of planning. With thousands of instructors conducting courses throughout the world, it would be impossible for either the AAP or the AHA to meet this requirement. In addition, the number of actual hours spent in the course can vary significantly, depending on the format used by the course directors. Consequently, the instructors seeking joint sponsorship of their NRP courses must work with accredited organizations closer to home, such as the continuing education department of a hospital, medical school, nursing school, or state medical or nursing organization.

How do I grant continuing education credits for my NRP course?

Requirements for continuing education credits vary from state to state and among professional disciplines (nursing, medicine, respiratory therapy, etc). Although the basic material to be submitted to the various governing bodies may be similar, the number of credits allowed and forms required will differ.

If you wish to offer continuing education credits to physicians, nurses, and respiratory therapists who attend your course, you need the course to be accredited by an organization that monitors the quality of continuing professional education. For physicians, the Accreditation Council for Continuing Medical Education (ACCME) is the accrediting agency that governs the quality of continuing education and grants category 1 continuing medical education credits to physicians. For nurses, the state nurses' association or a professional nursing organization may be the accrediting agency.

Instructors can begin the continuing education application process by considering the following points:

- Find out if your institution is accredited to grant continuing education credits to health care professionals. The education department or medical staff support office may be approved providers for education credit. This usually makes the application process easier than going through a state association or professional organization.

- Start your application process well before the course date. Submission deadlines can be up to 12 months before the offering.

- Use the continuing medical and nursing education staff at a hospital or training institution as helpful resources for this process.

- Ask whoever grants the continuing education credits for an application packet. A sample application is also helpful.

- Find a contact person who is available to answer your questions and screen your application prior to official submission, especially if you are inexperienced with continuing education applications.

- Check accrediting agency guidelines for the continuing education credits that may be available for your course. Be aware that states vary in what education courses qualify for continuing education credit.

- Many agencies allow you to submit one continuing education application that covers all NRP courses held at your institution for an entire year or longer.

> Instructors planning to conduct NRP courses internationally are encouraged to contact the AAP Life Support office. Staff can provide valuable information about translation of materials, copyright permission, current international activities, and program implementation.

Teaching the Neonatal Resuscitation Program Outside the United States: Things to Know

I teach NRP courses outside the United States. What should I know about planning this type of course?

If you plan to travel to another country to teach the NRP, please contact local authorities and network with local pediatric or neonatal organizations. The NRP Steering Committee recommends host country ownership of neonatal resuscitation training for the most effective dissemination and implementation of the NRP. Therefore, it is acceptable, and most likely necessary, to customize the NRP according to host country resources, policies, and practices. In resource-limited areas, it may be appropriate to use the Helping Babies Breathe curriculum (**www.HelpingBabiesBreathe.com**).

🖥www

Neonatal Resuscitation Program Provider Cards are not generally issued outside of the United States (one exception being for training that is led by the US military overseas). The primary rationale for this policy can be summarized as follows:

Although the educational principles of the AAP/AHA Life Support educational programs developed for use in the United States can be adapted for other countries, conducting the programs exactly as they are conducted in the United States may not be appropriate.

Appropriate health care organizations in other countries should be encouraged to develop a structure for implementing life support programs that will address educational needs unique to their country. This could include recognizing instructors, conducting training courses, awarding Course Completion Cards or certificates, and instituting a mechanism for tracking the number of people trained.

There is a concern that the ability to obtain a card issued by an American organization might serve as a disincentive for other countries to develop their own national structure. Inappropriate use of Course Completion Cards in the past also played a part in this decision.

Neonatal Resuscitation Program hospital-based instructors can receive credit toward maintenance of their instructor status for international Provider Courses they conduct by submitting a Course Roster in the usual manner. The course will be entered in their instructor file, but NRP Course Completion Cards will not be issued to participants.

Instructors planning to conduct NRP courses internationally are encouraged to contact the AAP Life Support office. Staff can provide valuable information about translation of materials, copyright permission, current international activities, and program implementation. A list of countries where the NRP has been implemented, as well as approved translations, can be found on the **NRP Web site at http://www.aap.org/ nrp/main.html (click on International).** ⌨www

If you wish to purchase materials for international teaching efforts, you can do so through the AAP Customer Service Department, which also may be able to put you in contact with a distributor in another country.

Instructor Q & A

Our unit has a long history of "checking off" NRP learners whenever they need to be renewed. We often checked off one learner at a time. For this reason, everyone is "due" at a different time, every month of the year. How can I get everyone onto a schedule where, for example, I could offer an NRP course for 9 staff members every month?
The introduction of the new NRP methodology and 6th Edition materials is an ideal time to take charge of time-consuming and resource-heavy methods of NRP compliance. Now, more than ever, the focus is on quality learning, not checking people off and handing out Course Completion Cards. Make a list of when all NRP providers are "due" for their next NRP course. Group them together as closely as possible by their renewal dates, bearing in mind that the most useful course will involve all members of the multidisciplinary team that resuscitates the baby together (MD, RN, NNP, RT, or various combinations of these disciplines). It does not matter that these learners' NRP provider status is not yet "due" for renewal; group them together and start fresh with a new schedule that is efficient for instructors and meets the learning objectives of course participants.

We have a medium-sized unit, but everyone has a different level of expertise when it comes to resuscitation. Expertise also varies by shift. Tailoring NRP courses to meet different learning objectives for different learners sounds like a nightmare. I want to do one course, the same way, every time, for every learner.

It is possible to do one standardized course for everyone while meeting differing learning objectives. If you do not know the levels of expertise of your learners, use the Experience Survey as a reference. Divide your course participants into teams, and attempt to place those with similar learning objectives and experience together.

Include *every* course component (eg, each Performance Skills Station) so that learners who need help have that opportunity. Your more experienced learners will want to move more quickly through most Performance Skills Stations; however, they may be surprised to learn that they, too, have things to learn about titrating oxygen with pulse oximetry, placing a laryngeal mask airway, etc. In this way, no learners feel bored (or rushed by other learners) as they move through the Performance Skills Stations and Integrated Skills Station.

The Simulation and Debriefing component comes after the Performance Skills Stations and Integrated Skills Station. The experienced group may want to proceed with simulation-based training without its less-experienced colleagues, and "get done" with the course. This puts both groups at a disadvantage. Try to put together resuscitation teams for Simulation and Debriefing that would normally occur in the work setting, and consider giving your quick learners and experienced NRP participants additional challenging activities while waiting for their colleagues to catch up. Set up a needle thoracentesis station and allow them to practice this skill while watching the "Needle Thoracentesis" Resuscitation Skills video on the textbook DVD at the station. They also can practice setting up for delivery room management of the extremely low birthweight (ELBW) newborn using the Resuscitation Skills video on the textbook DVD as a guide. If the Resuscitation Skills videos are used as a guide, these 2 stations do not require NRP instructor supervision. For additional activities, ask for suggestions about what procedures are infrequently performed at resuscitation, yet carry high stress and high risk. For example, do resuscitation team members know how to order blood and set it up in a hurry? Use this opportunity to discuss your protocol and simulate it, looking for work processes that could be improved and skills that need review. By the time your expert resuscitators and fast-moving course participants have been through the optional stations and have made notes about what they have learned and want to discuss later, the teams that needed more time for Performance Skills Stations will have caught up. For Simulation and Debriefing, you can now create resuscitation teams of people with varying skills who would typically work together to resuscitate babies in your birth setting.

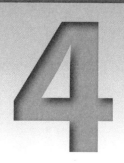

The Online Examination

The Neonatal Resuscitation Program™ (NRP™) course format now requires learners to study the material from the *Textbook of Neonatal Resuscitation, 6th Edition*, and take an online examination *before* attending their NRP course. Hospital-based instructors and regional trainers will also be required to take the online examination, as will applicants to any NRP Instructor Course.

In Chapter 4 you will learn about

- **Why the hard-copy examination format was eliminated.**
- **Advantages of the online format.**
- **Who takes the online examination.**
- **How to access the online examination.**
- **Components of examination design.**
- **A sample document to help inform learners about the online examination.**

"Instructor Self-assessment" for Chapter 4 begins on page 193.

After studying this chapter, complete the Chapter 4 questions, using the answer sheets that begin on page 188. Your regional trainer may ask you to bring the answer sheets to your NRP Instructor Course.

Why is the hard-copy format of the NRP examination no longer available with the 6th Edition after December 2011?

In the previous NRP course model, most instructors lectured about the Key Points of each lesson to a passive group of learners, then spent course time proctoring and correcting the examination. By self-studying the textbook or DVD and taking the examination prior to the NRP course, learners take responsibility for their own learning and valuable time is saved by eliminating lectures about textbook material that learners should have already mastered. The online examination also frees up course time for demonstration, discussion, hands-on practice, skills evaluation, and simulation and debriefing.

What are the advantages of online testing?

- The learner can take the online examination anywhere and at his or her own convenience, anytime during the 30 days before the scheduled NRP Provider Course.

- Continuing education credits for physicians, nurses, respiratory therapists, and EMS professionals are now available for online testing. Upon successful completion of the examination, learners will be able to print a certificate detailing the credits awarded.

- The online examination is financially advantageous for the institution. Previous NRP Provider Courses often involved hours of slides and lectures about textbook material and considerable time spent administering and correcting the hard-copy examination. Although NRP does not mandate how long a Provider Course should be, most instructors agree that the online examination shortens classroom time considerably.

- The NRP Steering Committee will be able to monitor how each question performs, quickly make needed adjustments to wording or illustrations, identify commonly missed questions, develop strategies to alert instructors to revised educational materials, and add audio and video clips to the questions.

- Online testing gives facilities and their instructors the ability to access a list of who has completed the examination, as well as the date of completion.

Who takes the online examination?

All learners using the *Neonatal Resuscitation Program, 6th Edition,* are required to take the NRP examination online. The hard-copy examination will no longer be available to instructors or learners.

Provider Course participants are required to self-study the *Textbook of Neonatal Resuscitation, 6th Edition,* and take the online examination during the 30 days before their scheduled NRP Provider Course.

Hospital-based instructors and regional trainers are required to complete the NRP online examination every 2 years, beginning in 2013, based on their renewal date. For example, an instructor with a renewal date of March 1, 2011, must complete the online examination by March 1, 2013, and every 2 years thereafter. However, instructors do not need to wait for their renewal date to approach after January 1, 2013, to take the online examination. The examination will be provided at no charge to instructors once per calendar year beginning in Spring 2011. Every time an instructor passes the online examination, continuing education credit will be offered; however, continuing education credits are valid only once every 2 years. Studying the 6th Edition of the textbook and taking the online examination may be part of the lead instructor's or regional trainer's requirement for an instructor update to the 6th Edition materials or as a requirement for an annual update to ensure instructors' proficiency with the content knowledge.

Neonatal Resuscitation Program *Instructor Course candidates* must have taken and passed Lessons 1 through 9 of the online examination during the 30 days before their Instructor Course or Regional Trainer Course. There is a fee for the examination in this case.

Why are Hospital-based instructors and regional trainers now required to take the online examination?

Many NRP instructors achieved their instructor or regional trainer status many years ago. The NRP has never required any evidence that instructors are knowledgeable about the current practice of neonatal resuscitation. Requiring instructors to take the online examination not only familiarizes them with the online examination that we ask all learners to take, but helps ensure that instructors and regional trainers have current knowledge for teaching their courses. This requirement is part of an ongoing effort by the NRP Instructor Development Task Force to ensure the quality of NRP instruction.

When should the learner take the online examination?

The learner preparing for an NRP Provider Course should take the examination during the 30 days before the scheduled NRP course.

Providers should successfully complete all relevant lessons of the online examination **prior** to the expiration date on their existing Provider Card. The NRP is able to send out reminders to those NRP providers nearing their expiration dates so that learners can take a Provider Course prior to their expiration date. The policy regarding what happens if an NRP provider's status expires is determined by each institution.

The NRP provider who is preparing for an NRP Instructor Course should take the examination during the 30 days before the Hospital-based

Instructor or Regional Trainer Course. This helps ensure that instructor candidates have recently reviewed all 9 lessons of the textbook.

Who takes which sections of the NRP online examination?
Instructors and those preparing for Instructor Courses take all 9 Lessons of the online examination.

Depending on professional roles and responsibilities, learners in NRP Provider Courses may take all 9 lessons, or the minimum NRP Provider Course requirement of Lessons 1 through 4 and Lesson 9, or the instructor may require learners to take Lessons 1 through 4 and Lesson 9 plus additional assigned lessons determined by hospital policy.

What if something unexpected happens online during testing?
HealthStream Customer Service is available from 7:00 am to 7:00 pm CST, Monday through Friday (except major holidays) at **customer. service@healthstream.com.**

How are people with disabilities taking the online examination accommodated?
The online examination is compatible with many types of Assistive Technology. If you or your learners require further accommodations, please contact the American Academy of Pediatrics (AAP) Life Support office at

American Academy of Pediatrics
Division of Life Support Programs
141 Northwest Point Blvd
Elk Grove Village, IL 60007
Phone: 847/434-4798
Fax: 847/228-1350
E-mail: lifesupport@aap.org
Web site: **www.arp.org/nrp**

How do learners access the NRP online examination?

The NRP has partnered with HealthStream, an online learning provider, to host the online examination.

If your institution is a HealthStream customer, your facility's HealthStream administrator contacts HealthStream and adds the NRP online examination to your facility's already established list of offerings. Then you may need to work with your facility's HealthStream administrator about making the NRP online examination available to your NRP learners, including physicians and others who access NRP training through your facility but are not necessarily hospital employees. Your facility's HealthStream administrator will purchase and deliver the course to your students in the same way that other online courses are currently delivered to your HealthStream system. Although your facility must purchase the examination from HealthStream for online use, there is no additional setup fee and no additional per-student fee.

If your facility uses a different Learning Management System than HealthStream, but would like to have the NRP examination delivered via your current Learning Management System, HealthStream can work with your facility's information technology (IT) staff to establish this access. There is no additional cost. Visit **www.aap.org/nrp** for more information.

🖥**www**

If your facility is not a HealthStream customer and wishes to purchase a "batch" of examinations to take advantage of bulk order discounts, go to **www.aap.org/nrp** and click Online Examination.

Bulk orders can be made for 10 or more licenses at a time. When you purchase batches of examinations as needed, HealthStream will build a Web site for your faculty, where your course participants will access the online NRP examination through a Web link.

- There are 2 ways to enter students into HealthStream so that they can access their examination:
  1. At some point, a list of your course participants can be sent to HealthStream. This can be done using the data file option (best for large classes where you have the names already in a spreadsheet and you know who is attending).

  OR

  2. Manually enter the student information over a period of time as students register for your course or come due for their examination. The instructor or other designated administrator provides the student with a simple username and password for access to the examination.

- Learners have the option to receive an e-mail reminder prior to their NRP provider expiration. They will need to visit the NRP Web site online examination section, and opt in to receive notification.

If you are an individual purchaser of one NRP examination (paying for the examination with a credit card), access the online test at **www.aap. org/nrp** and click on the "Online Examination" symbol.

🖥**www**

You will be asked to register with a user name and a password. You will receive a reminder e-mail in 2 years if you choose to provide a valid e-mail address (your personal e-mail address is usually the most reliable over time).

Instructor Q & A

One advantage of online testing includes the ability to access Advanced Tracking and Performance data from HealthStream. I know that hospitals who are already HealthStream customers have

access to this service. However, my facility is not a HealthStream customer but we would like Advanced Tracking and Performance data about our learners. How can we arrange this?

HealthStream will work with a representative from your institution's IT Department to create a HealthStream Express site that would allow the NRP instructor to enter student data. Your HealthStream Express site will then be set up to retrieve data about who has completed the online examination, and on what date. There is no additional cost for setting up the HealthStream Express site. Visit **www.aap.org/nrp** for more information.

🖥**www**

I'm surprised to learn that the online examination requires either the hospital or the NRP learner to pay a fee. Budgets are tight!

We understand that requiring participants to pay a fee is a significant change. The NRP has never charged any fees for the development or administration of this comprehensive international program. However, the expertise required to develop and maintain the online examination requires the use of a commercial vendor. We have made every effort to keep the fee as low as possible. Please be assured that the online examination is not a profit-making venture for the NRP.

We hope that our advance notice of this change (beginning in 2009 through articles in the *NRP Instructor Update,* in the online notice on the NRP Web site, and at our many NRP presentations at national and regional conferences) helped prepare hospitals and educational systems to make the necessary adjustments to their budgets. We believe that the required fee is small in comparison to those charged by other continuing education programs.

Taking the Online Examination

When logging in and beginning the online examination, the student will be asked if an instructor has been identified to provide the in-person components of the NRP course. An NRP instructor is not obligated to conduct an NRP course if the learner has not made these prior arrangements with the instructor. This contact between the learner and instructor is also important so that the learner knows the process for accessing the online examination, which will vary by facility, depending on how the facility gains access to the online examination for its learners.

How is the online examination scored?

- Online testing is arranged in sections, starting with Lesson 1.

- The questions and distracters are randomized, so the questions and distracters are never in the same order. New questions may be piloted through the system as well. Members of the NRP Steering

Committee have the ability to review questions to ensure that all questions are valid and reliable.

- The learner may skip questions within a lesson and come back to them. The learner also may change answers on any question until the lesson is submitted for grading.

- The learner must hit the submit button to submit his or her answers for scoring.

- The learner must receive a minimum passing score (80%) in each lesson for which he or she is being tested.

- If the learner fails one or more lessons, the test section can be retaken one time. Lessons can be retaken immediately, or a lesson can be retaken on a different day, within 14 days of the original purchase date. After 14 days, the unfinished online examination becomes invalid, and the learner needs to pay the fee and begin again. The original examination fee is not refunded.

- If the learner fails a second time, the learner needs to pay the examination fee again and retake the entire examination. (See Remediation Plan section.) The original examination charge is not refunded.

- The online examination program determines that the learner is finished when the tests for Lessons 1 through 4 and Lesson 9 are completed. If the learner is testing on more than Lessons 1 through 4 and Lesson 9, the learner should take those additional lessons prior to completing all the examination sections for Lessons 1 through 4 and Lesson 9. To prevent ending the examination prior to finishing all desired examination sections, you may wish to instruct learners to take Lesson 9 last, so that they are not shut out of the examination prior to finishing all the lesson examinations they need to take for their course requirement.

- Forms to keep track of individual progress, and a master sheet to track course participants' progress through the program, are available in Appendix D.

Feedback on Examination Scores

If the learner passes, he or she will receive a cue for a one-time opportunity to print what questions were missed in that lesson. The learner may wish to discuss the results of the examination with the instructor and clarify any questions or concerns.

- The learner should review any questions he or she may have missed before the NRP Provider Course. If the learner does not achieve the minimum passing score on any lesson, he or she must retake that section of the examination. This learner does not see which questions were missed.

- Learners who initially fail to successfully complete an examination may retest anytime, at their own convenience, within 14 days of the original examination date.

- If, after retaking the lesson examination for a second time, the learner is unable to achieve a minimum passing score, the instructor and learner should work together on a remediation plan.

What does the learner need to do after completing the online examination?

After online testing is complete, the learner completes the post-examination and receives online examination verification delineating which lessons have been successfully completed and the date of completion (the online examination verification is valid for admission into an NRP course for 30 days after completion). The learner also may print the certificate of continuing education document if desired.

The learner presents the online examination verification to the instructor on the day of the course (within 30 days of completion) as evidence of having successfully completed the online testing. The instructor also may request to see the learner's copy of missed questions prior to the course for the purpose of assessing the learner's needs during the course. However, it is the learner's responsibility to review missed questions and understand the answers. The instructor is not responsible for teaching missed content. The instructor should be available to the learner prior to the course if the learner has lingering questions after the examination is complete.

If 30 days pass after completion of the online examination without completion of the NRP Provider Course, the online examination becomes invalid. The examination fee is not refundable. The 30 days start on the day that the learner takes the examination the first time.

How do instructors create a remediation plan?

Most learners who study the textbook know the correct answers to the review sections at the end of each lesson, and who know the Key Points for each lesson, have no trouble successfully passing the NRP examination. Participants should be expected to determine their own readiness for taking the online examination by using these study tools in each lesson of the textbook or on the accompanying textbook DVD.

Repeated failure requires a remediation plan. This plan may be individualized for each learner or be a standard policy developed by an institution.

- The learning requirements of the plan for each individual situation are at the discretion of the instructor and/or the institution.

- The plan should include additional time for study and test practice using the review sections for self-assessment and the summaries of Key Points in each lesson of the *Textbook of Neonatal Resuscitation, 6th Edition.* This approach places responsibility for learning on the participant rather than the instructor.

Each institution needs to develop its own policy for managing the financial implications of learners who require retesting and repayment of the online examination fee after failing the online examination.

What security precautions are in place?

Distracters and test questions are in different order; therefore, 2 learners sitting side-by-side will appear to have 2 different examinations and will find it nearly impossible to discuss answers as they test.

What if the learner comes to the NRP Provider or Instructor Course without having taken the online examination?

As a general rule, instructors who deny admission to students who have not successfully passed the online examination will achieve good compliance with pre-course examination and enjoy the benefit of learners who are prepared to spend course time with hands-on skills and simulation training.

Health care professionals who are inexperienced perinatal or neonatal providers will have difficulty with hands-on skills and resuscitation scenarios if the online examination has not been completed as part of the course learning. They should not be admitted to the course as a participant.

Rarely, an instructor must use his or her own discretion and make an exception to the rule. Health care professionals who have many years of NRP courses behind them may be able to do well with hands-on skills without having completed the online examination; however, they do not achieve NRP provider status until the instructor receives the examination verification of the online examination. The instructor must be willing to wait for the learner to submit the online examination verification before giving the learner the NRP Provider Card and submitting a Course Completion Roster. The learner has up to 1 month from the date of the NRP Provider Course to submit his or her online examination verification. (The instructor may set the examination deadline for a shorter time period than 1 month, if desired.) In this case, the instructor must be willing to spend the extra time and effort to keep track of this learner's progress and potentially submit a different online Course Roster with a different course completion date for this learner. Allowing the learner to take the course without having completed the online examination should happen only on rare occasions, and should not be presented as a routine option for learners.

SAMPLE LETTER TEMPLATE FOR NEONATAL RESUSCITATION PROGRAM COURSE PARTICIPANTS

(Tailor to fit the needs of your learners.)

Hospital logo

Welcome to the American Academy of Pediatrics/American Heart Association Neonatal Resuscitation Program™ (NRP™) course. While this course does not guarantee proficiency during an actual resuscitation, it lays the foundation of knowledge, technical skills, and teamwork and communication skills that enable participants to continue development of neonatal resuscitation skills. Successful completion earns the participant an NRP Provider Card. Neonatal Resuscitation Program provider status should be renewed every 2 years.

Prior to the course, you must read the *Textbook of Neonatal Resuscitation, 6th Edition* (or view the DVD that accompanies the textbook) and **pass the NRP online examination.** You may find it helpful to go to **www.aap.org/nrp** and read the resources under the Online Examination tab.

We are expecting you

Date: _____

Time: _____

Location: _____

This is a hands-on interactive course. You successfully pass the course after you

- Produce your online examination verification on course day. You are assigned

_____ *Lessons 1-4* and *Lesson 9*

_____ *Lessons 1-9*

_____ *Lessons 1-4,* _____, _____, _____, _____, and *Lesson 9*

- Demonstrate the above assigned neonatal resuscitation lessons within the context of a clinical scenario in correct sequence according to the NRP flow diagram, with correct timing and proper technique. Use the Integrated Skills Assessment Checklist (Basic or Advanced) in the textbook as your guide.

- Participate in simulation training and debriefing exercises.

Information About NRP Online Examination

Bring your online examination verification to your NRP Course.

To access the NRP online examination (instructor fills in information appropriate to the institutional process), _____

You must take the online examination at your convenience on any computer prior to your NRP course, during the **30 days before the course. You must finish testing within 14 days of your original start date. If you complete the examination more than 30 days before your scheduled course, the examination is invalid and you must pay to take it again.**

This test covers the material in Lessons 1 through 9 the *Textbook of Neonatal Resuscitation, 6th Edition.* The test is not difficult for learners who focus on each lesson's Key Points and know the correct answers to each lesson's Review section (practice test). Most new learners require several hours of study time. You may not agree with the NRP approach to every clinical scenario. We will allow discussion time at the course for these differences in opinion.

Please note: Lessons 1 through 4 and Lesson 9 are required Lessons. Once you complete the final required lesson, the examination is considered complete, and you will not have the opportunity to test on additional lessons. To prevent being shut out of the examination prior to taking all the required lesson examinations for your course, take the Lesson 9 examination last.

The average time to complete the full examination (all 9 lessons) is 55 minutes. The online test is arranged by lesson, in the same order as in the textbook. You may skip questions and come back to them. You may change your answers on any question until you submit the lesson for grading. The computer scores each lesson as you submit answers. You may stop testing after a lesson, and resume testing later.

If you do not attain a passing score (80%) for a lesson, you may retake that section immediately, or on a different day, **within 14 days** of the original testing date. After 14 days, the online testing becomes invalid and requires payment to begin again.

You may retake sections ONE time. If you fail a second time, contact _____ at _____ to make a new plan. If you do not finish testing or cannot pass the test prior to the course start time, you may practice hands-on skills at the course with other learners, but you will not receive your NRP provider status on this course day.

The registration for online examination will ask if you have designated an NRP instructor for the in-person components of the NRP Provider Course. The answer is YES. You do not need to name the instructor.

After completing the examination, you will receive online examination verification. **Bring this with you to the NRP course** and give it to the instructor. If you cannot produce this online examination verification, you cannot receive NRP provider status at this course.

If you have questions about this NRP course or online examination process, contact

_____ at _____ (phone) or

_____ (e-mail).

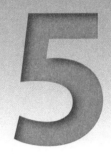

Organizing Supplies and Arranging the Classroom

A vital component of every Neonatal Resuscitation Program™ (NRP™) course is the instructor's skill at facilitating participant learning. The purpose of this chapter is to provide strategies for assembling, organizing, and setting up equipment for NRP practice, learning activities and evaluation, and simulation-based training. The instructor who spends time developing a system for keeping supplies and equipment organized and functional, and standardizes the work involved in setting up each course, saves countless hours "building" each course from scratch.

In Chapter 5 you will learn

- Supplies and equipment needed for a typical hospital-based training program

- How you may organize supplies, equipment, and written materials to facilitate course setup and administration

- How you may organize your classroom for an NRP Provider Course

"Instructor Self-assessment" for Chapter 5 begins on page 194.

After studying this chapter, complete the Chapter 5 questions, using the answer sheets that begin on page 188. Your regional trainer may ask you to bring the answer sheets to your NRP Instructor Course.

> The most successful and satisfied NRP instructors develop a system for organizing and maintaining NRP supplies and equipment and save time by standardizing the work involved in setting up each course.

What is meant by "standardizing" the work of your Neonatal Resuscitation Program?

Nothing is more frustrating than spending hours building the same NRP course every time a course is needed. If every course is fraught with time-consuming problems such as missing equipment, disorganized skills stations, paperwork that must be updated and collated, and confusion due to inconsistency in the way the classroom is arranged on course day, your training program may benefit from standardized work.

When you standardize this work, you eliminate the inconsistency and variability in the processes that cause wasted time and repetitive effort. For example, do you pull out your boxes or bags of NRP supplies a few days before every Provider Course and painstakingly sort through your piles to assemble skills stations? Do you discover items that are missing or broken, which necessitates a last-minute scramble for supplies? Although you will tailor each NRP course to meet the needs of your learners, many of the components of course organization and implementation are the same each time and can be organized so that the same work is not unnecessarily repeated for each course. This chapter makes suggestions for strategies that may help organize your equipment and paperwork, standardize your classroom setup, and save you hours of time setting up your NRP courses. If you plan your classroom layout, organize your paperwork and supplies, and take steps to ensure processes that keep you organized and well-supplied, you will also sustain these worthwhile efforts.

What equipment and supplies are needed for a Provider Course?

See the supply list for a typical Hospital-based NRP Course on pages 80-81, and pages 212-213. In addition to assembling supplies, an important part of getting organized is letting go of supplies that are not needed for an NRP Provider Course. It is tempting to save expired or surplus supplies "just in case," but supplies that are not needed for neonatal resuscitation (eg, disposable diapers, measuring tapes, and cuffed endotracheal tubes) create clutter and take up room. Every item in your supply area should have a purpose and a designated storage space.

The list of equipment and supplies for a hospital-based NRP is quite extensive. How can I assemble all those items?

To assemble all the needed items, you may need to be an equipment and supply scavenger at first. Notify everyone in the clinical area that you are looking for supplies that are opened but unused or unopened and about to be discarded. Many pieces of equipment can be cleaned for practice on manikins. These items are separated from patient use and designated for neonatal resuscitation practice and NRP courses.

Your hospital may need to purchase some equipment for your program, such as newborn manikins and neonatal intubation heads. Your hospital may be able to purchase equipment for you or may have a foundation that grants monetary requests for special projects.

Your regional outreach education program may have a loan program for NRP equipment. Check to see if you can borrow manikins, intubation heads, and other equipment.

Use every item for your NRP with reuse in mind. For example, endotracheal (ET) tubes can be reused many times for an NRP course simply by saving the original package and storing the ET tube in its plastic and paper wrapper. The end-tidal carbon dioxide (CO_2) detector also can be stored in its original package. Syringes and stopcocks can be used many times, as can suction devices and even umbilical catheters.

Expired drugs may go back to the manufacturer for a credit, but your hospital pharmacy might contribute them to your stock of NRP supplies. If necessary, medication vials and intravenous bags can be used repeatedly by refilling them with water. Mark these supplies "NRP use only" in bold marker and keep them well away from patient stock items so that they cannot be mistakenly used for patient care.

How can we get more organized and streamline our processes?

Standardize your written course materials.

If your course materials are the same for every course, you need not "build" the course from scratch every time. Collate written materials needed for every course and make packets for multiple courses at once, especially if you have numerous courses per year. Most courses entail the same handout materials each time. Most course materials can be printed on both sides of the page. The following list is one example of an NRP Provider Course syllabus.

- Agenda (See 2 samples in Appendix D and on pages 44 and 45.)

  - Do not date the agenda. You can use the same agenda for every course.

  - Do not write the actual time of day for each activity if your course times are variable (eg, if some of your courses occur in the morning and some occur in the afternoon). You may write the expected length of time for each activity, if that works for your course. Many NRP Provider Courses need a flexible timeline, which allows instructors to spend the appropriate amount of time needed to meet the learning objectives of their team.

- The NRP flow diagram (for learner reference if needed) (page 272)

- Provider Course Individual Recording Sheet (pages 41 and 245)

  - Ask learners to write in their name and the course date. If you need the learner's address for mailing the NRP Course Completion Card, the learner may write it here or write it onto an envelope for mailing.

- Integrated Skills Station Checklist (Basic and/or Advanced) (Appendix E)

- Provider Course Evaluation (ask learners to write in the course date and write in the instructors' names if needed for individual evaluations) (Appendix D)

- Confidentiality Agreement (sample in Appendix F)

Make reusable notebooks of Performance Checklists for the instructors at your course.
Printing each Performance Checklist for each learner in your course uses a lot of paper, and most learners do not need to keep a copy of this learning tool. Instead of printing many copies, consider printing each Performance Checklist, laminating each page, and putting all the laminated pages into a small, 3-ring binder. Use a dry-erase marker to write on the laminated pages for each learner, then wipe the page clean for the next learner. Each instructor needs this 3-ring binder of Performance Checklists during a course.

This binder also may include references to assist instructors, such as:

- Neonatal Resuscitation Program (NRP) Revisions 2011: A Brief Summary for Busy People

There are additional forms in Appendix F, such as:

- Ready, Set, Go: NRP Instructor Prep Sheet for Simulation and Debriefing

- Simulation Preparation, Tips, and Sample Debriefing Questions

- Neonatal Resuscitation Program Instructor Simulation and Debriefing Checklist

Organize written materials and course supplies in portable files or drawers.
Store all your forms and written handout materials in a portable file case or in plastic drawers. Assemble course handouts, staple written materials together, and keep the papers you use at each course supplied and organized. Initial setup of this system takes a bit of time, but it saves you a huge amount of time in the long run because you will not have to search for missing documents or assemble the paperwork for each course.

A Conference Room Setup

Standardize your classroom setup so that you and others can set up the classroom the same way each time. Make a diagram (Figure 5.1) so that assistants need little supervision to set up the classroom. The diagram below is one example of a possible conference room setup.

Components of the Conference Room Setup

Course check-in station

It is helpful to have a person at the check-in station to greet learners and answer questions. A typical check-in station includes the following items:

- Sign-in roster required by your facility or the continuing education accreditation organization

- Disclosure posting (if your facility or continuing education accreditation organization requires you to post any perceived or actual conflict of interest or co-sponsoring organizations)

- Size XL scrub top and cloth or cover gowns (to wear over clothing to simulate delivery room garb, and to protect clothing from simulated blood and meconium)

- Name tags and felt marker (may be unnecessary if all participants know each other)

- Handout materials

- Envelope for learner to write name and address for mailing NRP Course Completion Card, if necessary

Course checkout station

After all course participants have checked in, the table converts to a checkout station.

At the course checkout station, the course participant is instructed to

- Separate the Individual Recording Sheet from the packet of handouts and staple it to his or her online examination verification.

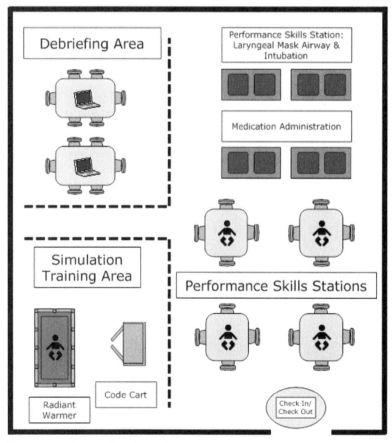

Figure 5.1. Diagram: Sample conference room setup

- Complete and turn in the Course Evaluation.

- Turn in the signed Confidentiality Agreement, if applicable.

- Take the NRP continuing education certificate, if you have provided continuing education at your course.

- If necessary, leave the self-addressed mailing envelope for the NRP instructor so that the NRP Course Completion Card can be mailed to the learner when it arrives from the American Academy of Pediatrics.

Performance Skills Stations

The diagram illustrates the classroom layout for a course with a maximum of 12 to 16 learners and 3 to 4 instructors. Under ideal circumstances, the ratio for the most efficient flow and least amount of waiting by learners to practice and demonstrate skills is 1 instructor for each table of 3 learners. Note that the Laryngeal Mask Airway Performance Skills Station (may also be used as the Intubation Performance Skills Station if the whole body manikin at each team's table cannot be intubated) and Medication Performance Skills Station are set up as separate and distinct stations to facilitate faster flow through these Performance Skills Stations. Because 4 neonatal intubation heads and 4 medication stations are set up on 2 separate tables, each 3- or 4-learner team may go to the station when ready and use its own equipment for practice. The alternative, which is to put one intubation head and one medication station at every team's skills station, means that the instructor coaches one person at a time through these skills, which slows everyone down. If learners must wait more than a few minutes for their opportunity to practice a skill, consider adding learning stations, applicable to your learners (see suggestions on page 73) to keep learners engaged and busy at all times.

Simulation Training Area

The ideal setting for simulation training is in the actual birthing area. However, this is not always possible. A radiant warmer, even in a conference room, is a powerful visual cue, but, if that is not possible, a conference room table will suffice. Attempt to make the simulation training area resemble the actual birth setting as closely as possible.

Debriefing Location

A comfortable and quiet place should be designated for viewing the film and debriefing your learners. Your setup will depend on your resources. Some facilities have chairs or couches and a viewing screen on the wall. Others will use chairs around a table and view the film on a laptop computer screen. The necessary elements for the debriefing location include places to sit, a method for viewing the film, such as a wall-mounted screen or a monitor, and privacy so that learners are comfortable viewing their scenario and discussing scenario events. You may find that a poster listing the 10 NRP Key Behavioral Skills is a helpful reference during debriefing.

Setting Up Equipment for Classroom Use

Ideally, your course participants can use the actual setting where newborns are resuscitated to practice and improve skills. However, this is not possible in every setting. Your simulated birth setting should contain key elements of your actual resuscitation area. Be sure to label supplies and equipment as NRP supplies to prevent simulation equipment from being used for actual patient care (eg, "NRP use only: Not for Patient Use").

How might I set up a radiant warmer and code cart?
If you cannot practice and evaluate resuscitation skills in the location where resuscitation takes place, try to set up an area that closely resembles the clinical setting. Borrow a radiant warmer from an unoccupied labor room or even better, procure a model that you can dedicate for NRP use that your hospital or a partner hospital is about to surplus. This radiant warmer can be used as a Performance Skills Station or reserved for simulation training.

This radiant warmer (Figure 5.2) is set up with all supplies and equipment for NRP use and is available in the unit conference room for practice anytime, and pulled into use for NRP courses when needed. It is set up in the same manner as every birthing room resuscitation area in this facility. Resuscitation supplies are kept in labeled pockets of the shoe bag on the side of the warmer (Figure 5.3). The "code cart" (Figure 5.4) contains the same supplies and equipment, but is an inexpensive plastic cart instead of a hospital-grade code cart. The emergency UVC and medications are on top of the newborn code cart during simulation training, or may be kept in their box inside the cart when the area is not in use.

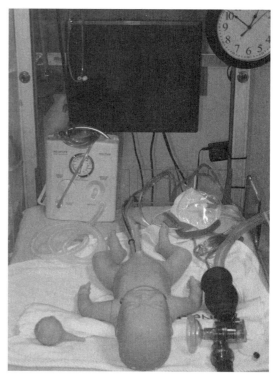

Figure 5.2. The manikin rests on a radiant warmer set up with supplies for initial steps and positive-pressure ventilation. The list used for Performance Checklist 1 (Equipment Check) and the table of targeted oxygen saturations are posted on the radiant warmer, out of photo view.

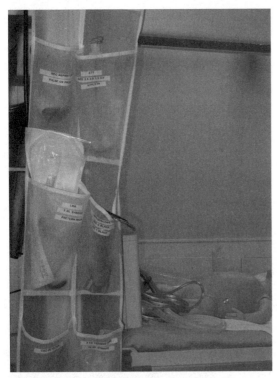

Figure 5.3. A shoebag hangs on the side of the radiant warmer and holds additional resuscitation supplies in labeled pockets

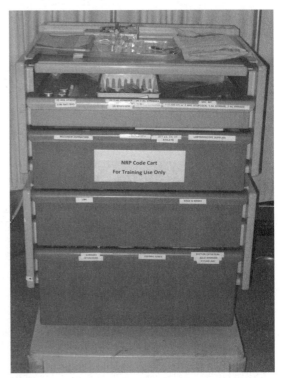

Figure 5.4. This inexpensive plastic cart functions as the neonatal code cart during simulation training, and is organized to be identical to the code cart used for patient care in this institution

Performance Skills Stations

Individual Performance Skills Station, such as Equipment Check, Initial Steps, and Positive-Pressure Ventilation are optional for your learners, depending on their learning objectives. While not every Provider Course will require learners to review and practice each skill in Lessons 1 through 6, equipping each learning station with supplies and equipment where participants can resuscitate a newborn through at least through Lesson 4 (chest compressions) enables the instructor to use the station to review any skill prior to administering the Integrated Skills Station (Basic) at that learning station. Airway supplies for intubation and laryngeal mask airway placement may be present at each learning station if resources allow or if the full body manikin is able to be intubated (as in Figure 5.5) and would permit evaluation through Lesson 5.

After all teams have reviewed and practiced at the separate airway skills station (Figure 5.7) and medication skills station (Figures 5.8 and 5.9), each team may move a Medication Skills Station box (and neonatal intubation head, if necessary) to its learning station for use during the Integrated Skills Station (Advanced) and for use during simulation training.

Setting up each Performance Skills Station in this way means that nearly every intervention may be practiced and evaluated at this station. When all equipment is present, all Performance Skills Stations and the Integrated Skills Station may be done in this same place. In most cases, this station also may be used for scenarios during simulation training. This integrates your equipment for the most efficient use possible. It also enables your instructors to meet every participant's unique learning needs.

If no birthing room is available for your course, and you do not have a radiant warmer, remember that the control board from *the Simply NRP* kit allows learners to simulate the hands-on action of pushing the "On" button for the warmer, adjusting oxygen flow and titrating oxygen concentration by interpreting oximetry, checking and adjusting wall suction, and pushing a Help button—all from a conference room table.

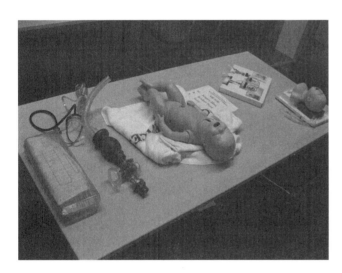

Figure 5.5. A complete Performance Skills Station in a conference room setting, including control board from the *Simply NRP* kit and a neonatal intubation head for laryngeal mask airway placement and intubation practice. The plastic supply box on the left contains supplies necessary for resuscitating the newborn (see Figure 5.6).

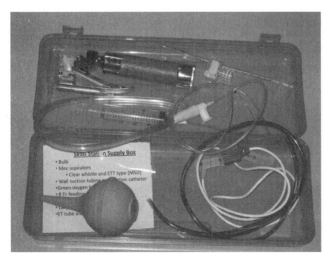

Figure 5.6. The plastic supply box (pictured on the left side of Figure 5.5) contains supplies used for resuscitating the manikin in the conference room resuscitation setting and can move to the radiant warmer for simulation training. Ideally, the ET tube would be kept "clean" inside its original packaging. Note the laminated supply list to help ensure that the supply box is re-packed correctly after each course. The box does not include supplies for laryngeal mask airway placement or medication administration.

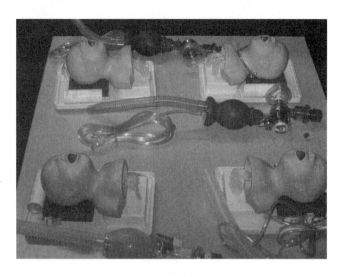

Figure 5.7. This NRP course is set up so that a team of 3 or 4 learners visits this separate table to practice laryngeal mask airway placement, which enables all learners to practice the skill at the same time. If the manikin at their Performance Skills Station table is not able to be intubated, this station would also serve as the Endotracheal Intubation Performance Skills Station. This separate table allows more effective use of time than having one neonatal intubation head at each team's learning skills station. A size-1 laryngeal mask airway fits the neonatal size intubation head and most electronic newborn simulator models.

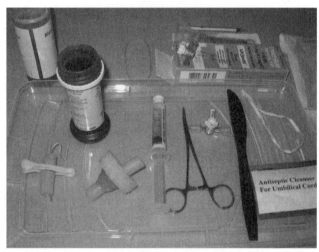

Figure 5.8. A table with 4 of these Medications Performance Skills Stations allows up to 4 learners at a time to practice preparing/assisting with or placing an emergency UVC, and drawing up and administering epinephrine and volume per UVC. Instructions for setting up the Medication Performance Skills Station are in Appendix C.

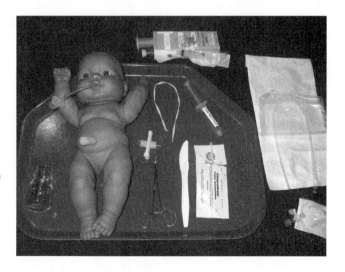

Figure 5.9. This is an alternate way to set up the Medication Performance Skills Station, using a plastic baby doll instead of a baby bottle and nipple. Four of these stations may be set up at the Performance Skills Station table, allowing up to 4 learners at a time to review and practice medication administration skills, including drawing up and administering epinephrine. Instructions for setting up this station are in Appendix C.

What other learning stations might be useful at an NRP Provider Course?

Your unit has specific equipment and protocols that resuscitators should know about. Consider adding learning stations that will help ensure optimal resuscitation outcome at your institution. These extra stations can be reviewed when learners are waiting for some component of the NRP course, such as their turn to participate in a scenario. Because these stations are not part of the NRP course elements, they do not require an NRP instructor as a learning facilitator.

Code cart orientation

- How does the code cart open? (Do not assume that everyone knows this. Physicians, as well as nurses and respiratory therapists, should know how to open the cart.)
- What is contained in each drawer?
- Where is the Code Documentation form?
- Who usually documents events on the Code Documentation form?
- Where is the list of medication dosages?
- Under what circumstances would the code cart be present at a birth?
- Where are the code carts kept on the unit?
- Who checks the contents of the code cart? How often?
- What is the process for re-stocking and re-securing the code cart?

Using the pulse oximeter

Learners may find it useful to view the Resuscitation Skills video for this skill (found on the DVD that accompanies the *Textbook of Neonatal Resuscitation, 6th Edition*). Post the table of "Targeted Pre-ductal S_{PO_2} After Birth" from the NRP flow diagram on the wall and discuss how to adjust the oxygen concentration with the blender based on the newborn's age and oxygen saturation.

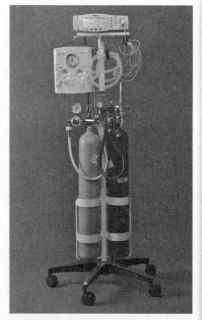

- Where are neonatal pulse oximeter probes located?
- How is the pulse oximeter attached to the newborn?
- What are some reasons a reliable signal may not appear on the oximeter?
- What is our hospital protocol for increasing and decreasing the oxygen concentration to meet the targeted oxygen saturation based on the newborn's age in minutes?

Using our "respiratory therapy on a stick"

If your birth setting does not have the capacity to blend air/oxygen in the delivery room and does not have pulse oximetry available in every delivery room, a portable system, such as this "respiratory therapy on a stick" may be useful. In Figure 5.10, the air and oxygen tanks are connected to the T-piece resuscitator (a bag and mask could also be used) and an oxygen blender. In this system, the pulse oximeter is also attached to the rolling pole, which is moved into any delivery room where a newborn requires more than the Initial Steps of resuscitation.

DVD viewing station

Consider having one station where learners can review selected Resuscitation Skills videos, found on the Instructor DVD and on the DVD that accompanies the *Textbook of Neonatal Resuscitation, 6th Edition*. A list of titles is found in Table 5-2 on page 79.

Figure 5.10. This rolling pole provides portable accessibility to oxygen and air tanks, a blender, a PPV device, and pulse oximetry (photo courtesy of Swedish Medical Center, Seattle, WA)

How will I store my supplies and equipment?

The following section suggests strategies for organizing supplies and equipment for easy setup, course cleanup, and equipment maintenance. Your objective is to organize and store supplies to make them visible and accessible in a system that is easily maintained. Every instructor finds the system that works best for his or her particular setting.

Once you have your supplies and equipment, spend some time setting up a system that meets your needs. Make your own list of what you own (eg, selection of ET tubes and stylets), what you must borrow prior to each course (eg, laryngoscopes from the respiratory therapy department), and what you must purchase for every course. Some items will need to be re-purchased or replaced intermittently, as they wear out from use or get misplaced or lost.

Keep manikins in the manufacturer's storage bag.

Storing your manikin as a separate item helps ensure that the manikin is not damaged or smashed by other items that do not fit easily into the storage bag. The newborn in Figure 5.11 is wrapped in a blanket or towel that is used for "drying" the newborn at birth and a smaller towel to use as a shoulder roll. Items that are used for manikin use or maintenance, such as baby powder and manikin airway lubricant, may be stored in the bag.

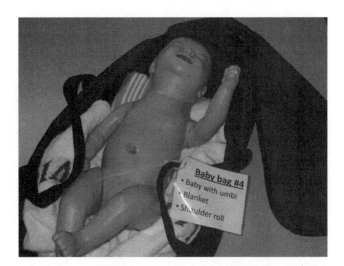

Figure 5.11. This manikin is stored in a numbered bag. Because the umbilical cord can come out of the manikin and be lost, the umbilical cord is listed on the bag's contents tag.

Keep resuscitation equipment and supplies in a Performance Skills Station bag.

Note that the skills station bag is numbered so that loaner bags can be traced back to the borrower, if necessary. Many of the supplies are stored in a plastic supply box (Figure 5.6) that fits inside the tool bag. (See Figure 5.12 for details.) The neonatal intubation head (Figure 5.13) fits inside this large bag. The stethoscope and self-inflating bag and mask are separate items that nestle inside the tool bag next to the small box of supplies and the intubation head.

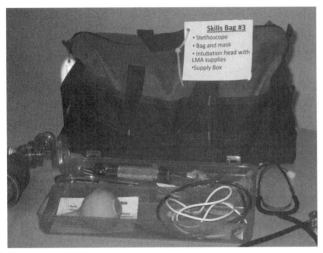

Figure 5.12. This bag (a large tool bag from a home improvement store) is large enough to keep all supplies and equipment needed for Lessons 1 through 5. The skills bag has a contents tag attached to its handle to ensure that all needed supplies are available when the bag is unpacked. The contents tag is also used to reload the supplies into the correct containers at the end of the course.

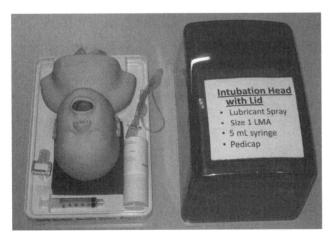

Figure 5.13. The supplies needed for inserting a laryngeal mask airway are kept in the box with this intubation head trainer (neonatal size). Note the contents label on the lid of the intubation head to help ensure that supplies are present when needed. This intubation head fits into the large equipment bag (Figure 5.12).

The Medication Performance Skills Stations are kept in separate identical boxes.

The Medication Performance Skills Station box contains necessary supplies and equipment to place an emergency UVC in a baby bottle/nipple setup (Figure 5.8) or medication doll (Figure 5.9). Each box's contents are written on a laminated list attached to the lid of the box. The tape keeps the box closed and indicates the date when the box was last checked for all items.

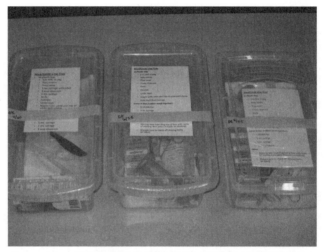

Figure 5.14. This facility has 3 Medication Station boxes ready for use at an NRP course. If set up at a separate table, up to 3 learners on a team may practice this skill at once (Figure 5.8). When teams are ready for the Integrated Skills Station and simulation, they may take a medication box to their simulation area for use during scenarios, if necessary.

Equipment for Filming and Viewing

Filming your scenarios during the Simulation component of the course and watching the film during debriefing enhances learning for your course participants. Keep your camcorder and tripod, and whatever equipment you use to view the scenario (laptop computer, LCD projector, or television and DVD player), in a secure location. Use this equipment to film mock codes on your unit. The same principles for simulation and debriefing (Chapters 7 and 8) apply to mock codes on the unit and keep your "filming and viewing" skills fresh. Appendix F includes information about conducting mock codes.

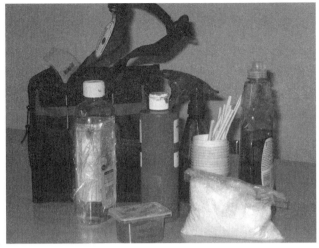

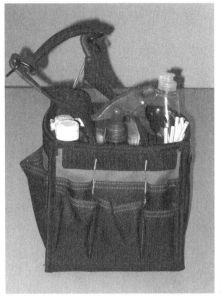

A

B

Figure 5.15A and 5.15B. Moulage supplies are shown next to the tool bag, and shown packed into the bag for easy portability.

Organize a Basic Moulage Kit.

Moulage is a French word for "casting/molding" and refers to the art of applying theatrical makeup and using theater techniques to provide visual cues for realism (such as blood, meconium, and vernix). Basic moulage supplies are necessary components for simulation-based learning.

Keep supplies needed to make fake blood, vernix, and meconium in one box or bag (Figure 5.15). Large bottles usually are not necessary for a Hospital-based NRP Course. Keep what you need in a portable container for easy use, and keep the large bottles (eg, the giant bargain store bottle of dishwashing liquid) on a shelf to refill the smaller containers.

See Table 5-1 for the supplies pictured in this bag. Recipes for making simulated blood, meconium, and vernix are located in Appendix F.

Table 5-1. Sample Supplies for Moulage Kit

Blood	Meconium
Red water-based paint	Small jars/cartons of pureed split pea or green beans baby food
Green water-based paint	
Blue dishwashing liquid	Baby oil or mineral oil
Baby oil or mineral oil	**Disposable wipes or towels for cleanup**
Vernix	
Heavy unscented hand cream	Paper cups for mixing and stir sticks
Mashed potato flakes (optional)	

Other ideas for organizing your resuscitation supplies and equipment

Organize by Purpose of the Item.

Categorize all your equipment and pull from each category to set up a Performance Skills Station. For example, put all suction items in one box or bag (transparent zipper bags work well) and all medication items in another box or bag. Then, when you need to set up a Performance Skills Station, select what you need from each category. This method enables you to see what supplies may be running low in each category (eg, it is easy to see if you are missing suction catheters or ET tubes), but it takes a considerable amount of time to "build" your Performance Skills Stations and set up a Provider Course. It is also time-consuming to put away all the supplies and equipment at the end of a course.

Organize by Individual Skills Performance Station.

Setting up individual Performance Skills Stations is discouraged because

- Individual stations require duplication of supplies and equipment and require an instructor at every station.

- Individual stations limit the learner's ability to practice more than one skill or practice several skills in sequence.

However, some Performance Skills Stations are not used at every course, or the Performance Skills Stations are separate stations, to help with the flow of students through the stations. (See Figures 5.7 through 5.9.)

To organize by individual Performance Skills Stations, put all supplies and equipment needed for each station in their own box or duffel bag. Mark the outside of this box or bag with the lesson number or name of the Performance Checklist. This way, you will always be ready to set up this station.

How can I help ensure that everything is put back into the bag or box after class, or know if items are now broken or missing?
Many different strategies exist for ensuring that supplies get back in place after an NRP course. However, no system will work if people do not use it. Make sure the people assisting you with setup and cleanup are oriented to your system. Make it easy to get skills stations back together by using lists or photos.

When something is found to be broken or missing, tag the item or the bag in a way that makes it easy for you or whoever maintains your equipment to see it. For example, a bright tag or piece of tape alerts instructors that this skills station needs attention before use (Figure 5.16).

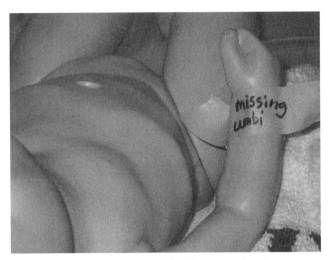

Figure 5.16. This institution uses bright green painter's tape to alert others that an item needs attention before the next NRP course

Table 5-2. Resuscitation Skills Videos

These short instructional videos can be found on the *NRP Instructor DVD: An Interactive Tool for Facilitation of Simulation-based Learning* and on the DVD that accompanies the *Textbook of Neonatal Resuscitation, 6th Edition.*

1. Equipment Check
2. Using a Meconium Aspirator
3. CPAP Administration
4. Using Pulse Oximetry
5. Using the T-piece Resuscitator
6. Positive-Pressure Ventilation With a Flow-inflating Bag
7. MR SOPA: Ventilation Corrective Steps
8. Orogastric Tube Placement
9. Endotracheal Intubation
10. Using an End-tidal CO_2 Detector
11. Endotracheal Tube: Emergency Tape Technique
12. Laryngeal Mask Airway Placement
13. Chest Compressions: Head of Infant Positioning
14. Preparing the Emergency UVC for Insertion
15. Placing an Emergency UVC
16. Securing and Safeguarding the Emergency UVC
17. Drawing Up and Administering Epinephrine
18. Needle Thoracentesis
19. The ELBW Baby: Aspects of Delivery Room Management

Basic Equipment and Supplies Needed for Most Neonatal Resuscitation Program Courses

- **Newborn manikin**   • **Neonatal intubation head or full-body intubation manikin**   • **Gloves**
- **Cover gowns or size-XL scrub tops to cover street clothing**

Optional: Simply NRP **kit control board to simulate radiant warmer power switch, wall suction, oxygen and blender, pulse oximetry, and "Help" button**

Warm	• Radiant warmer or simulation (tabletop) with surface area to hold equipment • Towels or blankets, including small towel or cloth diaper for optional shoulder roll For resuscitation of preterm newborn <29 weeks • Food-grade polyethylene bag (1-gallon size) or plastic wrap • Chemically activated warming pad (or simulated pad)
Suction	• Bulb syringe • Mechanical suction (or simulation) and suction tubing with 10F or 12F suction catheter • Meconium aspirator
Auscultate	• Stethoscope(s)
Oxygenate	• Oxygen tubing, mask, or flow-inflating bag and mask to deliver free-flow oxygen • Oxygen or air source with flowmeter and nipple adapter (required for use with flow-inflating bag or T-piece resuscitator) • Pulse oximeter probe for newborn use • Pulse oximeter device, such as on the *Simply NRP* control board, or simulated
Ventilate	• Self-inflating bag, flow-inflating bag, or T-piece resuscitator • Oxygen tubing • Face masks (preterm and term sizes) • Oxygen or air source with flowmeter and nipple adapter (required for flow-inflating bag and T-piece resuscitator) • 8F feeding tube and 20-mL syringe • Oral airways (various sizes)
Intubate	• Intubation head or full-body intubation manikin • Laryngoscope with straight blades, size 0 (preterm), size 1 (term), and size 00 (optional) • Endotracheal (ET) tubes sizes 2.5, 3.0, 3.5, and 4.0 • Stylets • Scissors • Tape or securing device for ET tube • End-tidal CO_2 detector • Size-1 laryngeal mask airway with 5-mL syringe

Medicate	• Equipment for emergency umbilical venous catheter (UVC) placement
	  – Umbilical catheters, 3.5F or 5F (preferred)
	  – 10-cc and 20-cc syringes (may be prefilled with non-bacteriostatic normal saline or simulate with water)
	  – Volume expander of choice (such as 100-mL bag of normal saline or prefilled syringes)
	  – Needle or puncture device to access volume expander, if needed
	  – Curved forceps or instrument to stabilize umbilical cord or catheter
	  – Three-way stopcocks and/or Luer lock connectors
	  – Antiseptic prep solution (may simulate with cotton-tipped applicators)
	  – Umbilical tape (may simulate with narrow, white cloth ribbon)

Basic Equipment and Supplies Needed for Most Neonatal Resuscitation Program Courses—*continued*

Medicate—*continued*	– Scalpel blade and handle – Securing device for UVC (optional) • Epinephrine 1:10,000 in 3-mL or 10-mL ampules (or substitute water in ampules) • 1-mL syringes, 5- or 6-mL syringes • Three-way stopcocks or Luer lock syringe connectors • Volume expander: normal saline (preferred), Ringer's lactate (or substitute water) • Assorted syringes, needles, or puncture devices/needleless system supplies • Medication labels and waterproof pen
Available for each course	• Silicone spray for use with some types of intubation heads • Extra balloons and rubber bands for intubation head "lungs" • Extra bulbs and batteries for laryngoscope • Oxygen regulator and key or wrench for oxygen or air tank, if used • Clock with second hand • Apgar timer or stopwatch to assess newborn's age in minutes

Simulate	• Metronome to simulate various newborn heart rates
	• Flash cards or dry-erase board to give learners physiologic feedback (optional for breathing, color, tone, oximetry)
	• Supplies for simulated blood, meconium, vernix
	  – Small cups for mixing, and coffee stirrer, spoons, and sections of drinking straws for stirring fluids
	  – Purchased simulated blood or red finger paint/green finger paint, OR ingredients for alternate recipe
	  – Baby oil or mineral oil
	  – Blue dishwashing liquid
	  – Meconium: Pureed baby food green beans or peas OR split pea soup OR ingredients for alternate recipe
	  – Vernix: unscented heavy hand cream, instant potato flakes OR ingredients for alternate recipe
	• Disposable wipes or alternate method for manikin cleanup
	• Spray bottle of simulated blood for towels and manikin, if needed
	• Camcorder
	• Tripod
	• Method for showing filmed scenario to viewers (TV monitor, computer screen, LCD projector)

Instructor Resources	Scenario template for creating scenarios Table of Pre-ductal Oxygen Saturation Targets (from NRP flow diagram) List of NRP Key Behaviors to post for reference during debriefing NRP Instructor Simulation and Debriefing Checklist and/or CAPE Debriefing Evaluation Tool Simulation Preparation, Tips, and Sample Debriefing Questions Ready, Set, Go: NRP Instructor Prep Sheet for Simulation and Debriefing Institution's Neonatal Code Documentation form
Optional	• Cardiac monitor/leads/alcohol sponges • Umbilical cord model for UVC placement (page 217) • Medication doll (page 218)

Administering Performance Skills Stations

The instructor plays a critical role in helping the Neonatal Resuscitation Program™ (NRP™) course participant understand the "when, why, and how" of resuscitation interventions, and evaluating the learner's knowledge and ability to perform these procedures. To be effective in resuscitating newborns, care providers must be able to perform hands-on technical skills in proper sequence using correct technique.

- The Performance Skills Stations give the learner an opportunity to practice or review hands-on resuscitation skills with assistance from an instructor, using each lesson's Performance Checklist as a reference to ensure correct technique.

- The Integrated Skills Station is a required Performance Skills Station where the provider demonstrates the steps in the NRP flow diagram using the proper sequence, timing, and technique without guidance or prompting from the instructor.

In Chapter 6 you will learn

- **How to facilitate skills development at Performance Skills Stations**

- **How to administer the Integrated Skills Stations (Basic and Advanced)**

"Instructor Self-assessment" for Chapter 6 begins on page 194.

After studying this chapter, complete the Chapter 6 questions, using the answer sheets that begin on page 188. Your regional trainer may ask you to bring the answer sheets to your NRP Instructor Course.

The Performance Skills Station and the Integrated Skills Station are both considered Performance Skills Stations. The first is for reviewing, practicing, and finally being able to perform the skill correctly and independently within the context of a scenario. The Integrated Skills Station is used to evaluate the learner's ability to correctly incorporate all relevant NRP resuscitation skills into a scenario without instructor assistance.

What is the difference between a Performance Skills Station and the Integrated Skills Station?

Both are considered Performance Skills Stations. However, the Performance Skills Stations for individual skills, such as Equipment Check, Initial Steps, Positive-Pressure Ventilation (PPV), Chest Compressions, and Intubation, are for the purpose of learning. The Integrated Skills Station is for evaluation. Both activities may occur at the same location (ie, the Performance Skills Station and the Integrated Skills Station usually occur at a fully equipped learning station, as pictured on page 71, Figure 5.5).

More About Performance Skills Stations

The individual Performance Skills Stations are learning opportunities where the participant is free to ask questions and practice hands-on skills with guidance from the instructor. Because the learner has already studied the textbook and passed the online examination, the instructor needs to clarify information only if needed and help the learner apply the cognitive learning to the hands-on skills.

Most NRP courses will include all Performance Skills Stations, but this is not required. The NRP instructor assesses the learning needs of the participants prior to the NRP course and determines which elements of the NRP course would best meet their learning objectives. (See Table 3-1 on page 39.) Even experienced learners whose course includes all 9 textbook lessons benefit from review and discussion of all Performance Skills Stations; however, the instructor who knows and works with the course participants who perform frequent complex resuscitation may choose to include only the unfamiliar or rarely practiced skills, such as laryngeal mask airway placement or medication administration. If the instructor determines that all participants are experts at neonatal resuscitation, it would be permissible to begin with the Integrated Skills Station. Be cautious. Even experienced providers may arrive at their course with previously unrecognized deficits in their skills that need to be corrected before the instructor allows the learner to proceed.

Performance Checklists (Appendix E) may be used to help the learner and instructor remember each step of the intervention. This practice continues until the instructor and learner agree that the learner can perform the skill correctly and smoothly and without coaching within the context of a short clinical scenario. Each scenario of a Performance Skills Station should build on the skills practiced in the scenarios before it, beginning with the Equipment Check and ending with the skill that is the focus of the Performance Skills Station.

More About the Integrated Skills Station

The Integrated Skills Station is a required component of every NRP Provider Course. Unlike the individual Performance Skills Stations, the instructor does not assist, coach, or interrupt the learner during the Integrated Skills Station clinical scenarios. Ideally, the learner has done multiple scenarios by this time in the course while practicing skills at Performance Skills Stations. Each scenario of a Performance Skills Station should build on the skills practiced in the one before it, so the learner is accustomed to the sequence and timing of neonatal resuscitation interventions by the time he or she is ready for the Integrated Skills Station.

The instructor may use one comprehensive clinical scenario or a series of increasingly complex scenarios to allow the learner to demonstrate all required skills for the NRP lessons assigned. The Integrated Skills Station Checklist is used to assess the learner's readiness to proceed to the Simulation and Debriefing component of the course. If the learner makes errors in the sequence, timing, or technical performance of the skills required to complete the scenario, the learner continues to practice in these areas, then tries the Integrated Skills Station again.

To enhance resuscitation knowledge and experience, learners may choose to learn about and practice skills that are not included in their regular job responsibilities. While learners may demonstrate these skills during the NRP Provider Course, individual health care institutions are responsible for evaluating the qualifications and competence of health care professionals before allowing them to perform procedures during an actual resuscitation.

Using the Performance Checklists

A Performance Checklist is the tool used at each Performance Skills Station. These checklists are found in both the *Textbook of Neonatal Resuscitation, 6th Edition,* and Appendix E of the *Instructor Manual for Neonatal Resuscitation.*

What is the purpose of the Performance Checklist?

Use a Performance Checklist to

- Provide the learner with a step-by-step outline of the procedure for use during the practice phase of the lessons at Performance Skills Stations.

- Furnish the instructor with a checklist to use in guiding the learner's performance of the skill and assessing readiness to move on to the Integrated Skills Station.

How can I facilitate learning at the Performance Skills Stations and Integrated Skills Station?

It is helpful to include an explanation for learners at the beginning of the Provider Course about how Performance Skills Stations work and how building these skills leads to the Integrated Skills Station Checklist. (See the following sample script.) When the instructor describes what to expect at the Performance Skills Stations, and then demonstrates a scenario for the Integrated Skills Station Checklist, the learner may have a clearer picture of the purpose and objectives of these course components. This type of learner orientation can lessen anxiety and promote learning.

Sample Script for Orienting Learners to Performance Skills Stations (Including Integrated Skills Station)

How Performance Skills Stations Work and Demonstration of the Integrated Skills Station

The Performance Skills Stations, where you and your instructor will use the Performance Checklists as your reference tool, are not tests where you are expected to do everything perfectly. This is a learning activity where you can ask questions, get help from your instructor, and refine your technique in preparation for the Integrated Skills Station and simulation exercises.

This is a Performance Skills Station. It has almost all equipment necessary for a complete resuscitation. If this newborn were to require medications and line placement, we would move the Medications Skills Station, which is a separate station in this room setup, next to our resuscitation area.

Before starting hands-on activities, you will have a discussion with your instructor about the intervention that is the focus of the Performance Checklist. Your instructor will ask you about when the intervention is indicated, how effectiveness is assessed, for how long the intervention continues, and indications for stopping the intervention.

Your instructor will tell you how you will know if the baby is breathing, what the heart rate is, and, if necessary, what the pulse oximeter reads. Your instructor also will tell you how to assess muscle tone, breath sounds, and other indicators as needed.

If you would like, your instructor will then demonstrate the procedure for you. The instructor talks through what he or she is thinking and actually demonstrates each step. Then, you will return the demonstration and your instructor will help you as much as needed. As soon as you can perform the intervention smoothly and quickly, with good technique, and without any assistance or coaching, your instructor will put the intervention in the context of a clinical scenario, so that you can practice the steps in the order of the NRP flow diagram. You may be given several different case scenarios to ensure that there is opportunity to demonstrate all the situations presented on the checklist.

Because you have all the supplies and equipment available for resuscitating a newborn at your station, each scenario will build on the one before it. By the time you are ready to demonstrate your last skill in a scenario (which may be Chest Compressions or Medications), you are ready for your Integrated Skills Station. The Integrated Skills Station is an assessment of your ability to put all the steps of the NRP flow diagram in correct order, using correct technique, before proceeding to Simulation and Debriefing. If you need coaching or make significant errors during the Integrated Skills Station scenario, you will determine what you need to practice more, and then try the Integrated Skills Station scenario again.

We would like to demonstrate one scenario from the Integrated Skills Station, so that you can see what is expected of you after completion of the Performance Checklists at each Performance Skills Station. Remember that more than one scenario may be used to evaluate your skills. This is the Basic Integrated Skills Station, which covers the technical skills in Lessons 1 through 4. The scenario begins with the Equipment Checklist and ends with Chest Compressions Performance Checklist.

> (Name) is the learner, (Name) is her assistant, and I am the instructor. The learner leads the decision making and performs the steps without interruption or coaching from the instructor. This is how you will know about the manikin's heart rate, breathing, tone, pulse oximetry, and color, if that is important. (Demonstrate how physiologic cues are relayed to the learner.)
>
> This is your scenario. (Reads scenario.)
>
> Do you have any questions?
>
> (Learners ask questions and perform scenario.)
>
> (Instructor ends scenario.)
>
> (Scenario concludes with Reflective Questions from the Basic Integrated Skills Station Checklist.)

Do you have any questions?

Then let's begin.

How do I begin with my learners at the Performance Skills Station?

- The instructor should assess the learner's cognitive knowledge by asking the questions on the Performance Checklist pertaining to why, when, and aspects of how the intervention is performed. These questions are found on the Performance Checklist under the heading, "Knowledge Check."

- The instructor must orient the learner to how information about the manikin's breathing, heart rate, tone, and, if necessary, oxygen saturation will be revealed to the learner. This is variable depending on your manikin and resources. See the table on simulation techniques (page 116) for suggestions about how to relay information to the learner, which also prepares the learner for the Integrated Skills Station and the Simulation and Debriefing exercise.

- The instructor may find that demonstrating the individual skill, such as PPV with a bag and mask, is helpful to the learner. The learner may then feel more confident about returning the demonstration so that the instructor can help refine technique if necessary.

How do I demonstrate the skill to a learner or a small team of learners?

Demonstrating the skills helps improve technique and encourages discussion.

- The instructor may first give directions and key points for proper technique while demonstrating the skill. Conversation may occur with the learner if the learner has questions during this demonstration.

- Next, the instructor discusses performing the skill within the context of a scenario. This is an opportunity to allow the learner to verbalize when the intervention is indicated, how effectiveness is assessed, and when to discontinue the intervention. If you demonstrate the procedure to the learner, model the following behaviors so that the learner is better prepared to return the demonstration:

  - Demonstrate each step and "talk through" what you are thinking so that other team members know what you are thinking.

  - Demonstrate the scenario in "real time." This means handling the manikin and performing procedures quickly and efficiently, with the same sense of urgency felt during an actual resuscitation. It also means that any procedure with a delineated time specification should be performed with that in mind (eg, perform PPV for a full 30 seconds before reevaluating breathing, heart rate, and oxygen saturation.)

  - Ask the learner to participate as a team member as you perform the intervention. This is the instructor's opportunity to help the learner understand how the intervention is done, what assistance is required, and what the assistant should do to help other team members.

What is my role when the learner practices the skill?
You may provide assistance as the learner practices the intervention. Allow the learner to ask questions. Avoid the temptation to demonstrate answers to the learners' questions with more instructor demonstration. It is the instructor's responsibility to facilitate hands-on practice. The Performance Skills Stations are not "tests." This is the learner's opportunity to practice and refine skills with your supportive assistance.

How do I provide feedback about the learner's performance?
Whenever possible, ask the learner reflective questions during and following the practice instead of giving direct feedback. In this way, the learner is more likely to connect the cognitive knowledge with the hands-on skill and remember it. Reflective questions follow each individual Performance Checklist and the Integrative Skills Stations Checklists.

Feedback	Reflective Question
You're bagging too fast.	What is the correct ventilation rate?
I don't see any chest movement.	How do you know ventilation is effective?
I can't *hear* you . . .	What are you thinking as you work?
You can stop now.	How do you know when to stop PPV?

How is the skill incorporated into a clinical scenario?

When you and the learner agree that the learner can perform the intervention smoothly and without assistance, incorporate the intervention into a clinical scenario. You may use the clinical scenario written on the Performance Checklist or create your own using the Scenario Builder. (See Chapter 7.) Use the Performance Checklist to help you assess the learner's technical proficiency.

- Each scenario builds on the scenario that precedes it. Your scenario always begins with the Equipment Check and includes all skills up to and including the skill that is your focus of the Performance Checklist. This repetition prepares the learner for the Integrated Skills Station and simulation training.

- Tell the learner why he or she has been called to attend the birth (read the scenario).

- As the learner performs the procedure, watch for

  - Steps performed correctly.

  - Steps performed incorrectly, performed with hesitation, performed out of sequence, or omitted.

- Check the box for actions performed correctly. Circle the box for all others. The checklist may be filled in as the procedure is being performed or at the conclusion of the clinical demonstration.

- The learner may perform the intervention as many times as necessary to achieve the objective. The checklist is not a scoring tool to determine a "passing" or "failing" grade. The checklist is a reference used to assess strengths and discover weaknesses that require more practice.

Assessing Readiness to Proceed to the Next Performance Checklist

All learners are asked reflective questions again, at the end of the scenario. These reflective questions are printed at the end of each Performance Checklist. You may ask additional reflective questions appropriate to the learner's performance, as needed. You can find additional questions on the Simulation Preparation, Tips, and Sample Debriefing Questions form in Appendix F1 of the *NRP Instructor DVD: An Interactive Tool for Faciliation of Simulation-based Learning* or in Appendix F of this Instructor Manual.

During the Reflective Questions, most learners can self-assess a satisfactory performance or the need for additional practice. Allow the learner to talk about his or her performance. Do not interrupt with your own comments until after the learner has finished speaking. It is helpful to then summarize the learner's comments and determine whether the learner is ready for the Integrated Skills Station, if the learner has not already determined this for himself or herself.

Positive reinforcement from the instructor is a motivating factor for many learners. The instructor may give direct feedback after the learner and instructor have finished assessing the performance. Comments should be honest and relate specifically to the individual's performance. To avoid interrupting the learner, offer positive feedback after the learner has completed the checklist and responded to reflective questions.

If the instructor and the learner agree that the learner can perform the intervention in correct sequence with proper technique without guidance or coaching, the learner may proceed to the next Performance Checklist. If not, the learner should continue to practice with the instructor's guidance.

Administering the Integrated Skills Station

The Integrated Skills Station assesses the learner's ability to integrate many of the cognitive, behavioral, and motor skills taught during an NRP course. The Integrated Skills Station is not a practice activity. Unlike the other Performance Skills Stations where the instructor may assist the learner, the instructor does not coach the learner or interrupt the demonstration. The instructor may evaluate the learner using one scenario, but often uses several increasingly complex clinical scenarios. Participants should be given an opportunity to demonstrate the skills from each lesson included in their course.

What happens when the learner proceeds directly to the Integrated Skills Station?
If the learner has practiced and reviewed skills prior to the NRP course, or if the learner is experienced and participates in complex newborn resuscitation often, the learner may be able to skip all Performance Skills Stations, such as Initial Steps and PPV, or learn or review only those that are unfamiliar (laryngeal mask airway) or infrequently practiced (placing an emergency umbilical venous catheter [UVC]). The learner who begins the NRP Provider Course with the Integrated Skills Station should clearly understand that the Integrated Skills Station is not a shortcut to skills review. If the learner cannot perform the skills in the context of scenarios beginning with the Equipment Checklist, the learner is directed to practice the skills that need review. When the learner and instructor are confident that the learner can perform the skills independently in NRP flow diagram sequence with proper timing and technique, the learner may attempt the Integrated Skills Station Checklist again. While technical skills can be refined

during the simulation component, significant deficiencies in technical skills interfere with the intended focus on teamwork and communication.

> Instructors who are highly skilled at planning simulation scenarios and have participants with well-established technical skills may choose to fully incorporate the Integrated Skills Station into their simulation and debriefing experience. This requires the instructor to plan multiple scenarios to observe each participant individually performing all the required technical skills with the proper sequence, timing, and technique during simulation-based training.

How do I use the Integrated Skills Station Checklist?

The Integrated Skills Station should be a positive experience for both the instructor and the learner. Both should be well-prepared by this point in the Provider Course. Because the learner has done multiple scenarios by now and incorporated the skills into a scenario in correct sequence and using correct technique, the Integrated Skills Station should not feel like a new or surprising experience or be presented as a frightening test for the learner.

The Integrated Skills Station tool includes only selected items from the Performance Checklists. This does not mean that other parts of the Performance Checklist are unimportant. Instructors are still expected to comprehensively evaluate the student's performance and give the learner feedback about skills that are incorrectly performed, even if they are not included on the Integrated Skills Station tool. If you would prefer to use a tool for the Integrated Skills Station that includes more detail than the Integrated Skills Station Checklists, use the Performance Checklist for Lesson 4 (this can serve as the Basic Integrated Skills Station Checklist) or the Performance Checklist for Lesson 6 (this can serve as the Advanced Integrated Skills Station Checklist).

Know what your learner needs to do during the Integrated Skills Station.

- If your learner is demonstrating skills through Lesson 4 (Chest Compressions), use the Basic Integrated Skills Station Checklist.

- If your learner is demonstrating skills through Lesson 6 (ie, intubation, laryngeal mask airway placement, medication administration, and emergency UVC preparation/placement), use the Advanced Integrated Skills Station Checklist.

If learners are completing lessons that include advanced skills, such as intubation or medication administration, the Integrated Skills Station should include skills consistent with the learner's job responsibilities.

If a nurse or respiratory therapist who does not intubate is completing Lesson 5, the Integrated Skills Station evaluation should evaluate the learner's ability to assist with intubation.

To assess skills in Lesson 6, the instructor should assess the learner's objectives and job responsibilities. If it is within the participant's learning objectives or clinical responsibilities, learners completing Lesson 6 should

- State the correct concentration and dosage of epinephrine for the intratracheal and IV routes, and draw up the correct volume of epinephrine (or fluid simulating epinephrine) for the intratracheal and/or umbilical venous route.

- Demonstrate administering epinephrine via the intratracheal route.

- Demonstrate administering epinephrine and volume via the umbilical venous route.

- Demonstrate how to prepare the umbilical venous catheter for insertion.

- Demonstrate assisting with UVC placement or demonstrate insertion of the UVC.

   Only those learners with clinical responsibility for inserting the emergency UVC must demonstrate the insertion procedure.

   At the instructor's discretion, the scenario may include components from Lessons 7 through 9, such as management of a pneumothorax or delivery room management of a premature newborn; however, those skills are not included in the Integrated Skills Station Checklist.

To enhance resuscitation skills and knowledge, every learner may choose to learn and practice any skill in the NRP course and demonstrate those skills at an Integrated Skills Station. Some learners, such as respiratory therapists, may never infuse medications at an actual resuscitation. However, depending on the student's learning objectives, instructors may teach all learners about these aspects of medication administration and allow them to have hands-on practice at a skills station. Knowing how to insert a UVC, even though it is not within the learner's scope of responsibility, may help to make the learner a more competent assistant during the procedure. Remember that learning the cognitive aspects of the skills and demonstrating them at a Performance Skills Station does not ensure competence or give the learner permission to perform the skills during an actual resuscitation. Successful completion of the course does not certify qualification or competence to perform that skill. Learners can demonstrate all the skills, if desired; however, each institution will need to decide which skills are required of learners, depending on job responsibilities.

Ensure that you and your learner understand the indicators for successful completion.

Successful completion requires that all steps appropriate to the learner's job responsibilities be carried out correctly, without prompting or undue hesitation. The learner should be able to direct assistants, if necessary, and work well as leader of the team.

Promote an environment that simulates an actual resuscitation.

During the Integrated Skills Station evaluation, instructors should stay on task and avoid social conversation. Do not prompt the learner or give hints for what the learner is to do next. Encourage the learner to proceed with the Integrated Skills Station in real time. This is important preparation for simulation-based learning. When the learner performs as a team member in a scenario during Simulation and Debriefing, the learner is expected to behave as if the scenario is an actual resuscitation.

Use more than one scenario, if needed.

The Integrated Skills Station often requires more than one clinical scenario. The instructor assesses the learner's skills using the Integrated Skills Station Checklist as the scenario proceeds. The amount of time required for an Integrated Skills Station performance varies, depending on the complexity of the scenarios and how quickly and competently the learner proceeds. Ideally, the Integrated Skills Station proceeds at nearly "real time," meaning that a complex Integrated Skills Station performance should be completed within approximately 10 minutes. If the learner does not need to perform intubation and/or medication administration, is well prepared, and proceeds through the steps skillfully and efficiently, the Integrated Skills Station Checklist may be finished in less than 10 minutes.

Stop the evaluation if the learner has significant deficiencies.

If the learner is unprepared or requires prompts or hints about what to do next, stop the evaluation. Ask reflective questions to help the learner self-assess deficiencies, and then send the learner back to appropriate Performance Skills stations for more practice. If necessary, allow the learner more time for practice and attempt the Integrated Skills Station Checklist on another day when the learner is more prepared.

> If someone is unable to pass a required component of the NRP course, such as the online examination, or cannot perform adequately at the Integrated Skills Station after a reasonable amount of time and supervised practice, the instructor should not feel compelled to "pass" the person simply because the person's job responsibilities require NRP provider status.

Evaluating the Integrated Skills Station

After each scenario, the instructor asks the learner reflective questions to promote self-assessment and determine whether the learner has met the objectives of the scenario. The Integrated Skills Station does not require a perfect performance. If, at any point, the learner makes significant errors in timing, sequence, or technique, the learner should return to the appropriate Performance Skills Station for additional help and practice. The learner may return to practice stations to practice and review skills with another instructor, and/or view the appropriate Resuscitation Skills videos on the DVD that accompanies the *Textbook of Neonatal Resuscitation, 6th Edition,* or the NRP Instructor DVD. Then the learner may attempt the Integrated Skills Station again.

Instructor Q & A

The recommendation for epinephrine administration necessitates that learners know 2 different routes with 2 different medication dosages. Why does the NRP continue to teach both routes? It would have been easier to learn only one route and one dosage.
This decision by the NRP Steering Committee was reached after extensive deliberations and careful consideration for both the 5th and 6th editions of the *Textbook of Neonatal Resuscitation.* Review of the best available scientific evidence still indicates that intravenous administration of epinephrine is more effective than endotracheal administration. The ideal dose for endotracheal administration is not currently known; however, the evidence suggests that the dose used for intravenous administration is NOT effective when given through the endotracheal tube. It is recognized that establishing umbilical venous access takes time and that most newborns will already be intubated at this point in the resuscitation. For this reason, the NRP Steering Committee decided that endotracheal epinephrine administration with an increased dose was a reasonable treatment option until umbilical venous access could be achieved.

Why is it important for the learner to draw up epinephrine during the NRP course?
Medication administration is infrequently required during neonatal resuscitation and, therefore, infrequently practiced. Actual resuscitations are high-stress events. Under stress, there is a greater risk that infrequently performed procedures will be performed incorrectly. Because there are 2 different doses of epinephrine, depending upon the route of administration (endotracheal vs intravenous), the potential for medication error is high. Preparing epinephrine gives the learner the opportunity to practice this infrequently used skill in a safe setting. In

addition, drawing up the epinephrine in the proper dose for endotracheal and/or intravenous administration demonstrates that the learner understands the important differences in routes and dosages and reinforces learning.

Why is it important for learners who take Lesson 6 to understand how to assist, or to actually demonstrate, preparation and insertion of the UVC and medication administration via the umbilical catheter?

Placement of a UVC is an infrequent event during neonatal resuscitation. If demonstration of this skill was not required during an NRP course, the learner may not have an opportunity to practice and demonstrate this skill for a long time. Years could pass between the Provider Course and the moment when the provider needs to perform UVC placement during an actual resuscitation. Review and evaluation of this skill at least every 2 years at an NRP Provider Course offers a valuable opportunity to practice a high-risk, low-volume procedure.

How "real" should the demonstration of UVC preparation, insertion, and medication administration be? Can the learner "talk through" the steps?

The demonstration should provide the learner with the opportunity to physically perform the steps of the procedure using essential supplies in proper sequence and with proper technique. Demonstrating this procedure takes several minutes, but steps should proceed at a brisk pace. All supplies used for the UVC insertion should be packaged together, precluding the need to decide what is needed and gather supplies. The learner may deduce from the presentation of the scenario that a UVC will be needed and draw up the normal saline, attach the 3-way stopcock, and flush the catheter before beginning the scenario, when given time to check and prepare equipment. If the neonatal manikin does not have an umbilicus for this purpose, the instructor can provide an umbilical model as described in Appendix C. The model should be placed next to the neonatal manikin, causing little or no interruption in the flow of the interventions.

I understand that the UVC placement is supposed to be a sterile procedure. In an actual code, does sterile procedure take precedence over getting the umbilical line placed? For example, if a minor break in sterile procedure occurs, does the team need to stop the procedure, get new equipment, and begin again?

The resuscitation team should strive to maintain sterile technique during emergency umbilical venous catheterization. Obviously, poor technique is unacceptable, and gross contamination of the catheter or equipment used to prepare or insert the catheter or medication mandates immediate remediation. However, no resuscitation is textbook perfect. Sterile procedure is the goal, but, if a minor break in sterile technique inadvertently occurs, the practitioner must use clinical judgment to decide if the risks of delaying administration of lifesaving volume or medication by beginning the procedure again outweigh the benefits of continuing the procedure.

I am a hospital-based instructor whose job responsibilities do not include intubation or emergency UVC placement. I feel nervous teaching these skills when I don't have experience or expertise performing them.

The NRP Provider Course presents basic theory for all lessons in the *Textbook of Neonatal Resuscitation, 6th Edition.* As an instructor, you are expected to be familiar with the material in all 9 lessons and facilitate the learning of your NRP course participants. It is necessary for instructors to reach a level of comfort with the material and convey a level of confidence that promotes self-efficacy in the learners. If you regularly assist with intubations and umbilical line placements, you should be able to present the important points. Consider the following suggestions:

- Teach with another instructor or a guest lecturer whose job responsibilities include these procedures.

- Integrate video instruction into your intubation, laryngeal mask airway placement, and Medication Performance Stations by using a laptop computer or LCD projector, such as the Resuscitation Skills videos that are included on both the NRP Instructor DVD and the DVD that accompanies the *Textbook of Neonatal Resuscitation, 6th Edition.* This can take the pressure off you having to demonstrate or describe a procedure that you do not perform.

- Ask a guest lecturer to give a brief presentation of strategies for intubation success (5 minutes) at some point during your NRP Provider Course. The guest lecturer should not be listed on the Course Roster submitted to the American Academy of Pediatrics, unless the lecturer is an NRP instructor.

Can the instructor be held liable for a former class participant's performance during actual neonatal resuscitation?

No, the NRP is not a certification course, and the instructor cannot be held liable for how information from an educational offering is applied in practice. However, it is important that the hospital use the most current NRP materials. It is also important to ensure timely communication about changes in guidelines for neonatal resuscitation to those who perform neonatal resuscitation.

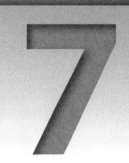

Simulation

Simulation-based training integrates cognitive, technical, and behavioral skills into an environment where learners "believe" the setting is real, act as they would in an actual resuscitation, and feel safe to make mistakes for the purpose of learning from them. While knowledge about newborn physiology and the ability to perform hands-on skills are important aspects of the Neonatal Resuscitation Program™ (NRP™), the Simulation and Debriefing components of the NRP course focus on teamwork and communication.

In Chapter 7 you will learn

- **The purpose of simulation-based NRP training**

- **How to create a useful scenario**

- **How to prepare the environment and the team for simulation-based training**

- **How to conduct an effective scenario**

- **About one program for improving teamwork and communication**

The *NRP Instructor DVD: An Interactive Tool for Facilitation of Simulation-based Learning*

One of the NRP instructor's most useful tools for learning about simulation and debriefing is the *NRP Instructor DVD: An Interactive Tool for Facilitation of Simulation-based Learning.* Although reading about simulation and debriefing is useful, the NRP Instructor DVD was developed by members of the NRP Steering Committee and simulation experts to help instructors incorporate this methodology into NRP courses. The DVD uses interactive media to bring you as close to "being there" as possible. Use the NRP Instructor DVD as a frequent reference because, as you learn and gain experience using simulation and debriefing, you will find different sections of the DVD useful.

"Instructor Self-assessment" for Chapter 7 begins on page 195.

After studying this chapter, complete the Chapter 7 questions, using the answer sheets that begin on page 188. Your regional trainer may ask you to bring the answer sheets to your NRP Instructor Course.

> Simulation and Debriefing focus on developing effective teamwork and communication. Simulation is meant to replicate the way that health care professionals actually behave in crisis situations, which may include unexpected or inappropriate responses. Neonatal Resuscitation Program Simulation and Debriefing provides team members with a safe setting in which to integrate cognitive and technical skills and a valuable opportunity to focus on team communication and patient safety.

In July 2004, The Joint Commission published a *Sentinel Event Alert* that influenced the ongoing evolution of the NRP.* The Joint Commission reported that communication issues played a role in nearly three-fourths of the perinatal death and injury cases reported to the Joint Commission during the reported time period. As a result, the Joint Commission recommended that organizations that deliver newborns conduct training to teach teamwork and communication. In addition, the Joint Commission recommended that organizations conduct drills for high-risk events, such as neonatal resuscitation, and include debriefings to evaluate and improve performance.

Simulation and Debriefing is a new component of the NRP Provider Course curriculum that addresses learning objectives for improved teamwork and communication.

We use scenarios all the way through the Performance Skills Stations, then again during the Integrated Skills Station. What makes the Simulation and Debriefing component of the NRP Provider Course different than what we have already done in the course? Can we skip this part?

The scenarios used for the Performance Skills Stations (eg, Equipment Check, Initial Steps, PPV, and Chest Compressions) are supervised and coached by an NRP instructor to help learners acquire technical skills. The Integrated Skills Station allows few errors. While knowledge of newborn physiology and the ability to perform hands-on resuscitation skills are important, *the focus of simulation training is teamwork and communication*. For this reason, the Simulation and Debriefing component of the NRP Provider Course is required.

*From The Joint Commission. (2004). Preventing infant death and injury during delivery. Retrieved from **http://www.jointcommission.org/sentinel_event_alert_issue_30_preventing_infant_death_and_injury_during_delivery/**. Accessed January 31, 2011.

What is simulation-based training?
(the following is adapted from **http://www.pediatrics.org/cgt/content/**   ⌨**www**
full/106/4/e45 with permission from *Pediatrics*)
A methodology for learning in which trainees

• Are immersed in an environment filled with realistic visual, auditory, and tactile cues

• Work through realistic, challenging situations

• Are provided the opportunity to reflect on their performance (debrief)

What are the advantages of simulation-based learning over traditional classroom learning?

• Adults learn better by active participation rather than by passive observation.

• Traditional training for health care professionals focuses on doing everything correctly. Often, the best learning comes from making a mistake. Therefore, simulation training pushes participants out of their comfort zones, allows mistakes, and provides learners the opportunity to reflect on their performance.

• Traditional classroom settings do not make trainees think and feel as though they are functioning in a real situation with consequences for their actions. When trainees are placed in a space with key visual, auditory, and tactile cues, they are able to "suspend their disbelief" and immerse themselves in the scenario, effectively re-creating real-life events.

• Simulation training promotes the use of decision-making skills in an environment similar to the clinical setting, where participants face unpredictable responses, complex team communication, time pressure, and high risk.

• Simulation training allows trainees to practice technical skills, rapid decision making, and problem solving during infrequently encountered crisis situations without endangering an actual patient.

> Technology is *not* the key to quality simulation and debriefing. The methodology, such as the auditory and visual cues used for realism, and the skills used by the instructor during debriefing, has more to do with the quality of the experience than the use of high-tech equipment.

I'm not sure our hospital can afford simulation training. It seems expensive.

Many NRP instructors believe that the NRP promotes the use of a sophisticated electronic simulator for this new methodology. While a state-of-the-art newborn simulator is a wonderful asset to a simulation center, it is not necessary to have one to make an excellent NRP course.

While having access to a state-of-the-art simulation center, along with the equipment, skilled staff, and many resources a simulation center offers, is a great thing, you also may conduct excellent simulation training in a conference room with a traditional plastic manikin. Both of these settings offer high-quality NRP learning. Technology is not the key to quality simulation and debriefing. The methodology, such as the auditory and visual cues used for realism, and the skills used by the instructor during debriefing, has more to do with the quality of the experience than the use of high-tech equipment.

Scenario Design

Creating a scenario for NRP participants takes preparation and forethought. The skilled NRP instructor strives to develop scenarios that meet the learning needs of NRP course participants and set the stage for the important learning that occurs during debriefing.

The instructor is responsible for setting up a simulation to seem as real as possible, by using or creating a realistic setting, using as much actual equipment as possible, and designing scenarios that learners believe could actually happen. In return, learners agree to "suspend their disbelief" and do their best to act as if everything is real.

A well-written scenario compels learners to integrate cognitive, technical, and behavioral skills while working under intense time pressure. An effective scenario is one in which the learning objectives are achieved.

How do I create scenarios for use during the Simulation and Debriefing component of my NRP course?

Before you can create a scenario, you must assess your learners' needs and formulate learning objectives. You may conduct a formal assessment prior to the course (see Experience Survey on pages 32 and 214), or you may ask your learners about their goals and objectives at the beginning of a course.

Assessment also enables you to find the learners who want to expand beyond the usual experience. Sometimes unit managers, clinical nurse specialists, and risk managers suggest scenarios based on previous clinical experiences that point out needed improvements in systems, processes, skills, and/or communication. Perhaps your learners would benefit from a scenario that involves a very preterm newborn, a congenital anomaly, or an unusual high-risk situation that demands expert communication and teamwork.

Neonatal Resuscitation Program scenarios usually involve information about

- A birthing mother

- A clinical complication with implications for the newborn

- A newborn who requires assessment and some degree of intervention

The scenario is the clinical situation used for simulation. Simulation sets the stage for debriefing, where the learning occurs. The scenario is based on 3 categories of learning objectives.

- Cognitive skills (knowledge about newborn physiology and evidence-based resuscitation practices)

- Hands-on skills (such as positive-pressure ventilation [PPV])

- Neonatal Resuscitation Program Key Behavioral Skills (see Table 7-1) that help ensure effective communication and teamwork

The list of Key Behavioral Skills if useful, but I have little training about team communication. Should I cover this in more depth?
Since 2004, when the Joint Commission recommended training in teamwork and communication, most hospitals have adapted strategic communication methods to meet this objective. The NRP instructor may incorporate hospital policies and protocols about communicating patient information and safety issues into NRP scenarios.

One effective strategy for improving teamwork and communication that partners well with NRP training is called "TeamSTEPPS." Developed by the US Department of Defense (DOD) and the Agency for Healthcare Research and Quality (AHRQ), this program is used nationally to improve team communication and improve patient safety. (See Table 7-2.) The DOD and AHRQ have now have teamed with the American Institutes for Research to build a national training and support network called the National Implementation of TeamSTEPPS Project. For more information, go to **http://teamstepps.ahrq.gov/index.htm.**   💻**www**

What tools are available to help instructors create scenarios?
1. Scenario Building Tool (page 110)
2. Scenario Template: One blank (pages 104-105), one filled in as an example (pages 106-107), and one with instructions and explanations for instructors about how to complete the template (pages 108-109)
3. The Scenario Template, in blank form and filled in, also can be found in the NRP Instructor DVD, Appendix D.

Table 7-1. Neonatal Resuscitation Program Key Behavioral Skills in Action

Neonatal Resuscitation Program Key Behavioral Skills*	Examples of the Behavioral Skill in Action[†]
Know your environment.	Learners perform Equipment Check before newborn arrives. Learners know location of code cart or how to access it. Learners know to call for help and who is available.
Anticipate and plan.	All learners listen to circumstances of scenario. Resuscitation team "huddles" and assigns roles and responsibilities. Team discusses action plan in event of potential complications.
Assume the leadership role.	Learners "huddle" and assign leadership role(s). Leader clearly articulates goals. Leader effectively uses resources. Leader delegates tasks, as appropriate. Leader uses call-outs to communicate critical information. Leader asks for input from team members. Leader enables team members to challenge the plan when appropriate. Leader promotes teamwork and resolves conflict. Learners discuss plan in the event leadership role must shift due to the leader becoming engrossed in a task or procedure. Leader includes family in communication.
Communicate effectively.	Team members call each other by name. All team members actively share information. Team member orders medications by name, dose, and route. Team members verify information that is communicated. Team members ensure that changes in information are shared with all team members.
Delegate workload optimally.	Team members do not duplicate work or use more resources than necessary. • One person holds endotracheal tube and positive-pressure ventilation device. • One person holds emergency umbilical venous catheter and flush syringe. Team members agree to change task assignments depending on skill sets and what is required at the moment. Team members protect each other from work overload.
Allocate attention wisely.	Team members maintain situation awareness by scanning and assessing at all times. Team members monitor one another's actions in context of patient safety.
Use all available information.	Team members ask about prenatal and intrapartum history, including presence of meconium-stained amniotic fluid prior to birth. Team members ask about newborn history, if newborn is being resuscitated after first minutes of life.
Use all available resources.	Know human resources available. Know supplies and equipment availability.
Call for help when needed.	Team members call for help in timely manner. Team members know process for getting assistance of the right kind.
Maintain professional behavior.	Team members use respectful verbal and nonverbal behaviors. Team members actively seek and offer assistance. Team members support and promote teamwork. All team members are equally valued and respected.

*NRP Key Behavioral Skills are from the Center for Advanced Pediatric and Perinatal Education (CAPE), Lucile Packard Children's Hospital at Stanford University. Available at: http://cape.lpch.org/courses/logistics/skills.html Accessed January 31, 2011.

†Selected information in column 2 derived from TeamSTEPPS™ Pocket Guide: Strategies & Tools to Enhance Performance and Patient Safety. Dept of Defense and Agency for Healthcare Research and Quality. *AHRQ.* Pub. No. 06-0020-2. Revised Nov 2008. Version 06.1.

Table 7-2. About TeamSTEPPS

(The following headings and bullets are taken from the TeamSTEPPS Web site at **http://teamstepps.ahrq.gov/about-2cl_3.htm**.)   💻**www**

TeamSTEPPS is a teamwork system designed for health care professionals that is

- A powerful solution to improving patient safety within your organization
- An evidence-based teamwork system to improve communication and teamwork skills among health care professionals
- A source for ready-to-use materials and a training curriculum to successfully integrate teamwork principles into all areas of your health care system
- Scientifically rooted in more than 20 years of research and lessons from the application of teamwork principles
- Developed by Department of Defense's Patient Safety Program in collaboration with the Agency for Healthcare Research and Quality
- TeamSTEPPS provides higher quality, safer patient care by:
  - Producing highly effective medical teams that optimize the use of information, people, and resources to achieve the best clinical outcomes for patients
  - Increasing team awareness and clarifying team roles and responsibilities
  - Resolving conflicts and improving information sharing
  - Eliminating barriers to quality and safety

How long does a scenario last?

Most scenarios run 3 to 5 minutes; a complex scenario with complex clinical interventions may take longer.

Why does NRP encourage the use of the Scenario Template? Why do I need to write it all down? Can't I simply create a scenario on the fly and then debrief the team based on what we all remember?

The Scenario Template gives the instructor a form for organizing an effective scenario based on the team's learning objectives.

By identifying learning objectives first, the instructor can create a scenario that sticks to those objectives.

- The Scenario Template gives the person who will debrief the team a place to make notes during or immediately after the scenario, which will help guide the debriefing.

- The Scenario Template helps your assistants set up for the exercise; know which visual, auditory, and tactile cues are important to include; and know what to expect from learners during the scenario.

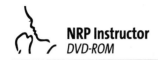

NRP Instructor
DVD-ROM

Title of Scenario: _____

Brief description for instructors: _____

_____

Learning objectives (cognitive, technical, and behavioral):

1. _____

_____

2. _____

_____

3. _____

_____

4. _____

_____

5. _____

_____

Pertinent history for learners:

Mother: _____ years old   G_____ P_____   estimated gestational age: _____ weeks

Delivery: ☐ vaginal birth   ☐ cesarean birth

Other (prenatal history, laboratory results, ultrasound results, pertinent maternal and social history, antepartum complications):

_____

_____

Scenario location:

☐ LDR   ☐ OR   ☐ ED   ☐ ambulance   ☐ parking lot   ☐ other _____

Necessary equipment and supplies:

☐ Complete resuscitation setup

☐ Variance in setup (list additional supplies or equipment required): _____

Manikin preparation:

_____

Initial condition of neonate:

Expected interventions during scenario:

Skills demonstrated (cognitive, technical, behavioral):

Cognitive

    1. _____

    2. _____

    3. _____

Technical

- ☐ Equipment check
- ☐ Initial steps
- ☐ Positive-pressure ventilation
    - ☐ Self-inflating bag   ☐ Flow-inflating bag   ☐ T-piece resuscitator
    - ☐ Management of oxygen concentration
    - ☐ Rate and pressure
    - ☐ MR SOPA
    - ☐ Assessment of heart rate
    - ☐ Assessment of breath sounds
    - ☐ Use of pulse oximetry
    - ☐ Administration of free-flow oxygen
    - ☐ Use of orogastric tube as necessary
    - ☐ Assessment of need for post-resuscitation care
- ☐ Chest compressions
- ☐ Endotracheal intubation (or assistance with intubation)
- ☐ Emergency umbilical venous catheter placement (or assistance with placement)
- ☐ Epinephrine administration (drawing up, routes, dosages)
- ☐ Laryngeal mask airway placement

Behavioral

- ☐ Know your environment.
- ☐ Anticipate and plan.
- ☐ Assume the leadership role.
- ☐ Communicate effectively.
- ☐ Delegate workload optimally.
- ☐ Allocate attention wisely.
- ☐ Use all available information.
- ☐ Use all available resources.
- ☐ Call for help when needed.
- ☐ Maintain professional behavior.

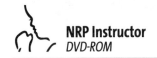
NRP Instructor
DVD-ROM

Sample Scenario Template

Title of Scenario: ___Resuscitation with Bag and Mask___

Brief description for instructors: ___This patient is born via vaginal delivery at 35 weeks' gestation___ ___& presents apneic; he begins to breathe spontaneously if bag-and-mask ventilation is properly administered.___

Learning objectives (cognitive, technical, and behavioral):

1. ___Identify the newborn who requires positive-pressure ventilation (PPV).___

2. ___Demonstrate correct technique for PPV, including placement of mask on the newborn's face,___ ___rate and pressure, and corrective actions (MR SOPA) for ineffective PPV.___

3. ___Demonstrate correct placement and interpretation of pulse oximetry.___

4. ___Recognize improvement during PPV by noting improvement in increased heart rate, color___ ___and oxygen saturation, muscle tone, and spontaneous breathing.___

5. ___Demonstrate pertinent key behavioral skills to optimize team performance.___

Pertinent history for learners:

Mother: __22__ years old   G_2_ P_1_   estimated gestational age: __35__ weeks

Delivery: ☒ vaginal birth   ☐ cesarean birth

Other (prenatal history, laboratory results, ultrasound results, pertinent maternal and social history, antepartum complications):

___none___

Scenario location:

☒ LDR   ☐ OR   ☐ ED   ☐ ambulance   ☐ parking lot   ☐ other _____

Necessary equipment and supplies:

☒ Complete resuscitation setup

☐ Variance in setup (list additional supplies or equipment required): ___none___

Manikin preparation:

___Blood, vernix___

Initial condition of neonate:

Limp, apneic, cyanotic, Heart rate (HR) 50 beats per minute (bpm)

Expected interventions during scenario:

Equipment check, including presence and function of PPV device, initial steps, assessment of heart rate and breathing, call for assistance, initiation of PPV, pulse oximetry, assessment of effectiveness of PPV, corrective steps, 30 seconds of effective PPV, recognition of improving HR, tone, pulse oximetry, cessation of PPV, administration of free flow oxygen, assessment of need for post-resuscitation care.

Skills demonstrated (cognitive, technical, behavioral):

Cognitive

1. Recognize the infant who requires PPV.

2. Recall indications for effective ventilation (rising HR, rising oxygen saturation, bilateral breath sounds, chest movement).

3. Interpret pulse oximetry & adjust oxygen concentration according to the newborn's age & SpO2 target range.

Technical

- ☐ Equipment check
- ☐ Initial steps
- ☐ Positive-pressure ventilation
  - ☐ Self-inflating bag   ☐ Flow-inflating bag   ☐ T-piece resuscitator
  - ☐ Management of oxygen concentration
  - ☐ Rate and pressure
  - ☐ MR SOPA
  - ☐ Assessment of heart rate
  - ☐ Assessment of breath sounds
  - ☐ Use of pulse oximetry
  - ☐ Administration of free-flow oxygen
  - ☐ Use of orogastric tube as necessary
  - ☐ Assessment of need for post-resuscitation care
- ☐ Chest compressions
- ☐ Endotracheal intubation (or assistance with intubation)
- ☐ Emergency umbilical venous catheter placement (or assistance with placement)
- ☐ Epinephrine administration (drawing up, routes, dosages)
- ☐ Laryngeal mask airway placement

Behavioral

- ☐ Know your environment.
- ☐ Anticipate and plan.
- ☐ Assume the leadership role.
- ☐ Communicate effectively.
- ☐ Delegate workload optimally.
- ☐ Allocate attention wisely.
- ☐ Use all available information.
- ☐ Use all available resources.
- ☐ Call for help when needed.
- ☐ Maintain professional behavior.

Instructions for Using the Sample Scenario Template

Sample Scenario Template Section	Instructions and Notes for Use
Title of Scenario "Resuscitation With Bag and Mask"	The Title of Scenario is the name you give the scenario so that instructors can easily find this in a file by title. We call this one "Resuscitation With Bag and Mask."
Brief Description "This patient is born via vaginal delivery at 35 weeks' gestation and presents apneic; he begins to breathe spontaneously if bag-and-mask ventilation is properly administered."	Brief Description is one sentence that tells Neonatal Resuscitation Program (NRP) instructors what occurs in the scenario.
Learning Objectives 1. Identify the newborn who requires positive-pressure ventilation (PPV). **(cognitive)** 2. Demonstrate correct technique for positive-pressure ventilation, including placement of the mask on the newborn's face, rate and pressure . . . **(cognitive and technical)** 3. Demonstrate correct placement and interpretation of pulse oximetry. **(cognitive and technical)** 4. Recognize improvement during PPV by noting improvement in increased heart rate (HR), color and oxygen saturation . . . **(technical)** 5. Demonstrate pertinent key behavioral skills to optimize team performance. **(behavioral)**	These describe what you expect the learners to know/do during the scenario when they successfully integrate the cognitive, technical, and behavioral skills. Each scenario should encompass about 2-5 learning objectives in each of the 3 categories depending on the length and complexity of the scenario. This is a short and simple scenario with 5 learning objectives which encompass 3 cognitive objectives, 3 technical objectives, and 1 behavioral objective. The behavioral objective is written in general terms to capture any Key Behavioral Skill listed on the second page of the scenario template form. Other skills may indeed be demonstrated, but only the most important are listed so instructors and learners alike know on which ones to focus. You may wish to use selected Learning Objectives listed on each Performance Checklist in the textbook or in Appendix E of this Instructor Manual.
Pertinent History for Learners Mother: *22* years old *G2 P1* Estimated gestational age: *35 weeks* Delivery: *x* vaginal birth Other: none	This section is more detailed than the Brief Description section above. Instructors need to know the details so they know how the newborn should respond (or not respond) to the learners' actions. The amount of information given to learners depends on the learning objectives. Sometimes a complete history is provided in the "Other" category, including maternal blood type, prenatal laboratory results, gestational age assessment methods, difficulties during pregnancy, ultrasound results, and pertinent maternal health and social issues. At other times, the learners are called to the delivery room, given limited information and limited time to prepare for the birth.
Scenario Location *X* LDR	Scenario location is usually the delivery room; however, the learning objectives may direct the birth setting to a different place such as the Operating Room, Emergency Department, ambulance, or parking lot.

Instructions for Using the Sample Scenario Template—*continued*

Sample Scenario Template Section	Instructions and Notes for Use
Necessary Equipment and Supplies *X* Complete resuscitation setup *X* Variance in setup: None	Scenarios that take place in the Delivery Room necessitate a complete resuscitation setup unless the learning objectives include improvisation or a work-around due to missing or malfunctioning equipment. "Variance in Setup" cues the instructor in the event that the usual setup is different, requiring either more or less equipment to match the learning objectives.
Manikin preparation Blood, vernix	Helps the instructor set the scene, especially if the newborn requires special effects besides blood, vernix, or meconium.
Page 2 of scenario template form	
Initial condition of the neonate Limp, apneic, cyanotic, HR 50 beats per minute (bpm)	Important to know so that learners begin the scenario with the correct physiologic feedback (eg, limp, apneic, cyanotic, HR 50 bpm in this case).
Expected interventions during the scenario Equipment check, initial steps, assessment of heart rate and breathing, call for assistance, initiation of PPV, pulse oximetry, assessment of effectiveness of PPV, corrective steps, etc	This is a list of what learners can be expected to do if they share the same mental model of the patient as the instructor, and if the learners perform resuscitation in a competent manner. The Expected Interventions section is essentially an outline of what the instructor can expect to happen if all goes according to plan. The learners may not necessarily perform these listed interventions, but, instead, take a different path that requires the instructor to be alert for unexpected learning opportunities.
Skills Demonstrated: **Cognitive, Technical, and Behavioral** **Cognitive:** 1. Recognize the newborn who requires PPV. 2. Recall indications for effective ventilation . . . 3. Interpret pulse oximetry and adjust oxygen concentration . . . **Technical** (complete list) **Behavioral** (complete list)	These are printed on page 2 of the form so that instructors have room to make notes on this page in preparation for the debriefing. Three cognitive skills are listed. The Technical and Behavioral Skills are listed on each Scenario Template in this way so you can indicate when an objective has been met in any scenario. Use this information to guide your debriefing. Technical: The form includes the complete list of technical skills for PPV because this is a critical resuscitation skill; the form also lists headings for additional technical skills. Behavioral: The form includes the complete list of Key Behavioral Skills because any or all would be appropriate.

Scenario Building Tool

Choose the gestational age, weight, and mode of birth. Select a risk factor. Choose or create other descriptions of the newborn's condition at birth. The newborn's condition suggests the resuscitation interventions the team must perform.

Note: Meconium-stained newborns should be term or post-term.

Gestational Age	Estimated Weight	Mode of Delivery	Risk Factor	Condition of Newborn at Birth	Procedures Indicated	Lessons Evaluated
Term, post-term	>3,500 g	Vaginal birth	Shoulder dystocia	Apneic, heart rate 40 beats per minute (bpm)	Equipment Check, Initial steps, positive-pressure ventilation, pulse oximetry, chest compressions	Lessons 1 through 4
					Baby deteriorates: Add intubation, epinephrine	Lesson 5 Lesson 6
Term, post-term	>3,000 g	Emergency cesarean birth	Failed vacuum extraction	Apneic, heart rate 50 bpm	Equipment Check, initial steps, positive-pressure ventilation, pulse oximetry, chest compressions	Lessons 1 through 4
					Baby deteriorates: Add intubation, epinephrine, +/- volume	Lesson 5 Lesson 6
Term, post-term	>3,000 g	Vaginal or cesarean birth	Meconium-stained fluid	Irregular breathing, limp, heart rate 80 bpm then 40 bpm after tracheal suction	Equipment Check, initial steps, intubation, positive-pressure ventilation, pulse oximetry, chest compressions, re-intubation, epinephrine	Lessons 1 through 5 Lesson 6
Choose appropriate gestation	Choose appropriate weight for gestational age	Cesarean birth	Placenta previa	Apneic, heart rate 50 bpm, limp	Equipment Check, initial steps, positive-pressure ventilation, pulse oximetry, chest compressions	Lessons 1 through 4 Lesson 8 if preterm
					Baby deteriorates: Add intubation, epinephrine	Lesson 5 Lesson 6 Lesson 9 may be applicable

Gestational Age	Estimated Weight	Mode of Delivery	Risk Factor	Condition of Newborn at Birth	Procedures Indicated	Lessons Evaluated
Choose appropriate gestation	Choose appropriate weight for gestational age	Vaginal birth in mother's bed on antepartum unit	Amnionitis	Apneic, heart rate 80 bpm then falls to 50 bpm	Equipment Check, initial steps, positive-pressure ventilation, pulse oximetry, chest compressions	Lessons 1 through 4 Lesson 8 if preterm
					Baby deteriorates: Add intubation, epinephrine	Lesson 5 Lesson 6 Lesson 9 may be applicable
		2-day-old found in bassinet in mother's room	Unknown	Apneic, heart rate 40 bpm	Modified initial steps, positive-pressure ventilation, pulse oximetry, chest compressions	Lessons 1 through 4
					Baby deteriorates: Add intubation, epinephrine, +/- volume	Lesson 5 Lesson 6
		Cesarean birth	Cord entanglement	Apneic, heart rate 40 bpm, pale	Equipment Check, initial steps, positive-pressure ventilation, pulse oximetry, chest compressions	Lessons 1 through 4 Lesson 8 if preterm
					Baby deteriorates: Add intubation, epinephrine, +/- volume	Lesson 5 Lesson 6 Lesson 9 may be applicable
		Vaginal or cesarean birth	Congenital malformations	Breathing then apneic, heart rate 90 bpm then 50 bpm, persistent cyanosis	Equipment Check, initial steps, positive-pressure ventilation, pulse oximetry, chest compressions	Lessons 1 through 4 Lesson 8 if preterm
					Baby deteriorates: Add intubation, epinephrine	Lesson 5 Lesson 6 Lesson 9 may be applicable

Create Your Own Scenarios

Choose the gestational age, weight, and mode of birth. Select or create your own risk factor. Describe the condition of the newborn at birth to create a scenario in which selected procedures are necessary to resuscitate the newborn.

Note: Meconium-stained newborns should be term or post-term.

Appropriate weights for gestational age

28 weeks = 800 to 1,500 g   30 weeks = 1,000 to 1,750 g   32 weeks = 1,250 to 2,000 g

34 weeks = 1,500 to 2,700 g   36 weeks = 2,000 to 3,200 g   38 to 40 weeks = 2,500 to 3,700 g

Gestational Age	Estimated Weight	Mode of Delivery	Risk Factor	Potential Conditions of Newborn at Birth	Procedures Indicated	Lessons Evaluated

Procedure	Criteria
Intubate and suction trachea	Meconium in amniotic fluid or on the baby's skin/baby with depressed respirations or tone, or heart rate <100 beats per minute (bpm)
Free-flow oxygen	Heart rate >100 bpm after initial steps, breathing with perceived persistent cyanosis, low target oxygen saturation for age in minutes confirmed by pulse oximetry
Positive-pressure ventilation (PPV)	Apneic/gasping, heart rate <100 bpm even if breathing, or persistent cyanosis after free-flow oxygen and low target oxygen saturation for age in minutes confirmed by pulse oximetry
Chest compressions	Heart rate remains <60 bpm after 30 seconds of effective assisted ventilation
Intubation	Tracheal suctioning of meconium for non-vigorous newborn, mask ventilation ineffective or prolonged, to facilitate coordination of chest compressions and ventilation, or as route for epinephrine pending establishment of emergency umbilical venous catheter (UVC)
Laryngeal mask airway placement	When ventilation is unsuccessful and intubation is not successful or not feasible
Placement of emergency UVC	When epinephrine or volume administration is indicated
Epinephrine administration	Intubated or UVC in place, heart rate <60 bpm after 30 seconds of effective assisted ventilation and another 45-60 seconds of coordinated chest compressions and effective PPV
Volume administration	Baby appears in shock and is not responding to resuscitation efforts or there is a history of a condition associated with fetal blood loss.

Preparing for Effective Simulation

The key to successful simulation training is thorough preparation. You already have laid much of the foundation for the Simulation and Debriefing component of the course by assembling and organizing your NRP supplies and equipment for Performance Skills Stations. Your Integrated Skills Station probably includes everything needed for a complete resuscitation. (The NRP course supply list is on pages 80-81, and pages 212-213) As you discover more about your trainees' learning objectives, you may wish to add additional items to your simulation training supplies.

Where should I conduct my simulation training?

Simulation means immersing the learner in the setting where the learning will occur. Effective simulation eliminates "pretending" whenever possible; therefore, it is ideal to conduct your scenarios in the setting where you actually perform neonatal resuscitation with the actual supplies and equipment used. In most cases, this means using an unoccupied delivery room, newborn stabilization room, or operating room where cesarean birth occurs.

I do not have reliable access to an actual birth setting for my simulation training. How can I set up a realistic environment that will help learners suspend their disbelief?

If an empty patient space is not available, set up a newborn resuscitation area that resembles the actual birth setting as closely as possible. Simulation does not require that every detail of an actual birth setting be present. Determine which visual, auditory, and tactile cues are most important for creating environmental and psychological realism. In most cases, the following strategies are helpful for NRP course simulation:

- A radiant warmer is a powerful visual and auditory cue for learners. Plug it in and allow learners to turn on the heat and operate the controls. On some models, the suction and oxygen equipment may be on the warmer.

- If you use a T-piece resuscitator, make it operational by connecting it to a gas source on the wall, or to compressed air or an oxygen tank.

- If you must perform resuscitation on a conference room table, try to set up visual cues for the heat source on a radiant warmer, suction and oxygen, and whatever system is used at your hospital to call for additional help. The control panel from the *Simply NRP* kit can be used on a conference room table. Although it is a simple model, it gives learners the opportunity to perform the steps of preparing for newborn resuscitation.

What additional visual cues are important for effective simulation?

- Learners should wear scrubs or a cover gown over their clothing. Size XL scrub tops or cloth-cover gowns fit almost everyone, and can be placed quickly over street clothes. For a surgical setting, learners also should wear a surgical mask and head covering.

- Gloves help learners feel as though they are participating in an actual resuscitation.

- Linen: Use hospital-issued baby blankets and towels that your learners will recognize as part of their hospital birth setting, not baby blankets or towels purchased from a department store.

- Phones and pagers: Use actual phones and pagers. Be sure that message recipients are aware that they are players in a simulation-based newborn resuscitation training exercise.

- Body fluids: Easy recipes for blood, vernix, and meconium, strategies for quick and realistic application, and clean-up information can be found in Appendix F.

How do we provide feedback to the learner who needs to know about the "baby's" breathing, heart rate, tone, and perhaps oxygen saturation?

This question points out another big change in the way experienced NRP instructors are accustomed to conducting a scenario.

Physiologic Cues: Using an Electronic Simulator

During a resuscitation scenario, the trainee talks through the interventions and performs the actions. For example, the trainee begins PPV and asks the assistant to listen for a rising heart rate, and then note bilateral breath sounds and chest movement. The person running the simulator assesses the trainee's technique and "makes" the manikin respond either with rising heart rate, chest movement, and bilateral breath sounds or, if the instructor wants to elicit the corrective ventilation sequence from the trainee, the instructor will not allow the simulator to respond to the initial attempt at PPV.

The manikin and the computerized oximetry device demonstrate physiologic cues for the learner, because the instructor pays attention to the interventions performed by the trainees and electronically controls the manikin's responses. When an electronic simulator is used, little or no conversation is required between the trainee and the instructor. The instructor does not wait for the trainee to ask, "Is the baby breathing? What is the heart rate?" to elicit the correct electronic response from the manikin. The manikin responds just as a live human newborn would respond, and it is the trainee's responsibility to continuously monitor the simulator's changing status.

> The learner who uses an electronic simulator does not need to ask the instructor about breathing, heart rate, oxygen saturation, or muscle tone. It is the instructor's job to listen to the team talk through the interventions, watch for these actions to occur, and make the simulator respond in real time. It is the trainee's job to continuously monitor the simulator's changing status, say aloud what is happening during the scenario, and perform the next appropriate steps.

Physiologic Cues: Using a Traditional Manikin
When the trainees use a traditional manikin, the instructor must emphasize the importance of the trainees talking through their actions so that the instructor can reveal the physiologic responses to the trainee's interventions. This requires a combination of questions and answers between the instructor and the trainee, and may be done in a variety of ways.

The goal is to synchronize the manikin's responses to the trainees' interventions (or lack of intervention). In many ways, the instructor must "be" the manikin and be ready to reveal the physiological responses based on cues from the learner.

Heart Rate
When the scenario begins and the newborn arrives at the radiant warmer, experienced NRP learners are accustomed to asking the instructor to announce the heart rate. You may be surprised to learn that many health care professionals have difficulty assessing heart rate by counting the pulse for 6 seconds and multiplying by 10. When the instructor announces the heart rate, the learner misses an opportunity to practice this skill.

Instead of announcing the heart rate, watch the learner and give the auditory cue for the newborn's heart rate only when the learner palpates the umbilicus or places the stethoscope on the manikin's chest. The newborn's heart rate can be simulated in a few different ways.

- Tap out the heart rate on the tabletop. Be sure to use a clock with a second hand to ensure that you can accurately tap out the intended heart rate.

- Use a metronome. Visit a music store and try out different models. Consider a handheld digital model that does not take up a lot of storage room. Choose the least expensive model that fits your needs so that you can replace it, if necessary. Consider the size of the numbers for easy viewing, the speed and responsiveness of the metronome when you want to increase or decrease the heart rate, the ability to mute the heart rate sound (the heart rate is audible only when the learner listens with the stethoscope or palpates the umbilicus), and the tone and volume of the pulse. Some metronomes have a very high pitch with more emphasis on the first "beat of the measure." Work with a variety of metronomes so that you can make a good purchase. Compare notes with other NRP instructors and share what you have learned.

- Download a metronome with adjustable tempos onto your laptop. Search the Internet for "download a metronome" to find numerous choices.

- Your cell phone may have a metronome application. Simulation training can get noisy, so be sure the volume is loud enough to be heard by learners in action.

> Watch the learner and give the auditory cue for the newborn's heart rate only when the learner palpates the umbilicus or places the stethoscope on the manikin's chest.

Breathing, Muscle Tone, Oxygen Saturation, and (Sometimes) Color
The goal is to limit interaction between the resuscitation team and the instructor during the scenario. However, interaction is unavoidable when the learners must depend on the instructor for physiologic cues, such as breathing, oxygen saturation, muscle tone, and, in some scenarios, color. The instructor must orient the learners to how physiologic cues will be revealed to them during the scenario. A practice scenario is a good way to orient learners to your system. Walk through a scenario, and stop and discuss how they will get information about breathing, heart rate, muscle tone, and pulse oximetry, if indicated.

Table 7-3. Physiologic Cues From a Traditional Manikin

Physiologic Cue	Learner's Action	Instructor's Action
Breathing	ASK instructor. Put stethoscope on baby's chest and state what is being assessed: "I'm assessing breath sounds."	Give information about respiratory status ONLY when the learner indicates breathing is being assessed. TELL THE LEARNER. USE FLASH CARDS. USE DRY ERASE BOARD. USE COMPUTER SCREEN.
Heart Rate	ASK instructor. Put stethoscope on baby's chest and state what is being assessed: "I'm assessing heart rate."	Indicate heart rate ONLY when the learner auscultates the chest or palpates the umbilical pulse. USE METRONOME. TAP IT OUT.
Muscle Tone	ASK instructor. Lift and drop baby's extremities and indicate that tone is being assessed.	Indicate muscle tone ONLY when the learner asks for this information. TELL THE LEARNER. USE FLASH CARDS. USE DRY ERASE BOARD. USE COMPUTER SCREEN.
Pulse Oximetry	ASK instructor. (The pulse oximeter probe must be attached to the newborn's right hand or wrist before asking for information.) Encourage use of the Apgar timer on the radiant warmer (or use stopwatch to begin scenario at birth) so that learners can aim for "Target Pre-ductal SpO_2 After Birth" on the NRP flow diagram.	Indicate pulse oximetry value ONLY when the learner asks for this information. TELL THE LEARNER. USE *SIMPLY NRP* CONTROL BOARD PULSE OXIMETER. USE FLASH CARDS. USE DRY ERASE BOARD. USE COMPUTER SCREEN.
Color*	ASK instructor.	Indicate color ONLY when the learner asks for this information. TELL THE LEARNER. USE BLUE EYE SHADOW AROUND EYES AND MOUTH.

*Routine assessment of color is not stressed because visual interpretation of oxygen saturation is unreliable. Color is usually assessed along with use of an oximeter. Color is an important cue if the scenario involves color as a cue intended to elicit an intervention, such as persistent pallor that may indicate the need for volume administration.

How does the instructor simulate resuscitation of a newborn with a special need or congenital defect? For example, I would like our staff to begin incorporating the laryngeal mask airway into our scenarios as a rescue airway. I also would like to create challenging scenarios for experienced providers who may need to manage a newborn with a congenital defect.

- A photo on a laptop screen or a hard-copy photograph may be used to show important patient information that is not otherwise possible due to constraints of your resources. If you want your team to resuscitate a newborn with a special clinical situation (eg, Robin syndrome or a large cleft palate), begin the scenario by showing the learners a photo or image of a newborn with this condition. The photo will cue the learners to manage the resuscitation with this additional information.

- Congenital anomalies for your manikin can be purchased.

- Some congenital anomalies can be "do-it-yourself" projects made from common household items. (See Appendix F.)

- If the scenario is intentionally scripted to progress past the initial resuscitation period, vital signs, x-rays, and laboratory results that are added to the scenario template may be used to guide the team's post-resuscitation interventions.

Filming the Scenario

Taping a scenario is not absolutely necessary, but is not difficult, and enhances the learning experience for both the learners and the instructor.

- Videotape provides an objective record of who said and did what and when it occurred.

- When use correctly, videotape assists with debriefing.

- Most learners agree that video debriefing is a valuable educational experience, unmatched by any other learning experience.

- Videotaping saves a lot of time during debriefing, because learners do not need to recount each event out loud.

Equipment needed includes a camcorder, a tripod, cables, and some method of playing back the video for participants. You may use a TV monitor, a laptop, an LCD projector, or other device. If you are unfamiliar with the equipment, practice video recording and viewing the film, stopping and starting at various segments, until you are efficient at using film during debriefing.

Preparing the Team for Effective Simulation Training

Learners who are in their actual birth setting, using their own equipment with familiar team members, and who just completed the Performance Skills Stations and Integrated Skills Station may require little orientation to how simulation-based training works. However, most teams benefit from basic orientation and a "warm-up scenario" that allows learners to ask questions and clarify expectations before proceeding with the Simulation and Debriefing component of their NRP course.

Supplies and Equipment

Allow the learners to find the equipment and handle it, as needed. This is critical if they are not resuscitating in their usual birth setting with their own familiar supplies and equipment. Performing the Equipment Check by using the Quick Pre-resuscitation Checklist at the end of Lesson 1 of the *Textbook of Neonatal Resuscitation, 6th Edition* (and in Appendix I), will help learners find essential items needed for resuscitation in any setting.

Physiologic Feedback

How will the learners know the newborn's heart rate, or if the newborn is breathing? If you are using an electronic simulator, take the simulator through its capabilities and let the learners palpate the umbilicus, listen to heart rate and breath sounds, and feel the differences in muscle tone. It is important that learners have an opportunity to see, hear, and feel the physiologic capabilities of the simulator before beginning a simulation exercise.

If you are using a traditional manikin, familiarize learners with your system for conveying the newborn's physiologic status. Demonstrate the use of the metronome, and make sure learners understand that, in most instances, information such as heart rate, breathing, tone, and oxygen saturation will not be revealed until the learner performs the appropriate assessment action (eg, listens to the chest with a stethoscope) and/or asks for the information.

Team Member Orientation and Role Designation

Allow time for introductions if learners do not know each other. Learners should wear visible name tags with their designated role. This is especially important if participants are expected to act outside their usual role (eg, a nurse filling the role of a physician or a respiratory therapist). Remind learners that acting in a role different than their everyday role (eg, if a nurse needs to play the role of a physician), does not authorize the learners to perform interventions outside their scope of practice in their real-life professional setting.

Confidentiality

The assurance of a safe and supportive learning environment includes the learner's right to confidentiality. Consider using a confidentiality agreement (see sample on pages 120 and 309) and assure the learner that

- All events are confidential. This protects the integrity of the learner *and* protects the confidentiality of the scenarios so that future learners do not know what scenarios to expect during simulation training.

- The events of a simulation and debriefing exercise are not used as part of a learner's performance evaluation.

- If the exercise is filmed, the tape is erased at the end of the course, unless the learner has given written permission for its additional use.

Instructions and Expectations

Go over the "rules of the game." You may find it more interesting for participants to come up with their own Ground Rules or behavioral expectations than to read them a list. (See the sample Ground Rules on pages 121 and 308.) The following are additional important principles of simulation-based learning:

- Mistakes are acceptable; in fact, the best learning may come from an error. The goal of simulation and debriefing is learning, not perfection.

- Laughing and joking are not acceptable during resuscitation. Observers who have side conversations or laughter are asked to leave the room. If the instructor is professional and focused on the exercise, learners usually will follow that lead.

- The instructor never "tricks" the learners. For example, if learners check the presence of supplies and equipment prior to beginning the scenario, it is inappropriate for the instructor to then remove or sabotage equipment unless this is a learning objective built into the scenario to develop improvisation and teamwork.

- Learners need to think out loud so that the other team members and the instructor know what learners are thinking and why they are doing what they are doing. This is important to ensure that the team and the instructor have the same "mental model" of what is happening during the scenario.

- Learners need to actually perform the actions, not simply say that they are doing something. The exception to this rule is that liquids of any kind should not be administered into the electronic simulator's airway (eg, epinephrine). In this case, epinephrine can be drawn into the syringe and first expelled onto the bed linen, then "administered" through the endotracheal tube.

- Everyone participates during a simulation, and team members may help each other in any way that is plausible to the scenario. Communication and teamwork are encouraged and expected during the scenario.

- The instructor, not the learners, indicates when the scenario has ended.

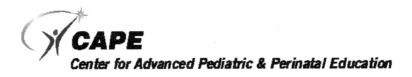

CONFIDENTIALITY AGREEMENT

During your participation in training in a simulated medical environment at the Center for Advanced Pediatric and Perinatal Education (CAPE) at Lucile Packard Children's Hospital at Stanford you will be both an active participant in realistic scenarios and an observer of others immersed in similar situations (either in real time or on videotape). The objective of this training program is to train individuals to better assess and improve their performance in difficult clinical situations. It is to be understood that the scenarios to which you and your colleagues will be exposed are designed to exacerbate the likelihood of lapses and errors in performance. Because of these issues you are asked to maintain strict confidentiality regarding both your performance and the performance of others, whether witnessed in real time or on videotape. Failure to maintain confidentiality may result in unwarranted and unfair defamation of character of the participants. This could cause irreparable harm to you and your colleagues and would seriously impair the effectiveness of this simulation-based training program.

While you are free to discuss in general terms the technical and behavioral skills acquired and maintained during training at CAPE, you are required to maintain strict confidentiality regarding the specific scenarios to which you are both directly and indirectly exposed. The development of challenging scenarios is extremely labor intensive and any foreknowledge by participants of what is to be presented to them will defeat the purpose of this type of training.

The bottom line: All that takes place in the simulator, stays in the simulator.

By signing below, you acknowledge having read and understood this statement and agree to maintain the strictest confidentiality about the performance of individuals and the details of scenarios to which you are exposed.

Signature: _____ Date: _____

Print name: _____

E-mail: _____

From the Center for Advanced Pediatric and Perinatal Education (CAPE), Packard Children's Hospital at Stanford University (**http://www.cape.lpch.org**).

Allow a "warm-up" scenario.
Give inexperienced learners the opportunity for a short "warm-up" scenario where it is permissible to pause and ask the instructor questions and where the instructor can clarify expectations. For example, you may need to say, "I want you to actually ventilate the newborn for a full 30 seconds, as you would in an actual resuscitation." A warm-up scenario often allows learners to work through their initial nervousness and mentally prepare for the serious work ahead.

Table 7-4. **Sample Ground Rules for Simulation and Debriefing**

The NRP instructor will	• Create a plausible scenario based on the participants' learning objectives. • Create a learning environment that resembles the birth setting as closely as possible, given the constraints of available resources. • Orient learners to supplies and equipment and how physiologic responses are demonstrated. • Promote learning in a safe and supportive environment where mistakes are considered an important part of the learning process. • Assume that learners are intelligent, doing their best, and striving to improve. • Maintain confidentiality. A learner's performance is never discussed outside the event, videotape is deleted after debriefing unless the instructor has each participant's written permission to use the film for a specified purpose, and aspects of a learner's performance are never used for an evaluation with a supervisor.
Neonatal Resuscitation Program learners will	• Participate fully in simulation and debriefing and maintain confidentiality as instructed. • Suspend disbelief and behave as they would during an actual resuscitation. • Think out loud and talk through interventions so that everyone knows what is happening. • Help each other in any way that is plausible to the scenario. Teamwork is expected. • Perform the actions. Pretending or "saying" the action without doing it is not acceptable. • Maintain professional behavior. Giggling and joking are not acceptable during resuscitation. • Treat others with respect. Support everyone's learning, even when it occurs by making mistakes. • Agree to play a role other than one's real-life professional role, if necessary, remembering that the NRP does not certify or authorize learners to perform interventions outside their designated scope of practice.

Instructor Roles During a Scenario

- It is sometimes difficult for one instructor to do everything during a scenario. Usually one instructor will watch the scenario unfold, give the appropriate physiologic feedback from the manikin or simulator, listen to what the participants are saying, and watch the participants performing interventions.

- It usually takes another instructor to take notes about what occurred and plan for what may be discussed during debriefing.

Conducting a Scenario

Learners benefit most from participation in more than one scenario. After the participants have agreed to the ground rules and have been oriented to the location of supplies and equipment and how vital signs will be conveyed, begin with a short, simple scenario. Progress to more complex scenarios where learners are pushed outside their usual comfort zones.

1. Prepare the manikin with the appropriate visual cues, such as vernix, blood, and meconium, if indicated.
2. Agree on the instructors' responsibilities (giving physiologic feedback from the manikin, taking notes, filming, etc).
3. Read the scenario.
4. Allow learners to ask about relevant perinatal history. (What is the gestational age? Is the amniotic fluid clear? How many babies are expected? Is there anything else I should know?)
5. Allow learners to designate roles (assign leaders and tasks), check supplies and equipment, and ask additional questions, if needed.
6. Announce when the scenario has begun.

Depending on the complexity of your scenario setup, you may include the obstetrical cues for birth, such as a mother crying out as she gives birth, her partner's excitement or anxiety about the birth, and comments or instructions from the obstetrical providers. The manikin may be carried from another area and set on the warmer or conference room table, or the manikin may be present already and covered with a towel until the scenario is ready to begin.

Once the scenario has begun, stay out of the way as much as possible. If using an electronic simulator, you may be able to leave the room. If using a traditional manikin, you probably need to stay present to give physiologic indicators, such as the metronome heart rate, and convey information about breathing, breath sounds, chest movement, muscle tone, and oxygen saturation. For complex resuscitation scenarios, be prepared to answer questions about confirmation of endotracheal tube placement (color of end-tidal carbon dioxide [CO_2] detector, mist in the tube, etc) and other resuscitation indicators. Do not give hints or additional information beyond what participants must ask to continuously assess their actions.

Allow the learners to take the scenario down the path they choose. Do not interrupt, coach, or give more feedback than necessary during the scenario.

Preparing for the Debriefing as the Scenario Unfolds

As you watch the scenario unfold, use your Scenario Template form to take notes. Filming the scenario helps during debriefing; however, you will want to remember which segments of the film are valuable and avoid viewing long, uneventful segments of the film, searching or waiting for the moments your team wants to discuss. Check off the interventions that were performed as expected, and make a note of unanticipated occurrences. Make a quick note to remind yourself of behavioral objectives that were met by participants and how that was done so that you can guide that discussion during the debriefing.

Note participants who are especially dominant and those who are more submissive. Those participants will influence the strategies you use during debriefing to ensure overall participation in the discussion.

Managing the Unexpected

Just as in real life, the unexpected may occur during a scenario. Equipment may be accidentally dropped on the floor, medication errors may occur, or participants may not share the instructor's mental model of the patient and take the scenario down a totally different or far more complex and time-consuming path than the instructor anticipated.

Sometimes these events present the opportunity to discuss unanticipated but equally valuable learning objectives as those that were intended. If the event could occur in real life, such as missing or malfunctioning equipment or a participant who stops the resuscitation to answer a pager, the participants should continue the scenario and solve the problem. If the event is not plausible (eg, if the manikin's head falls off), the participants may fix the problem or deal with it as well as they can and continue the scenario.

If the scenario has continued for some time and the participants seem lost and far afield of the learning objectives, instructors must think quickly and use their best judgment to decide if the scenario should continue or if the instructors should end the scenario short of successful resuscitation of the newborn. It is permissible for an instructor to end the scenario by saying something such as, "Let's end the scenario here." The debriefing might include a different set of learning objectives than originally planned. It is perfectly alright for the scenario to veer off course as long as the instructor can use debriefing skills to help the participants relate the scenario events to real life, if possible, and learn from the experience.

May the instructor send in a "confederate" to help with a problem or redirect the scenario?

A confederate is someone (usually not a learner) the instructor directs to enter the scenario to play a certain role for a specific purpose. For example, if a learner cannot stop giggling during the scenario, the instructor may send in "the baby's grandfather" to remedy the problem with minimal interference in a scenario that is well underway (eg, "I'm this baby's grandfather and I'd like to know what is so funny. This looks like a pretty serious situation to me.").

Some scenarios are extremely complex, involve many players, and need to stay fairly close to the anticipated "script" to meet multidisciplinary learning objectives. When learners take these scenarios down a path that changes the medical roles, equipment, or procedures, the instructor may send in an "attending physician" or other health care professional to give "new" information and help redirect the scenario to meet the original learning objectives as written. Newborn resuscitation scenarios are rarely this complex and it would be unusual to send in a confederate to redirect learners.

May the instructor end the scenario with the "newborn's" death?

That depends on the learning objectives of the scenario. If the scenario includes learning objectives that address ethics, discontinuing resuscitation efforts, and disclosure of bad news to parents, then ending the resuscitation portion of the scenario with the newborn's death would be appropriate.

What if the scenario did not have any aspect of newborn death as a learning objective? A team that works well together and is highly experienced in simulation-based training may understand and learn from the death of the newborn if an egregious error is made during their scenario. However, the instructor never ends the scenario with the newborn's death to "punish" the resuscitation team for errors made during the scenario.

Ending a Scenario

End the scenario with an objective statement, such as, "That ends your scenario. Let's debrief now." The instructor does not end the scenario with a judgmental statement, such as, "That was great" or "Well, okay. We have a lot to talk about." Debriefing should occur as soon as possible after the scenario has ended. Debriefing is covered in Chapter 8.

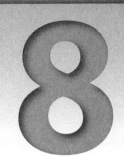

Debriefing

Debriefing is a facilitated, interactive discussion about events that just occurred during the resuscitation scenario. Debriefing is where the learning occurs. The skills of the debriefer are critical to the learning experience of the participants.

In Chapter 8* you will learn about

- **What debriefing is and what it is not**
- **Tips and strategies for facilitating an effective debriefing**
- **Using film to enhance debriefing**
- **Tools to help you conduct an effective debriefing**

The *NRP Instructor DVD: An Interactive Tool for Facilitation of Simulation-based Learning*

One of the Neonatal Resuscitation Program™ (NRP™) instructor's most useful tools for learning about simulation and debriefing is the *NRP Instructor DVD: An Interactive Tool for Facilitation of Simulation-based Learning.* Although reading about simulation and debriefing is useful, the Instructor DVD was developed by members of the NRP Steering Committee and simulation experts to help instructors incorporate this methodology into NRP courses. The DVD uses interactive media to bring you as close to "being there" as possible. Use the Instructor DVD as a frequent reference because, as you learn and gain experience using simulation and debriefing, you will find different sections of the DVD more useful.

"Instructor Self-assessment" for Chapter 8 begins on page 196.

After studying this chapter, complete the Chapter 8 questions, using the answer sheets that begin on page 188. Your regional trainer may ask you to bring the answer sheets to your NRP Instructor Course.

*Much of the information in this chapter comes from McDonnell LK, Jobe KK, and Dismukes, R Key. (1997). Facilitating LOS Debriefings: A Training Manual. National Aeronautics and Space Administration, NASA Technical Memorandum 112192.

> Debriefing is a facilitated interactive discussion about a prior series of events. The instructor guides the discussion with open-ended questions and allows reflection and self-discovery. Debriefing is when learning occurs.

Many NRP instructors are accustomed to the "score sheet" method of evaluation—focusing on what interventions should have occurred during a scenario, giving direct feedback to individuals on what is needed for improvement, and determining if individuals "pass" or "fail." Learners who have taken numerous NRP courses in the past expect to be scored by the instructor and told about the strengths and weaknesses of their performances. With the addition of the Simulation and Debriefing component to the NRP course, both the instructor and the course participant must learn a different set of skills.

What is debriefing?

Debriefing is a facilitated, interactive discussion of the events that just occurred in the resuscitation scenario. Debriefing is conducted by an NRP instructor whose goal is to facilitate a discussion where learners talk mostly with one another, analyze the situations that confronted them during the scenario, and evaluate how well they managed those situations.

The debriefing component of simulation-based training allows adult learners to actively participate and make their own analyses rather than listen passively to instructor feedback. The goal is for learners to self-evaluate how the team managed the events, what went well, what did not go well, and how to improve. Through active participation in the scenario and debriefing, it is hoped that learners will draw upon this information in the future and perform effectively when faced with the real-life situations they encountered in the scenarios.

Does every NRP instructor need to be a skilled debriefer?

The ideal debriefer has relevant resuscitation experience, content expertise, and hands-on expertise. Not every NRP instructor will be comfortable or good at debriefing.

- If you are a solo NRP instructor in your institution, you will be the debriefer. Use the form titled "Simulation Preparation, Tips, and Sample Debriefing Questions" (page 137) or the "Ready, Set, Go" checklist (page 136) to get started and use one of the Self-assessment Checklists on pages 138 and 140 to strengthen your skills.

- If you are one of several instructors, allow the instructors who are most interested in debriefing to practice this skill. Debriefing can be done by more than one debriefer at a time, but at least one of these instructors will need to attend your NRP courses. If debriefing does not seem to be your strength, you may find another area in which to excel, such as creating scenarios or facilitating the Performance Skills Stations.

What are the attributes of an effective debriefing?

- Debriefing is a team-centered discussion, not an instructor-centered discussion. Learners talk mostly to each other, not to the instructor.

- An effective debriefer facilitates the discussion by asking questions, not making comments or giving feedback. The effective debriefer uses a ratio of about 3 questions to every statement.

- An effective debriefer does not give immediate feedback or lecture to learners about what needs improvement. A skilled debriefer enables the learners to figure it out for themselves. When this occurs, they are more likely to learn from their mistakes and carry these lessons into real-life situations.

- The best debriefing allows learners to link their simulation experience to personal real-world experience. This helps the learner remember the experience and draw upon lessons learned when the experience is faced again in real life.

- An effective debriefing focuses on teamwork and communication. The debriefer guides learners into discussing which Key Behavioral Skills helped them manage or could have helped them manage the events during the scenario.

How do I begin a debriefing?

Set the stage.

If possible, conduct the debriefing in an area somewhat removed from the scenario. This helps reduce the emotional load participants may be feeling and enables their more objective analysis of the events. Seating should be arranged in a conversational way so that all participants can see one another and there is no perceived "head of the table." If the group is watching the filmed replay of the scenario, everyone needs to be able to see the screen.

While instructors and learners are new to simulation methodology, it may be helpful to orient learners about how the instructor and learners are expected to participate in the debriefing.

Review the NRP instructor's role.*

- Outline the process for the debriefing and help establish an agenda for complex scenario analysis. Tell the learners about how long the debriefing is expected to last (usually about 3 times as long as the scenario).

- Help the learners identify topics and facilitate discussion as necessary.

- Act as a resource for teamwork/communication and NRP issues.

- Keep the discussion learner-centered rather than instructor-centered.

- Ensure that the scenario objectives are met.

Review the NRP learner's responsibilities.*

- Raise issues and initiate discussion.

- Discuss issues directly with each other rather than only with the instructor.

- Discuss Key Behaviors used during the scenario and how they affected performance.

- Critically analyze the situations that were encountered and how the learner attempted to manage those situations.

- Evaluate how things turned out and why.

- Discuss what, if anything, the learner would do differently in the future.

If the scenario became complex and you anticipate too many issues to discuss in the time allotted, set an agenda with your learners.

- Begin by reviewing the learning objectives of the scenario. It is helpful to have these written on a large piece of paper or dry-erase board.

- Ask the learners to identify the issues they wish to discuss. These may be unanticipated learning objectives that presented during the scenario. Remind learners that positive events are valuable discussion points, as well as things that need to be improved. Make a list of these issues so that all critical issues are covered.

What questions should I ask to help facilitate the discussion? My mind is a blank.

Debriefing questions are based on the learning objectives of the scenario. In addition, unique events may have occurred during the scenario, presenting unanticipated learning objectives. Finally, team members may have their own ideas about what is important to discuss.

*Adapted from McDonnell LK, Jobe KK, Dismukes R Key. Facilitating LOS Debriefings: A Training Manual. National Aeronautics and Space Administration, NASA Technical Memorandum 112192; 1997: p 9.

Use the debriefing questions on the form "Ready, Set, Go: Neonatal Resuscitation Program Instructor Prep Sheet for Simulation and Debriefing" (page 136) to get you started.

- Often, the first question is, "Tell me in a few sentences about this baby" or "When you heard the history and initially assessed the baby, what did you think you would need to do?"

- Avoid asking learners, "How did you *feel* about this experience?" This question distracts learners from focusing on behaviors that helped (or did not help) meet the learning objectives.

- Direct the first questions to the most submissive learners. If the most authoritative person speaks first, the quieter participants are unlikely to contradict or offer different perspectives on events.

- Notice that questions are not phrased to elicit "Yes" or "No" answers. Questions begin with "What, How, and Why?"

- Use strategies to encourage more in-depth discussion, such as

  - "Tell us more about that."

  - "What would have happened if…?"

  - "What caused the disagreement?"

  - "Why don't you talk about that for a moment?"

  - "Who else observed this behavior? What did you notice and what were you thinking about?"

  - "Why was that helpful?"

  - "How could your team have helped you at that point?"

What if I ask a lot of questions but no one is participating?

Your questions are used to guide the discussion and encourage analysis by the learners. Your role is not to ask a continuous string of questions, as if interrogating learners about their performance. Your role is to ask questions that help identify topics and encourage in-depth discussion among learners.

Try these strategies to encourage participation:

- Direct questions to people by name.

- Post visual aids in the debriefing area, such as the NRP flow diagram and the Key Behavioral Skills. Referring to these concepts during debriefing can help promote discussion: "Which of these Key Behavioral Skills did Laura use to help the team when things got busy?"

- Try a question that has no right or wrong answer: "Laura, how effective was the team in responding to the problem with the bag-and-mask ventilation?"

- Redirect a question to a quiet person: "Tom, talk a little about the initial steps and the team's first assessment of the newborn. What went well for you during that phase of the resuscitation?"

What if I have long lapses of silence?

Use silence to your advantage. Remember it takes most learners a few seconds to formulate a confident and well thought-out response. Sit back, look relaxed, and be patient.

- Give learners at least 3 or 4 seconds before you intervene—more time if possible. Do not panic and answer the question for them.

- If silence continues, ask someone to elaborate (eg, "What do you think about what Tom just said?" or "Sarah, how do you think this intervention worked out?").

- If no one can elaborate further, provide positive feedback about the issue before moving on to a different topic (eg, "That was a complex situation and everyone was trying their best. Your discussion points out where you might improve next time.").

What other learner behaviors might I encounter during a debriefing and what strategies can I use to improve the experience for everyone? (See Table 8-1.)

Table 8-1. **Managing Behaviors During Debriefing**

Learner Behavior	Debriefer's Strategy	Notes
Too quiet	*Poll participants directly:* "Kathy, what happened next?" *Ask for more information:* "Steve, which Key Behavioral Skills might have been useful to help manage the situation Sarah was discussing?" *Accentuate the positive:* "Laura, what helped you most in that difficult part of the scenario?"	Participants who are very quiet during debriefing may fear criticism or negative feedback about their performance. They may be introverted and uncomfortable in a group. However, the instructor's role is to draw all participants into the discussion. Nod, smile, make eye contact, sit forward, and look genuinely interested in the discussion.
Sensitive, crying *"This is too upsetting for me."*	*Inquire:* "You seem to be especially affected by this. Tell me what's going on." *Encourage learner to problem solve:* "How can we help you through this debriefing?"	Is the learner reliving an experience that was especially difficult? A personal loss? A professional error that resulted in an adverse outcome? Be supportive, but the group probably cannot use the debriefing to resolve this learner's issues.
Defensive *"I did not ventilate the baby at a high rate. You don't know what you're talking about."*	Use videotape to review the performance. *Acknowledge:* "We all feel defensive because we want to do a good job." Or "We've all been there. Most of us begin by ventilating too fast." *Inquire:* "What is the ventilation rate during positive-pressure ventilation?" "Do you see why your teammate asked you to slow down to a rate of 40 to 60?"	The instructor should try to let the team manage its own defensive team member, especially if the team works together in real life. Most defensive team members are insecure about their skills. Use videotape to review events, stick to the objectives, and balance criticism with questions that focus on the positive.

Table 8-1. Managing Behaviors During Debriefing—*continued*

Learner Behavior	Debriefer's Strategy	Notes
	It's not personal: "Team members monitor one another's actions in the context of patient safety." *It's NRP:* "We do it this way because it's the AHA guideline for neonatal resuscitation." *Balance criticism with the positive:* "What helped you do such a good job in this part of the scenario?"	
Unable to suspend disbelief. *"This is so fake. What a waste of time."*	*Give the learner a chance:* "We can't replicate everything exactly as it is in the delivery room. Can you try to believe that these scenarios are real?" *Point out the link to real-life events:* "Has (name a scenario event) ever happened to you in real life?" *Ask the learner to leave:* "It's important for your teammates to believe that this is an actual resuscitation. Your behavior is ruining the experience for others, so you need to leave.	Most learners willingly engage in simulation-based training and debriefing. Skeptics soon recognize the value of the experience and fully participate. Orient learners to simulation methodology before beginning the exercise, which includes the learners' agreement to suspend disbelief. Learners who refuse to suspend their disbelief and whose behaviors are disruptive during the scenario and/or debriefing need to leave the event. Because the learner did not complete requirements of the course, it may be necessary to involve this learner's supervisor in the remediation plan.
Learner fixates on the cognitive and technical skills. *"I've made a quick list of all the clinical errors I noticed. Let's discuss those first, starting with how she forgot to remove the wet linen."*	*Remind learner that simulation and debriefing focuses on teamwork and communication.* "Your list is important to our discussion, but let's use it in the context of teamwork. How can team members help each other when they notice a hands-on skill that needs improvement?"	It is easier and more familiar for experienced NRP learners to focus on cognitive and technical skills than teamwork and communication. Review the learning objectives and acknowledge that clinical skills affect outcome; however, the team needs to focus on teamwork.
Too much to say. *"This scenario reminds me of those twins born on Christmas Eve, 1988........."* *"Remember when we used to...."* *"I read an article that talked about ....."*	*Acknowledge the link to real life:* "By remembering that delivery in 1988, you're making the link from that event to the scenario that just occurred. Tell us about what you think went well in the scenario we just went through." *Refocus on the learning objectives:* "Your experience is valuable to the team. What Key Behavioral Skill did you use during that part of the scenario that helped the team accomplish its goal?" *Request silence:* "Let's hear from the rest of the team now."	Some learners dominate the conversation. Acknowledge the learner's comments and refocus the learner on the current scenario and learning objectives. It may become necessary to apologize and interrupt a long monologue to redirect the debriefing. It may become necessary to ask for the learner's cooperation by asking to hear from others on the team, or, if necessary, taking this team member aside during a break and asking for his cooperation in allowing others to participate more fully.

What if everything went well during the scenario?

A well-run scenario does not mean that debriefing is cut short or deemed unnecessary. The team who performed well benefits from analyzing its scenario and figuring out why it went so well. Which Key Behavioral Skills were used that resulted in a positive performance? The team who knows why it works well together can transfer these skills to other scenarios where teamwork is more challenging.

Using Film During Debriefing

It is often difficult to remember exactly what transpired during a stressful event. Filming the scenario is helpful for reminding learners what and when events occurred. Viewing segments of the video allows your learners to self-assess their behaviors with some emotional detachment, because watching video makes learners feel more like observers than participants.

These are the most important points to remember.

- Know how to use the equipment. Your learners will lose interest quickly if they must wait while you problem solve the technology.

- Show video segments so that learners can discuss important aspects of the performance. Do not show long video segments that will not be discussed.

- Introduce each video segment. Set the scene and tell viewers what you want them to analyze (eg, "This segment begins as the team decides to begin chest compressions. Watch your performance and think about what went well here, and what could be improved.").

- Pause the tape when asking a question, or when someone is making a point.

When can I finally give my perspective and provide feedback to the learners?

The debriefer holds his or her own opinion and feedback until the team has finished its discussion. At the end of the debriefing, the instructor may summarize what was discussed and next steps. The instructor may offer the team a chance to repeat the same scenario to make corrections.

The debriefer may need to assist the team if it becomes obvious that the team is overlooking an important discussion point. This is when you are required to blend your roles of facilitator and instructor. Use every possible strategy to guide the team toward self-discovery. When the team has finished its analysis, you can reinforce the positive points of the performance. If necessary, fill in any important points the team has missed and make sure the learning objectives have been met.

How does the debriefing end?

A debriefing usually lasts about 3 times as long as the scenario. As soon as your team has covered the learning objectives and discussed any additional critical issues, you may conclude the debriefing. You may summarize the main points, ask each learner what he or she learned from the experience, or ask for a summary of the team's next steps for improvement. Some teams want an opportunity to repeat the scenario and use what they have learned. Then the debriefing would occur again.

Conclude on a positive note. The goal is learning, not perfection.

What can I do to become more skilled at debriefing? We have only 1 or 2 NRP courses per year, and that's not enough practice to get good at this.

- When you are ready to begin practicing debriefing, review the *NRP Instructor DVD* often and use the media that is most useful for your stage of learning. In addition, use the tools on the following pages.

- Film your debriefing and use other instructors to "debrief the debriefer." If you are the only instructor available to assess your performance, film your debriefing and then self-assess your debriefing skills using the forms on pages 136, 137, or 140.

- Use the sample questions to get started. Film yourself conducting a debriefing and use the assessment tools to improve your next debriefing. Debriefing is a critical skill that takes practice, but it is well worth the work to ensure that your team has the best possible learning experience.

Debrief After Every Mock Resuscitation, Actual Resuscitation, or High-Risk Event

Remember that debriefing should occur after every mock resuscitation and actual resuscitation, or after any high-risk procedure or unusually stressful event in your setting. Make an agreement with your colleagues that the leader at every resuscitation or high-risk procedure will conduct a debriefing after the event and all team members will participate.

Ready, Set, Go: Neonatal Resuscitation Program Instructor Prep Sheet for Simulation and Debriefing

READY

- ❏ Scenario is based on learning objectives, is plausible, and useful to these learners.
- ❏ Instructors have agreed on responsibilities (eg, vital signs, filming, taking notes).
- ❏ Instructors have prepared the setting with key visual, tactile, and auditory cues.
- ❏ Learners have been oriented to
  - a. Location of supplies and equipment
  - b. Each other (names and usual roles during a resuscitation in their birth setting)
  - c. How they will know the manikin's heart rate, breathing, tone, pulse oximetry, etc.
- ❏ Learners are given a chance to touch and handle the supplies and arrange them as desired.
- ❏ Learners are given a chance to do a short "practice" scenario with instructor's guidance.
- ❏ Learners understand that they
  - a. Think out loud.
  - b. Do the actions, not pretend them.
  - c. Act as a team and help each other.

SET

- ❏ Learners' roles are designated based on the needs of the scenario (as determined by the instructor) or their usual team composition. Learners wear name tags designating roles (eg, RN, MD, RT, NNP, etc).
- ❏ Begin filming the scenario.
- ❏ Instructor reads the scenario.
- ❏ Instructor (or "obstetric provider") provides additional information if learners ask questions.
- ❏ Learners may appoint a leader, determine the plan of care, and delegate tasks.
- ❏ Learners may check equipment, if not already done.

GO

- ❏ Obstetric provider arrives at radiant warmer with the newborn, or gives the newborn to a resuscitation team member. If manikin must be on the radiant warmer during learner preparation, cover the manikin with a towel until the scenario begins.

- ❏ Instructor gives vital signs information only if cued by the learner (when learner auscultates or palpates heart rate) or when learner asks about breathing, tone, etc, if necessary.
- ❏ Instructor stays out of the way and allows the learners to take the scenario down its own path.
- ❏ Instructor signals the end of the scenario without judgment (eg, "That ends your scenario. Let's debrief now."). Learners do not end the scenario.
- ❏ **Instructor does not lecture or give feedback. The instructor guides self-discovery and discussion among team members.**
  - a. Tell me in a few sentences about this baby. What did you think you would need to do?
  - b. What were your objectives? Which objectives were met? Not met?
  - c. What was your thought process when . . .
  - d. Who was the leader? How did you know?
  - e. What key behavioral skills did you use? Give examples. How did that help?
  - f. What could have gone better? What would you do differently next time?
  - g. What did you learn? Any additional comments?
- ❏ Instructor uses strategies to encourage more in-depth discussion, such as
  - a. "Tell us more about that."
  - b. "What would have happened if . . . ?"
  - c. "What caused the disagreement?"
  - d. "How would that sound? What could he or she have said to make it more clear for you?"
  - e. "Who else observed this behavior? What did you notice and what were you thinking about?"
  - f. "Why was that helpful?"
  - g. "How could your team have helped you at that point?"
  - h. How can you help when a team member's performance needs improvement?

Appendix F1
Simulation Preparation, Tips, and Sample Debriefing Questions

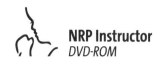
NRP Instructor
DVD-ROM

I. Prepare the Learners for Simulation Training

a. Orient to supplies and equipment and manikin's abilities as a simulation tool.

b. Learners must "get into it" and "think aloud."

c. Learners can't say they are doing something – they must actually do it.

d. The instructor sets up the scenario but does not coach, guide, or interrupt.

e. The instructor determines when the scenario is over. Most scenarios last 2-5 minutes.

II. Debriefing is NOT feedback from the instructor. Keep the discussion team-centered.

a. Self-discovery is key. Team members do most of the talking to EACH OTHER.

b. For complex debriefing, help team develop an agenda. What issues will be covered?

c. Link simulation to real-life practice.

d. Question: Statement ratio is 3:1. Ask WHAT, HOW, and WHY questions.

e. Use active listening – this is not an interrogation. Look and sound interested.

f. Use silence/pauses to encourage participation. Reword the question; do not give the answer.

g. Debrief constructively – hold your teaching points until team has finished. The debriefer enables the team to figure things out; then enhances understanding of the points they might have missed.

h. Maintain confidentiality. What happens here STAYS here.

i. A complex debriefing can last up to 30 minutes. You probably have 5-10 minutes. Choose the most important objectives to discuss. You may not be able to cover everything.

III. Sample debriefing questions

a. Tell me in a few sentences what happened to this baby.

b. What were your objectives? Which objectives were met? Not met?

c. What was your thought process when …

d. What did the group do well? How did (those behaviors) help the team?

e. Who was the leader? How did you know?

f. What key behavioral skills did you use? When did you use (a behavioral skill)?

g. What could have gone better? What would you do differently next time?

h. How can you help when a team member's performance needs improvement?

i. What did you do to help the team? How did that help?

j. What did you learn?

k. Any additional comments?

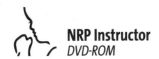

NRP Instructor
DVD-ROM

CAPE Debriefing Evaluation Tool©

Scenario description: _____

Before scenario:	• Reviews learning objectives and anticipated actions.
During scenario:	• Takes notes: performance of cognitive, technical, and behavioral skills.
After scenario:	• Briefs regarding performance issues/items on debriefing checklist.
Debriefing:	• Determines whether trainees share same mental model of patient.
	• Facilitates self-reflective learning.

Scenario start time: _____   Debriefing start time: _____

Scenario end time: _____   Debriefing end time: _____

Scenario length: _____   Debriefing length: _____

Time between end of scenario and start of debriefing: _____ min

Time when tape first rolls during debriefing: _____ min

Percentage of scenario covered during debriefing: _____ %

Percentage of learning objectives covered during debriefing: _____ %

Length of debriefing : Length of scenario ratio: _____

Number of times tape paused during debriefing: _____

Length of tape segments played: _____

Instructor Questions:	**Instructor Statements:**	**Trainee Responses:**
1. ☐☐☐☐☐☐☐☐☐☐	☐☐☐☐☐☐☐☐☐☐	☐☐☐☐☐☐☐☐☐☐
2. ☐☐☐☐☐☐☐☐☐☐	☐☐☐☐☐☐☐☐☐☐	☐☐☐☐☐☐☐☐☐☐
3. ☐☐☐☐☐☐☐☐☐☐	☐☐☐☐☐☐☐☐☐☐	☐☐☐☐☐☐☐☐☐☐
4. ☐☐☐☐☐☐☐☐☐☐	☐☐☐☐☐☐☐☐☐☐	☐☐☐☐☐☐☐☐☐☐
5. ☐☐☐☐☐☐☐☐☐☐	☐☐☐☐☐☐☐☐☐☐	☐☐☐☐☐☐☐☐☐☐
6. ☐☐☐☐☐☐☐☐☐☐	☐☐☐☐☐☐☐☐☐☐	☐☐☐☐☐☐☐☐☐☐
7. ☐☐☐☐☐☐☐☐☐☐	☐☐☐☐☐☐☐☐☐☐	☐☐☐☐☐☐☐☐☐☐
8. ☐☐☐☐☐☐☐☐☐☐	☐☐☐☐☐☐☐☐☐☐	☐☐☐☐☐☐☐☐☐☐
9. ☐☐☐☐☐☐☐☐☐☐	☐☐☐☐☐☐☐☐☐☐	☐☐☐☐☐☐☐☐☐☐
10. ☐☐☐☐☐☐☐☐☐☐	☐☐☐☐☐☐☐☐☐☐	☐☐☐☐☐☐☐☐☐☐
11. ☐☐☐☐☐☐☐☐☐☐	☐☐☐☐☐☐☐☐☐☐	☐☐☐☐☐☐☐☐☐☐
12. ☐☐☐☐☐☐☐☐☐☐	☐☐☐☐☐☐☐☐☐☐	☐☐☐☐☐☐☐☐☐☐
13. ☐☐☐☐☐☐☐☐☐☐	☐☐☐☐☐☐☐☐☐☐	☐☐☐☐☐☐☐☐☐☐
14. ☐☐☐☐☐☐☐☐☐☐	☐☐☐☐☐☐☐☐☐☐	☐☐☐☐☐☐☐☐☐☐
15. ☐☐☐☐☐☐☐☐☐☐	☐☐☐☐☐☐☐☐☐☐	☐☐☐☐☐☐☐☐☐☐

Instructor question : Instructor statement ratio: _____

Trainee responses : Instructor questions + statements ratio: _____

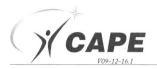

Instructions for Use of
CAPE Debriefing Evaluation Tool

Overview: This tool is designed to evaluate a debriefing following a simulation or drill. The tool can be used for self-evaluation when reviewing a taped debriefing session or by evaluators as the debriefing occurs.

Scenario Description: Indicate the name of the scenario as it is named on the Scenario script. Identifying the scenario gives the evaluator the option to review the written scenario during or after evaluation for specifics such as learning objectives.

Bulleted Items: These describe the role and activities of the instructor/debriefer.

Scenario/Debriefing Times and Length: The debriefing usually lasts about three times the length of the scenario. Shorter debriefing sessions should be evaluated to ensure that learning objectives were discussed. Long sessions should be evaluated to make sure time allotted for simulation was used effectively.

Time between end of scenario and start of debriefing: The recommended time period is 5-10 minutes. This short waiting period keeps learners engaged in the scenario and reduces anxiety of waiting for the tape to be viewed.

Time when tape first rolls during debriefing: A *brief* discussion before rolling tape is optional, use video to discuss major learning objectives and incidental or unanticipated findings.

Percentage of scenario covered during debriefing: Majority of scenario should be reviewed but covering the learning objectives adequately is the main priority which is captured in the next area.

Percentage of learning objectives covered during debriefing: A copy of the scenario with learning objectives should be available to the evaluator during completion of this tool.

Length of debriefing: Length of scenario ratio: Calculation based on times listed in box at top of tool.

Number of times the tape is paused during debriefing: Each time the tape is paused place a tic mark. The tape should be paused to discuss learning objectives, other areas of interest for discussion or if the learners are talking among themselves while the tape is playing.

Length of tape segments played: The tape should be stopped at least every 90-120 seconds to keep learners engaged in the scenario.

Instructor Questions: The number of questions the instructor/debriefer asks is captured by checking a box for each question.

Instructor Statements: The number of statements the instructor/debriefer makes is captured by checking a box for each statement.

Trainee Responses: Each response from a trainee is counted by checking a box in this category. A response is considered an answer to a question or a question that is posed by a trainee. For example, if three trainees respond, three boxes are checked. If a trainee poses a new question during discussion, another box is checked.

Instructor question Instructor statement ratio: The instructor/debriefer guides the discussion, not dominate it. The ratio of questions to statements should be high with significantly more questions noted than statements.

Trainee responses Instructor questions + statements ratio: Add the debriefer's questions and statements together. That number is then compared to the number of trainee responses. Ideally, the trainees will be doing most of the talking with the instructor/debriefer guiding the discussion by asking questions designed to further discussion among the trainees.

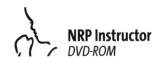

NRP Instructor
DVD-ROM

NRP Instructor Simulation and Debriefing Checklist

Scenario start time: _____ Scenario end time: _____ Length of scenario: _____ min

Debrief start time: _____ Debrief end time: _____ Length of debrief: _____ min

Component	Yes	Notes About Variance

Scenario Development

The scenario is based on learning objectives tailored to learners' needs. _____ _____

The scenario is plausible. _____ _____

Supplies and equipment are present that enable learners to resuscitate the newborn with correct technique. _____ _____

Learner Orientation

Learners introduce themselves and describe their roles, if necessary. _____ _____

Learners receive orientation to manikin and its functions. _____ _____

Learners receive orientation to location and function of supplies if necessary. _____ _____

Learners receive orientation to how they will get feedback pertaining to manikin's breathing, heart rate, muscle tone, pulse oximetry, color, or special circumstances. _____ _____

Instructor reviews learner responsibilities (suspend disbelief, think out loud, perform actions instead of pretending actions). _____ _____

Instructor allows the learners a few minutes to practice using the supplies and equipment before beginning. _____ _____

Instructor tells learners the cue for beginning the scenario and reminds learners that the instructor will end the scenario. _____ _____

During the Scenario

The instructor allows the learners to proceed through the scenario without coaching, interference, or assistance. _____ _____

The instructor takes notes about performance of cognitive, technical, and behavioral skills. _____ _____

The instructor ends the scenario without judgmental comments or feedback. _____ _____

Component	Yes	Notes About Variance

Debriefing

Instructor begins by ensuring a shared mental model of the patient (learners are asked to describe the clinical situation they faced).

Instructor assists the team to formulate a discussion agenda if necessary for a complex scenario.

Instructor promotes discussion about what went well, and what could be improved, and how.

Instructor allows silence after asking a question; if no response, instructor rephrases the question.

Instructor is sincere, approachable, uses active listening, uses open body language.

Instructor keeps the discussion positive and constructive.

Instructor keeps the learners focused on the learning objectives. Instructor encourages learners to list their objectives: cognitive, technical (hands-on) and behavioral.

Instructor involves quiet learners by asking them questions directly.

Instructor encourages learners to talk to each other, not to the instructor.

Instructor helps learners link scenario to real-life experience.

Instructor encourages learners to talk about what they were thinking as they made decisions and performed interventions.

Instructor asks learners to discuss how they were affected by each others' actions.

Instructor shows video segments for purpose of discussion.

Video paused when instructor asks questions and during comments and discussion.

Instructor ends scenario by briefly summarizing important issues and clarifying any plans for follow-up.

Instructor uses at least 3 questions: 1 statement.

Comments: _____

_____

_____

_____

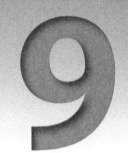

Instructor Courses

As you know, the revised Neonatal Resuscitation Program™ (NRP™) Provider Course is an interactive course that includes little or no lecture about textbook content, uses course time for skills stations and supervised practice, and uses simulation and debriefing as an important part of the learning experience. Following the same methodology, the revised NRP Instructor Course moves the regional trainer away from using a lecture-based format to an interactive, hands-on, team-oriented environment. In addition, regional trainers and hospital-based instructors are asked to be more aware of instructor eligibility requirements, course prerequisites and self-study, and new requirements for maintaining instructor status. These changes will help ensure a consistent level of instructor quality and competency and yield a better experience for instructors and learners.

In Chapter 9 you will learn about

- **Who is eligible to be an NRP instructor***

- **Two NRP instructor levels: Hospital-based instructor and regional trainer**

- **Requirements for maintaining instructor status**

- **Desirable attributes of an NRP instructor**

- **Principles of adult learning**

- **New regional trainer responsibilities for ensuring that only eligible applicants gain admittance to Instructor Courses and ensuring that registered participants know about course prerequisites**

- **Components of a Hospital-based Instructor Course**

- **Components of a Regional Trainer Course**

"Instructor Self-assessment" for Chapter 9 begins on page 197.

After studying this chapter, complete the Chapter 9 questions, using the answer sheets that begin on page 188. Your regional trainer may ask you to bring the answer sheets to your NRP Instructor Course.

*In this chapter, the term "instructor" refers to both hospital-based instructor and regional trainer, unless otherwise specified.

The NRP Instructor Course teaches instructor candidates how to be better facilitators of the learning process. Through a totally interactive course, instructor candidates become more responsible for their own learning and the regional trainer becomes their coach. This yields a much better experience for instructors and learners at all levels of NRP training.

Since its inception in 1987, the NRP has had 2 important goals. The first goal is to have one person present at every delivery whose primary responsibility is the baby and who is capable of initiating resuscitation. Either that person or someone else who is immediately available should have the skills required to perform a complete resuscitation. The second goal is to have an NRP training program available in every hospital that provides obstetrical services.

This edition of NRP introduces new education goals: To help learners take responsibility for their own learning, and to help instructors become skilled facilitators of the learning process.

Who is eligible to be an NRP hospital-based instructor or regional trainer?

NRP hospital-based instructors and regional trainers are *physicians, registered nurses, respiratory care practitioners, and physician assistants* who have experience in the hospital care of newborns in the delivery room, newborn nursery, or newborn intensive care setting. Ideally, the NRP instructor has ongoing delivery room experience and current educational or clinical responsibility within a hospital setting. Instructors are selected for their experience in newborn care, good interpersonal skills and self-confidence working with all levels of professionals, and ability to implement and maintain the NRP enthusiastically in their institution.

Instructor Training Levels and Responsibilities

The NRP supports 2 levels of instructors: The hospital-based instructor and the regional trainer. The different responsibilities for each type of instructor are outlined on page 145.

Neonatal Resuscitation Program training is made accessible to hospitals regardless of size and geographic location. Instructors for NRP courses must meet the training requirements outlined on page 145.

Persons who are not NRP instructors may be used to present content such as orientation to the unit's code cart, intubation tips, or how to use unit-specific respiratory therapy equipment. Guest lecturers cannot replace the NRP instructor and should not be listed on the Course Roster form submitted to the American Academy of Pediatrics (AAP).

Hospital-based Instructor	Regional Trainer
Provides information and skills required to develop, implement, and maintain a Neonatal Resuscitation Program (NRP).	Helps hospitals identify a need for an in-house NRP.
Plans, coordinates, and facilitates NRP courses for those desiring NRP provider status.	Trains NRP hospital-based instructors and regional trainers, and trains NRP providers as needed.
Maintains the NRP in the instructor's institution.	Oversees implementation of provider programs in assigned hospitals in his or her region.
Follows course documentation procedures.	Provides ongoing support for hospital-based instructors and maintains ongoing interaction with providers, hospital-based instructors, and other regional trainers.
Interacts with regional trainer(s) to ensure that the hospital's NRP needs are met.	Acts as crucial link between local programs and the American Academy of Pediatrics (AAP) Life Support staff.
Teaches or assists with at least 2 NRP Provider Courses during the 2 years for which the Instructor Card is valid.	Teaches or assists with at least 2 NRP courses during the 2 years for which the Instructor Card is valid. (At least one course must be a Provider Course.)
Beginning January 2013, instructors are required to complete the NRP online examination every 2 years as part of instructor renewal.	Beginning in January 2013, instructors are required to complete the NRP online examination every 2 years as part of instructor renewal.

Course Level	Instructor Must Be
Provider Course	Hospital-based instructor or regional trainer.
Hospital-based Instructor Course	Regional trainer. (Hospital-based instructors may assist, if needed.)
Regional Trainer Course	Regional trainer. (Hospital-based instructors may assist, if needed.)

What are AAP requirements for maintaining instructor status?
1. Every hospital-based instructor and regional trainer must teach or assist with at least 2 NRP courses during the 2 years for which his or her Instructor Card is valid. For a regional trainer, at least one course during the 2-year period must be a Provider Course. Instructors do not need to maintain a separate NRP Provider Card.
2. As it is essential that instructors possess mastery of the knowledge and skills presented in the Provider Course, beginning in 2013, instructors will be required to complete and pass all 9 lessons of the NRP online examination every 2 years, based on their renewal date.

For example, an instructor with a renewal date of March 1, 2011, must complete the online examination by March 1, 2013, and every 2 years thereafter. The examination will be provided at no charge to instructors renewing their instructor status.

3. Every instructor who has attained hospital-based instructor status or regional trainer status before January 1, 2012, must watch the *NRP Instructor DVD: An Interactive Tool for Facilitation of Simulation-based Learning* by January 1, 2012.

4. Instructors who attain instructor status after January 1, 2012, are required to watch the *NRP Instructor DVD: An Interactive Tool for Facilitation of Simulation-based Learning* as a prerequisite for attending the Hospital-based Instructor or Regional Trainer Course.

All NRP instructors who have not met the minimum teaching requirement will receive notice approximately 6 months before their Instructor Card expires. *No grace period is allowed beyond the expiration date (month and day) of the card.* If the maintenance requirements are not met by the expiration date on the card, instructor status is lost. To regain instructor status, a person is required to retake the Provider Course and the NRP Instructor Course.

Can institutional policies for maintaining NRP instructor status be more stringent?

The NRP Steering Committee believes that NRP instructors in any setting can meet the current requirements. However, some hospital administrative teams feel that because NRP instructors carry major responsibilities for providing current information and expertise in neonatal resuscitation, their hospital-based instructors and regional trainers should be required to meet more requirements to maintain instructor status within their institution.

The policies for maintaining NRP instructor status may be made more stringent by the institution in which these instructors are providing NRP provider services. The institutional requirements for instructors should be based on the population served and the needs of the providers. For example, the institutional policy may require that the NRP hospital-based instructor teach or assist at 3 or 4 or more Provider Courses in 2 years or that the NRP instructor pass the NRP online examination annually. The institution would be responsible for monitoring adherence to additional requirements. If the instructor failed to meet the institutional requirements to maintain NRP instructor status, the institution would be responsible for determining the instructor's status, which might include termination of the instructor's role within the institution. The AAP would not revoke the instructor's status unless the instructor failed to meet the AAP/American Heart Association (AHA) requirements to maintain NRP instructor status.

The Effective Neonatal Resuscitation Program Instructor

While the mastery of knowledge and skills necessary to perform neonatal resuscitation is essential for becoming an instructor, so, too, is the ability to teach and communicate the NRP material effectively. Many of the attributes necessary for effective performance during neonatal resuscitation apply to the characteristics of a good NRP hospital-based instructor and regional trainer.

What are desirable characteristics of an NRP instructor?

- Strong interest in the art and science of neonatal resuscitation

- Complete and correct understanding of the origin of neonatal resuscitation guidelines and premise for the education methodology of the NRP

- Professional credibility

- Desire to continuously improve knowledge and skills

- Excellent communication skills, including the ability to listen, paraphrase to show understanding, and correct errors in a supportive manner

- Ability to create a safe and supportive learning environment

- Ability to manage the technology that supports the learning process

- Ability to motivate learners and keep them engaged in the learning process

- Ability to facilitate different learning styles

- Ability to see stressful situations as positive challenges

- Ability to be creative and innovative

How does the instructor contribute to a quality NRP course?

Know the information.

- In the past, NRP instructors have been encouraged to study each new edition of the *Textbook of Neonatal Resuscitation* and self-assess their knowledge by taking the hard-copy NRP examination. Beginning in 2013, instructors are *required* to pass the online examination every 2 years to maintain instructor status.

- View the *NRP Instructor DVD: An Interactive Tool for Facilitation of Simulation-based Learning* and use the information to incorporate simulation-based training into NRP Provider Courses.

Know your participants' learning objectives.
If the students are unfamiliar to you, consider having them complete an Experience Survey (pages 32 and 214) so that you can customize your course to meet their needs. You should have clearly stated objectives

that are flexible enough to meet the needs of a multidisciplinary audience.

Know how to build and implement a quality course.

Your course needs to be well-organized and professionally presented. Many of your students will have other professional commitments, so it is important that your course operates within the stated time period. To maintain the learner's interest, the learning activities should be tailored to the needs of the students.

Know how to engage learners in the process.

It is the instructor's responsibility to ensure that the classroom is a safe, a supportive, and an interesting learning environment. The astute instructor understands that learners expect material to be hands-on, engaging, and facilitated by instructors who are professionally credible, experienced, and entertaining. The instructor must not only convey the skills and information, but also must do so in a manner that keeps the learners alert, motivated, and engaged in the learning activities. This is hard work—good instructors report total exhaustion and exhilaration at the end of a successful NRP course.

What Motivates Adult Learning?

Adult learners are motivated to learn in areas that have a direct impact on their lives. Three important motivations for learning include the following:

1. **Achievement and competence.** These are probably the best motivations for learners. Successful completion of the online examination allows for a sense of achievement. However, positive feedback to comments, questions, and answers during the practice and review component of the Performance Skills Stations also provides learners with a sense of proficiency. Learners who are unsure of themselves and their abilities benefit from beginning with the least complex skills because they have a high probability of success. An increasing sense of competence, coupled with positive feedback from the instructor, strengthens self-efficacy as the learners approach more complex assignments. By the time learners have passed their Integrated Skills Station, they are ready for the challenge of simulation training, where their experience and own abilities to critically think through complex clinical situations without fear of reprimand or embarrassment sets the stage for debriefing, and where learning occurs through self-discovery and team-centered discussion.

2. **Curiosity.** Adults have a need to know and understand a concept thoroughly. Their curiosity builds when they are challenged by concepts related to something already familiar to them. Many adults enjoy this aspect of simulation training because it involves a new experience with a more hands-on and creative method of learning. Many learners are curious about their own abilities to "suspend disbelief" and immerse themselves in a "real" resuscitation.

3. **Reciprocity.** Adults enter the learning process with previously developed self-esteem and self-concepts. They bring experience in decision-making, problem-solving, and learning strategies. Effective debriefing (where the learners, not the instructors, assess the strengths and weaknesses of the team) enables each learner to become a valued resource and contribute to everyone's learning.

Hospital-based Instructor Course

Hospital-based instructors are the foundation of the NRP. Their educational efforts increase the confidence and career satisfaction of professionals who believe in their capabilities, can manage the unexpected, and support each other's efforts during neonatal resuscitation.

> Regional trainers have a responsibility to ensure that course participants are eligible to become NRP hospital-based instructors. Regional trainers also must ensure that instructor candidates have the information they need to gain admission to the course and complete course prerequisites.

Course Eligibility

The hospital-based instructor candidate must submit the following items to NRP regional trainer to apply for admittance into the course:

- Evidence of current licensure as an RN, MD (or DO), Respiratory Care Practitioner, or Physician Assistant

- Evidence of current NRP Provider Card (Lessons 1 through 9)

- Evidence that the instructor candidate is supported and recommended by his or her institution as a person who has the necessary skills and abilities to be a hospital-based instructor

How can the regional trainer be sure that participants who want to attend the Instructor Course meet these eligibility requirements?

The regional trainer is required to screen candidates for the Hospital-based Instructor Course by corresponding and confirming eligibility. The recommended method is to send an e-mail* or letter notifying the candidate that you have received the candidate's intent to register for

---

*When sending e-mail with essential information to course registrants, it is recommended that the sender use the "read" receipt to ensure that the recipient receives the e-mail and opens it. Often, e-mail from an institution will be sent to a recipient's spam or junk folder instead of the inbox.

the course. See the Eligibility Confirmation form on page 157. This correspondence between the regional trainer and the instructor candidate confirms the applicant's intent to attend the course and also confirms eligibility. In addition, the letter of support (see page 158) is highly recommended so that the regional trainer knows that the institution recommends the candidate and endorses him or her as an instructor for its institution.

Sometimes ineligible applicants are upset by exclusion from the Instructor Course. It is important for these people to know that the eligibility requirements are those of the AAP and the AHA, not the institution sponsoring the Instructor Course.

Course Prerequisites

After eligibility is confirmed, the applicant receives confirmation of acceptance into the course. See the sample letter for course confirmation on page 159. This correspondence clearly outlines the course prerequisites.

If the following course prerequisites are not completed by the time the course begins, applicants may not participate in the course:

- Self-study the *Textbook of Neonatal Resuscitation, 6th Edition.*

- Take and pass the NRP online examination, Lessons 1 through 9, *during the 30 days before* the Instructor Course. This ensures that the candidate has recently studied the textbook.

- View the *NRP Instructor DVD: An Interactive Tool for Facilitation of Simulation-based Learning* during the 30 days before the Instructor Course date.

- Study the *Instructor Manual for Neonatal Resuscitation*. The regional trainer cannot possibly cover every point in the Instructor Manual at an Instructor Course and should not waste time lecturing about material that learners can master through self-study.

- Take the NRP Instructor Self-assessment (page 187) prior to the Instructor Course (strongly recommended).

Admission Into the Course on the Course Date

The regional trainer collects the following documents from instructor candidates at the Instructor Course (and keeps these documents as part of each learner's course records):

- Examination verification of the 6th Edition online NRP examination (Lessons 1 through 9)

- Certificate of completion for viewing the Instructor DVD

- A copy of the completed NRP Instructor Self-assessment answer sheet (strongly recommended)

What course materials are required?

- *NRP Instructor DVD: An Interactive Tool for Facilitation of Simulation-based Learning.* Each instructor candidate must own his or her own DVD, which offers continuing education credit.

- *Textbook of Neonatal Resuscitation, 6th Edition,* **and** an *Instructor Manual for Neonatal Resuscitation.* Individual purchase of these 2 books is not required. However, access to the textbook and Instructor Manual is necessary to fulfill course prerequisites.

Sample Course Curriculum and Agenda

The Hospital-based Instructor Course can be designed and implemented in a number of ways. Just as the NRP instructor needs to assess the abilities of the course participants prior to a Provider Course, the NRP regional trainer needs to assess the abilities of the hospital-based instructor candidates. Most regional trainers e-mail or speak with hospital-based instructor candidates prior to the course and assess learning needs. If you administer numerous Hospital-based Instructor Courses, you may want to require instructor candidates to return an Experience Survey similar to the survey used for Provider Course participants.

What is the recommended course length?

Participants should study the *Textbook of Neonatal Resuscitation, 6th Edition,* take and pass all 9 lessons of the NRP online examination, view the NRP Instructor DVD prior to the course, and study the *Instructor Manual for Neonatal Resuscitation* and take the NRP Instructor Self-assessment; therefore, extensive lecturing is unnecessary. The recommended length for the Hospital-based Instructor Course varies, depending on the experience and learning objectives of the participants. To cover all the components of the "new" NRP curriculum and methodology, an 8-hour course is usually required. If instructor candidates must learn some of the skills (such as laryngeal mask airway placement, intubation, and placement of the emergency umbilical venous catheter [UVC]), the course will take more than 1 day.

What is the recommended instructor:participant ratio?

If the curriculum involved giving information in a lecture format only, one instructor could suffice for a large number of participants. However, a potential hospital-based instructor also must learn to demonstrate the Performance Checklists and the Integrated Skills Station Checklist of the NRP Provider Course and to evaluate others performing these procedures. Teaching simulation and debriefing skills must be orchestrated in small groups with extensive facilitation by an instructor. Because of the need to evaluate personal instructional skills of course participants, **one instructor for every 3 to 4 participants** is usually required.

How are Course Completion Cards distributed?

- The course instructor must submit the completed Course Roster to the AAP.

- The AAP mails each course participant an AAP/AHA Hospital-based Instructor Card that is valid for 2 years. The regional trainer who teaches the Hospital-based Instructor Course does not receive the Instructor Cards.

Components of the NRP Hospital-based Instructor Course

1. *Self-study Prior to the Course* (required):
   - Self-study the *Textbook of Neonatal Resuscitation, 6th Edition*.
   - Take and pass the NRP online examination, Lessons 1 through 9, during the 30 days before the Instructor Course.
   - View the *NRP Instructor DVD: An Interactive Tool for Facilitation of Simulation-based Learning* during the 30 days before the Instructor Course.
   - Self-study the *Instructor Manual for Neonatal Resuscitation, 5th edition*.
   - Take the NRP Instructor Self-assessment found on page 187 (strongly recommended).

2. *Neonatal Resuscitation Program Skills Review and Practice* (*regional trainer decides which skills need review and practice*) Many NRP providers have never experienced hands-on practice for intubation, laryngeal mask airway placement, medication/volume administration, or emergency UVC preparation and placement. In addition, using pulse oximetry to titrate oxygen concentration is a new skill for many NRP providers. For this reason, the regional trainer must decide if a review and practice of hands-on skills would be beneficial for the Hospital-based Instructor Course participants. After all, it is difficult for the instructor to serve as a credible resource to others if the instructor is unfamiliar, unsure, or misinformed about procedures.

   The Hospital-based Instructor Course gives the regional trainer an opportunity to ensure that all potential instructors have correct and complete information about resuscitation interventions. Most Hospital-based Instructor Course participants benefit from review and practice of resuscitation skills within the context of learning to administer the Performance Checklists and Integrated Skills Station Checklists.

3. *Administration of Performance Skills Stations and Performance Checklists*
   Instructor candidates learn how to administer Performance Skills Stations and practice this Provider Course component with other instructor candidates.

4. *Administration of Integrated Skills Station Checklists*
   Instructor candidates learn how to administer the Integrated Skills Station Checklist (Basic and Advanced) and practice this Provider Course component with other instructor candidates.

5. *Facilitation of Simulation and Debriefing*
   Instructor candidates review the basics of creating and facilitating a scenario and conducting a debriefing.

The following course curriculum allows time for review and practice of all neonatal resuscitation skills—from the Equipment Check through Medication Administration and UVC placement. If you can be sure that your hospital-based instructor candidates do not need to review and practice every Performance Checklist, select the skills that would be most beneficial for review and practice.

Hospital-based Instructor Course Sample Curriculum

1. **Welcome and Introductions**
   Lead regional trainer asks hospital-based instructor candidates if there are any questions about the NRP Instructor Self-assessment content.

2. **Group Skills Review (all learners together)**
   Lead regional trainer talks through important points and demonstrates
   • Equipment Check
   • Initial Steps
   • Positive-Pressure Ventilation with a bag and mask, T-piece resuscitator if applicable to learners' needs, and use of pulse oximetry and MR SOPA
   • Chest Compressions

   The lead regional trainer may choose to show Resuscitation Skills videos from the NRP Instructor DVD or the DVD that accompanies the *Textbook of Neonatal Resuscitation, 6th Edition*, especially to help ensure standardized and accurate information about the least familiar procedures, such as use of pulse oximetry, laryngeal mask airway placement, and emergency UVC placement.

3. **Practice Session in Teams:**

   Learners break into groups of at least 2 learners and no more than 4 learners. Each team is coached by a regional trainer or hospital-based instructor who is an experienced assistant instructor for the course.

   Each learner practices and demonstrates these skills at a complete skills station
   - Equipment Check
   - Initial Steps
   - Positive-Pressure Ventilation with a bag and mask, T-piece resuscitator (if applicable to learners' needs), and use of pulse oximetry and MR SOPA
   - Chest Compressions

4. **Group Skills Review (all learners together)**

   Lead regional trainer talks through important points and demonstrates laryngeal mask airway placement, intubation, UVC preparation and insertion, and medication administration. The regional trainer also may lead a discussion about how to incorporate additional aspects of neonatal resuscitation into the Provider Course (management of the preterm newborn, special resuscitation circumstances, and ethics).

5. **Practice Session in Teams**

   Performance Skills Stations are set up so that 3 to 4 learners may practice the skill at a time. Learners rotate to each station with their team and assistant instructor.
   - Laryngeal mask airway placement
   - Intubation
   - Umbilical venous catheter preparation and insertion
   - Medication administration

6. **Group Skills Review (all learners together)**
   - Review use of Experience Survey. Discuss NRP Provider Course agenda development to ensure that hospital-based instructor candidates understand the core elements of an NRP Provider Course and how to choose optional elements to meet the course participants' learning objectives.
   - Review purpose of and how to administer Performance Skills Checklists and Integrated Skills Station Checklist.
   - Review how to convey physiologic feedback (heart rate, breathing, muscle tone, oximetry). If using an electronic simulator, orient learners to the simulator capabilities. If using a traditional manikin, remind hospital-based instructor candidates that physiologic cues are not revealed using a traditional manikin unless the learner palpates the umbilicus or auscultates the apical

pulse for heart rate, or listens to breath sounds, or asks about muscle tone and oxygen saturation.

- Observe a demonstration of the Basic Integrated Skills Station Checklist, including Reflective Questions.

7. **Practice Session in Teams**

Teams return to complete skills stations. With coaching and feedback from the assistant instructor, the team members practice administering the Performance Skills Stations Checklists to one another and end by administering the Integrated Skills Station to one another, using the Advanced Integrated Skills Station checklist and asking Reflective Questions.

Simulation and Debriefing

8. **Group Skills Review (all learners)**

Lead regional trainer introduces how Simulation and Debriefing Training session works.

- Review use of Scenario Template and discuss how to design a scenario.
- Each team designs a scenario for the practice session.
- Lead regional trainer or assistant hospital-based instructor demonstrates basic moulage techniques for blood, meconium, and vernix. This "Baby Prep" station includes supplies for making and applying the appropriate body fluids, and for cleaning up the manikin between scenarios.
- Lead regional trainer or assistant hospital-based instructor points out the key cues at the Simulation area.
  A. Radiant warmer (or conference room table with *Simply NRP* kit control board or other visual cues to make the setting resemble the birth setting as closely as possible)
  B. Scrub tops or cover gowns and gloves for participants
  C. Metronome for heart rate when learner listens or palpates for heart rate in a traditional manikin
  D. Pulse oximetry (per *Simply NRP* kit control board, flash cards, dry-erase board, etc)

9. **Simulation and Debrief Practice**
  - Lead regional trainer appoints
    A. Team 1: Learners who act as instructors and facilitate the scenario, prepare the newborn with simulated blood, etc, and debrief the learners.
    B. Team 2: Learners who are the resuscitation team.
    C. Team 3: Learners who operate the camera and film the team, then prepare the video for group viewing.
    D. Team 4: If there are additional hospital-based instructor candidates, they are assigned to watch the team facilitate the scenario and debrief the learners, using a tool that works for you (pages 136-141).

Teams rotate roles until all hospital-based instructor candidates have had a chance to facilitate and debrief a scenario, be part of the resuscitation team, operate the video camera and set up to view the film, and, if possible, debrief the debriefers, using the tool you prefer on pages 136-141.

10. **Group Discussion (all learners)**
    At the conclusion of the Simulation and Debriefing practice, the lead regional trainer
    - Reviews high points of the day.
    - Polls learners about what they found most valuable about the course.
    - Recommends that novice hospital-based instructors co-teach at least one Provider Course with an experienced instructor or regional trainer to further develop their instructor skills, if possible.
    - Reminds learners that the regional trainer is available to answer questions and serve as a resource in the future. (See sample letter on page 161.)
    - Reminds hospital-based instructor candidates that their NRP Instructor Card will come to them in the mail from the AAP. At that time, the new instructor must go online and register as an instructor. This is important for being able to complete NRP Provider Course Rosters and receive information about NRP from the AAP Division of Life Support.

11. **Course Conclusion**
    Course participants
    - Turn in their completed course evaluations
    - Takes resource letter from regional trainer (optional, see page 161)

Lead Regional Trainer

- Completes online Course Roster for the Hospital-based Instructor Course as soon as possible after the course. See the form on page 172 for what information the regional trainer needs to know about each course participant to complete the online Course Roster form.

- Summarizes course evaluation results and sends to appropriate people

SAMPLE LETTER "Eligibility Confirmation"

Hospital letterhead or logo

We have received your *intent* to complete registration requirements for the American Academy of Pediatrics Neonatal Resuscitation Program™ (NRP™) Hospital-based Instructor Course scheduled for **(date) and (time).**

DO NOT DELAY completing your registration prerequisites. Your space in this course is not confirmed until you have submitted the items listed below.

Class size is limited. If the class fills to capacity with registrants who complete all registration materials before you finish submitting your required materials, you will not have a space in the course. You will be given the option of being placed on the waiting list in the event of a cancellation on this date, being moved to the next course date, or receiving a full refund of your registration fee. Refunds cannot be issued for purchased books or DVDs.

To complete your course registration, submit the following items immediately:

- Photocopy of both sides of your current NRP Provider Card (Lessons 1 through 9)

- Photocopy of verification of your professional licensure as an RN, MD or DO, RT, or PA

- Letter of support from your manager or supervisor (link to this form at _____ _____) or see the form on the following page

Fax or mail these 3 items to: (name, contact information)

After your registration is complete, you will receive a confirmation letter with driving/parking directions. The NRP Instructor Course requires the following prerequisites, which must be complete on the course date:

- Self-study the *Textbook of Neonatal Resuscitation, 6th Edition.*

- Take and pass the NRP online examination, Lessons 1 through 9, *during the 30 days before* the Instructor Course. You will be sent directions for how to access the online examination after your 3 course registration items have been received and registration is complete.

- View the *NRP Instructor DVD during the 30 days before* the Instructor Course.

- Self-study the *Instructor Manual for Neonatal Resuscitation.*

- Take the NRP Instructor Self-assessment (page 187 of the *Instructor Manual for Neonatal Resuscitation*).

For additional course content information, contact _____ at _____. For registration information/assistance, contact _____ at _____.

SAMPLE Hospital-based Instructor Course

Letter of support from applicant's manager/supervisor/hospital administrator

This letter supports the intent of _____

(Print applicant's name)

to become a Neonatal Resuscitation Program™ (NRP™) hospital-based instructor for

_____

(Print name of institution, city)

The applicant meets eligibility requirements:

❑ Current NRP Provider Card, Lessons 1 through 9

❑ Current licensure as an RN, MD or DO, RT, or physician assistant

❑ Experience working with newborns in a hospital setting

❑ Current educational or clinical responsibility within a hospital setting

I am confident that this applicant

• Will implement our hospital Neonatal Resuscitation Program enthusiastically

• Will demonstrate good interpersonal skills and the self-confidence necessary to work with all levels of health care professionals

• Will meet the time commitment necessary to implement NRP in our institution

I am aware that course prerequisites include purchasing the *NRP Instructor DVD* for this individual and passing the online NRP examination during the 30 days before the Instructor Course.

My institution will provide administrative support for a hospital-based Neonatal Resuscitation Program, including components such as space, resources, and personnel.

_____   _____

Print name   Signature

_____   _____   _____

Title   Date   Phone Number or E-mail

Return this form to: _____ at _____ or fax to _____

SAMPLE LETTER "REGISTRATION CONFIRMATION IN INSTRUCTOR COURSE"

Hospital letterhead or logo

Thank you for completing your registration prerequisites for the NRP Hospital-based Instructor Course.

We are expecting you: **Date:**   **Time:**   **Location:**

See the attached information for driving directions and parking information.

Lunch on your own (brown bag encouraged due to short time for lunch; a microwave is available).

These course prerequisites must be complete by the course date:

- Self-study the *Textbook of Neonatal Resuscitation, 6th Edition.*
- Take and pass the Neonatal Resuscitation Program™ (NRP™) online examination, Lessons 1 through 9, *during the 30 days before* the Instructor Course.
- View the *NRP Instructor DVD during the 30 days before* the Instructor Course.
- Self-study the *Instructor Manual for Neonatal Resuscitation.*
- Take the NRP Instructor Self-assessment (page 187 of the *Instructor Manual for Neonatal Resuscitation*).

To gain admittance to the course, you must bring your:

- Examination verification for the NRP online examination, Lessons 1 through 9
- Certificate of Completion for the *NRP Instructor DVD*
- Copy of the completed NRP Instructor Self-assessment Answer Sheet

This is a hands-on interactive course. You successfully pass the course after you

- Identify core components of a Provider Course and accompanying administrative duties.
- Demonstrate the ability to facilitate participants' learning at the Performance Skills Stations.
- Demonstrate the basic steps of creating a scenario and conducting a simulation and debriefing.
- Identify resources for NRP instructor assistance and continued learning.

Neonatal Resuscitation Program course attendance does not guarantee successful course completion and attainment of NRP instructor status. If a participant cannot demonstrate basic abilities to perform and evaluate critical skills of neonatal resuscitation with adult learners, the learner may be asked to repeat the Instructor Course at a later date.

If you have questions about this NRP course, contact: _____

Neonatal Resuscitation Program

Hospital-based Instructor Course
SAMPLE Individual Recording Sheet

Name: _____ Credentials: RN   MD   DO   RT   PA

Work Phone: _____ **Home Phone (optional):** _____

Address (the American Academy of Pediatrics [AAP] will use this address to correspond with you and mail Neonatal Resuscitation Program™ [NRP™] Provider Course Completion Cards):

_____

E-mail address: _____

Institution: _____ Department: _____

> For Regional Trainer Use:
> _____
> _____ Evidence of current licensure as RN, MD, DO, RT, or PA (required)
> _____ Evidence of current NRP provider status, Lessons 1 through 9 (required)
> _____ Letter of Support from supervisor or administrator (required)
> _____ Examination verification for NRP online examination, Lessons 1 through 9 (required)
> _____ Certificate of Completion for *NRP Instructor DVD*
> _____ NRP Instructor Self-Assessment (strongly recommended)

At the end of this course, you should be able to demonstrate

• Technical skills at all Performance Skills Stations and at the Integrated Skills Station
• Excellent communication skills and ability to facilitate the student's learning
• Developing skills at creating and conducting a scenario and facilitating a debriefing

❑ Set up Performance Skills Stations (Performance Skills Stations and Integrated Skills Station).

❑ Communicate indications for each skill and facilitate learning for participants.

❑ Equipment check   ❑ Initial steps

❑ Positive-pressure ventilation including use of oximetry   ❑ Chest compressions

❑ Intubation   ❑ Laryngeal mask airway   ❑ Emergency umbilical venous catheter

❑ Medication administration

❑ Ability to ask reflective questions and help learners improve performance.

❑ Demonstrate administration of the Integrated Skills Station Checklist.

❑ Create a scenario for simulation-based training based on learning objectives.

❑ Set up and prepare for a scenario including construction of visual and auditory cues.

❑ Prepare learners for simulation-based training (ground rules, orientation, method of giving physiologic feedback from manikin) and conduct a scenario.

❑ Conduct a debriefing and demonstrate developing debriefing skills.

❑ Observe demonstration or discuss how to submit a Provider Course Roster to the AAP.

SAMPLE LETTER of Resources

For participants who successfully completed the Hospital-based Instructor Course

Hospital Logo or Letterhead

Thank you for attending our Neonatal Resuscitation Program™ (NRP™) Hospital-based Instructor Course.

As your regional trainer, I'm happy to assist you with NRP questions or topics anytime.

You can reach me at: _____

The American Academy of Pediatrics (AAP) will mail you an AAP/American Heart Association (AHA) Hospital-based Instructor Card that is valid for 2 years.

Maintain your instructor status by

- Teaching or assisting with at least 2 NRP courses during the 2 years for which your Instructor Card is valid.

- Taking and passing all 9 lessons of the NRP online examination every 2 years as part of instructor maintenance, beginning in January 2013.

American Academy of Pediatrics Resources for Hospital-based Instructors

Be the first to receive broadcast information about new educational programs, administrative updates, new NRP course materials, program revision information, and much more.

NRP broadcast e-mail list: www.aap.org/nrp

Share your views with other NRP instructors.

NRP discussion groups: www.aap.org/nrp

Receive the *NRP Instructor Update* newsletter, which is your primary source of current NRP information.

***NRP Instructor Update*: www.aap.org/nrp**

Let the AAP Life Support staff know if you change your hospital base or home address.

Begin at **www.aap.org/nrp,** click on "Courses and Instructors," then "Instructor Only." Click on "Update Info."

Regional trainers play a pivotal role in the AAP/AHA Neonatal Resuscitation Program by training instructors, serving as a resource for hospital-based instructors, and, in some cases, overseeing implementation of provider programs in a region. Therefore, regional trainers must be experts in all aspects of the NRP.

The Neonatal Resuscitation Program Regional Trainer

When the NRP was launched in 1987, the term *perinatal regionalization* meant that hospitals were categorized into service levels designated as Level I, II, or III, depending on the complexity of the maternal and newborn patients. At that time, the most acutely ill patients were cared for in university medical centers. The AAP established the first groups of national and regional NRP trainers in those university medical centers in the late 1980s, and they trained hospital-based instructors who established the NRP in their community hospitals. The regional trainers acted as resources and advocates for the hospital-based instructors, and regional trainers knew which community hospitals were within their perinatal "region."

Since the 1990s, the concept of regionalized care has come to mean different things, depending on the region of the country. Some states continue to offer regionalized neonatal and perinatal care, and some regionalized care programs and perinatal networks still include state-funded education for health care professionals. In other states, it is difficult for an NRP regional trainer to identify his or her "region."

Because the concept of "region" has changed so much in the past 20 years and differs widely across the country, it is now difficult for the NRP Steering Committee to describe the role and specify responsibilities of a regional trainer. As the role of all NRP instructors shifts into our new education methodology, the NRP Steering Committee will re-examine the role of the regional trainer.

For this edition of NRP education, some regional trainer responsibilities will be clearly defined. Other responsibilities may not "fit" the context of the role in certain parts of the country, and the experienced regional trainers in this situation will need to use discretion to determine how to use their regional trainers in the best interests of the NRP community they serve.

How is the regional trainer's role different from that of the hospital-based instructor?

Regional trainers must have full command of all NRP roles because they teach and interact with providers, hospital-based instructors, and other regional trainers.

A major difference between the regional trainer and the hospital-based instructor is that the regional trainer has the authority to conduct Instructor Courses. In other words, the regional trainer can "produce" NRP hospital-based instructors and additional regional trainers. In large medical centers, the main responsibility of the regional trainer is to ensure that there are enough NRP instructors to maintain the NRP provider status of all perinatal and neonatal staff.

On a broader scale and in keeping with the original concept of the role, the regional trainer is responsible for

- Facilitating regional implementation of the NRP

- Training hospital-based instructors and regional trainers

- Providing a crucial link between local programs and the NRP Steering Committee

The regional trainer is responsible for providing ongoing support to hospital-based instructors who request assistance. Activities may include the following:

- Responding to NRP and resuscitation-related questions from hospital-based instructors

- Assisting hospital-based instructors with NRP-related problem solving

- Assessing the stage of NRP development (if any) attained by each hospital within the trainer's scope of responsibility and creating strategies for enhancing existing programs.

- Developing a process for recognition and reinforcement of hospital-based instructor efforts at hospitals across a region

The regional trainer may serve as a resource for hospitals initiating an NRP. Activities may include assisting hospitals to

- Define resuscitation responsibilities of staff.

- Identify resuscitation training needs.

- Implement initial NRP courses.

- Develop a process for evaluation and selection of resuscitation equipment for the hospital.

The regional trainer may be called upon to assist hospital-based instructors when interacting with their administration. Activities may include the following:

- Determining benefits of NRP training to the hospital

- Identifying strategies to encourage physician involvement

How many regional trainers are needed in a region?

The size of the region, number of hospitals, and other responsibilities of regional trainers will determine the number of regional trainers needed in a particular region. Where there is more than one regional trainer, or regional trainers in numerous hospitals, every effort should be made to coordinate efforts. It is not uncommon for regional trainers from more than one region or hospital to sponsor Hospital-based Instructor and Provider Courses jointly.

Who can become a regional trainer?

Persons who wish to become NRP regional trainers **must meet the following eligibility requirements:**

- Have current licensure as a physician (or DO), registered nurse, respiratory care practitioner, or physician assistant with current newborn training or experience.

- Have a current Hospital-based Instructor Course Completion Card. If the regional trainer candidate is not an experienced hospital-based instructor, he or she must complete an NRP Instructor Course prior to becoming a regional trainer.

- Be available to assume leadership responsibilities at the request of the NRP Steering Committee.

Does the instructor have the ability to decline applications from persons not meeting the eligibility criteria to be a regional trainer?

Regional trainers have the highest level of responsibility for the NRP at the regional level, including training NRP hospital-based instructors. Persons conducting the Regional Trainer component of the NRP Instructor Course may decline to accept course applicants who do not meet the criteria to be a hospital-based instructor and who do not have regional educational responsibilities.

What are important attributes of a regional trainer?

The qualities and capabilities described previously for the hospital-based instructor are also applicable to the regional trainer. In addition, regional trainers should

- Be comfortable communicating with medical, nursing, and administrative staff of the various hospitals within the region.

- Know the differences between basic, specialty, and subspecialty perinatal services in terms of responsibilities, types of patients, equipment, and staff.

- Have experience working as an educator or know principles of adult learning.

- Have the ability to commit the time necessary to implement and oversee the NRP on a regional level.

Regional Trainer Course

See the sample "REGISTRATION CONFIRMATION IN REGIONAL TRAINER COURSE" letter (page 170).

Course eligibility

- Evidence of current licensure as an RN, MD, respiratory care practitioner, or physician assistant

- Evidence of current NRP Hospital-based Instructor Card

Course prerequisites

After admission into the course is confirmed by the regional trainer, the regional trainer candidate completes the following prerequisites:

- Self-study the *Textbook of Neonatal Resuscitation, 6th Edition* (required).

- Take and pass the NRP online examination, Lessons 1 through 9, during the 30 days before the Instructor Course (required).

- View the *NRP Instructor DVD* and bring a copy of the completion certificate to the course (certificate may indicate a previous viewing).

- Study the *Instructor Manual for Neonatal Resuscitation*. The regional trainer cannot possibly cover every point in the Instructor Manual at an Instructor Course. This course covers the most essential information needed to lead an NRP Provider Course and focuses on the technical skills needed to facilitate the learning activities of participants in an NRP Provider Course.

- Take the NRP Instructor Self-assessment in on page 187 (strongly recommended).

Admission into the course on the course date
The regional trainer collects the following documents from regional trainer candidates at the course (and keeps these documents as part of each learner's course records):

- Examination verification for NRP online examination, Lessons 1 through 9

- Copy of the Certificate of Completion for the *NRP Instructor DVD* (certificate may indicate a previous viewing)

- Completed copy of the NRP Instructor Self-assessment Answer Sheet (strongly recommended)

What is the recommended instructor:participant ratio?
Only a regional trainer may teach the regional trainer component of an NRP Instructor Course. Because participants will not need to work in small groups at performance stations, a single regional trainer can teach the Regional Trainer component. The training experience can be enhanced, however, if several regional trainers are available. This will provide a wider variety of perceptions, experiences, and ideas related to the role of the regional trainer.

What is the recommended course length?
Course length will depend on the experience of the participants. Those who have had considerable experience working with hospital-based instructor and provider programs and the hospitals in their region may already have developed many of the skills necessary to be a regional trainer. Enough time must be allotted to sufficiently cover the objectives that fit the community standard for what regional trainers are responsible for doing in that specific region. The content may be covered via telephone in some cases or at a networking meeting of regional trainers. The course coordinator can be creative in accomplishing the goal of relating regional trainer responsibilities to qualified participants.

What materials are required for a Regional Trainer Course?

- *Textbook of Neonatal Resuscitation, 6th Edition*

- *Instructor Manual for Neonatal Resuscitation, 5th Edition*

- *NRP Instructor DVD: An Interactive Tool for Facilitation of Simulation-based Learning*

How are Course Completion Cards distributed?
After successful completion of the Regional Trainer component of the NRP Instructor Course, individuals will be issued an AAP/AHA NRP Regional Trainer Card that is valid for 2 years. After receiving a complete Course Roster form, the AAP will mail the Regional Trainer Card directly

to the new regional trainer. See the form on page 172 for what information the Regional Trainer needs to know about each course participant to complete the online Course Roster form.

Regional Trainer Course Curriculum

The regional trainer plays a pivotal role in the NRP by training instructors and overseeing implementation of provider programs in assigned hospitals within his or her region.

The NRP Regional Trainer Course can be modified to meet the needs of the learners and the geographic region. Because the NRP education methodology and course components are new with the 6th Edition materials, most regional trainer candidates will benefit from participating in most components of the NRP Hospital-based Instructor Course (pages 153-156). The regional trainer candidate may need only a review of how the Performance Skills Stations and the Integrated Skills Station work, and may focus most of the course on learning about Simulation and Debriefing. Use the sample Individual Recording Sheet on page 171 to document course requirements.

> The regional trainer candidate needs to know everything a hospital-based instructor knows, plus the information specifically needed by a regional trainer. Therefore, the regional trainer who conducts a Regional Trainer Course designs the course to include all elements of the Hospital-based Instructor Course, or tailors the Regional Trainer Course curriculum to the learning needs of an experienced hospital-based instructor who is now a regional trainer candidate.

What are the criteria for successful completion of the Regional Trainer Course?

- Learner meets AAP eligibility and training requirements to become a regional trainer.

- Learner can identify and discuss the role as conceptualized by the AAP.

- Learner demonstrates abilities (or developing abilities) to plan and implement all levels of NRP instruction, if this is a region-specific expectation of the role.

- Learner demonstrates knowledge of NRP in his or her region and can explain the expectations of the role.

- Learner demonstrates excellent interpersonal skills, demonstrates the ability to facilitate learning to a diverse group of learners with different learning styles and abilities, and is ready to represent his or her region's NRP as an expert resource and respected leader.

Potential Learning Objectives for the Neonatal Resuscitation Program Regional Trainer Course	
1. Describe the role of the Regional Trainer.	The Neonatal Resuscitation Program (NRP) regional trainer's role is to • Help hospitals identify a need for an in-house NRP. • Train NRP hospital-based instructors. • Oversee implementation of NRP within the region. • Train NRP providers, if needed. • Provide ongoing support for hospital-based instructors. • Act as a liaison between AAP Life Support staff and hospital-based instructors.
2. Identify core elements of an NRP Provider Course and the purpose of each.	• Self-study of *Textbook of Neonatal Resuscitation, 6th Edition*. • Take and pass NRP online examination during the 30 days before attending the NRP course. **Purpose:** Learner takes responsibility for own learning; moves instructor away from lecture format; frees up course time for hand-on skills and simulation training. • Review/demonstrate skills at Performance Skills Stations. **Purpose:** (1) Instructor can assist, coach, help with technique and (2) ensure learner can perform specific skills without instructor assistance prior to Integrated Skills Station. • Demonstrate skills per the Integrated Skills Station Checklist. **Purpose:** Learner demonstrates specific skills in correct order of the NRP flow diagram with proper technique and without assistance from instructor. The Performance Skills Stations are learning stations; the Integrated Skills Station is an evaluation station. Although cognitive and technical skills can be remediated during Simulation and Debriefing, this distracts from the focus of simulation-based learning, which is teamwork and communication. • Practice skills and teamwork during simulation and debriefing. **Purpose:** Simulation replicates the actual neonatal resuscitation experience and allows learners to work through high-risk situations in a safe learning environment. It allows students to actively engage in the learning process. Debriefing is an instructor-facilitated team discussion that allows learners to reflect on the experience and critically evaluate their actions. Simulation training is dependent on good methodology, not technology; therefore, expensive simulators and equipment are not necessary.
3. Identify components of a successful hospital-based NRP.	A hospital may choose to offer NRP on site to • Improve the quality of neonatal resuscitation. • Meet performance expectations or attain hospital privileges for staff. • Serve as a quality improvement strategy. • Meet regulatory agency requirements for evidence of an education program that supports competency-based practice of neonatal resuscitation. • Save money by being able to use its own instructor rather than sending all providers off site for NRP instruction. • Allow instructors to collaborate with care providers to customize information to their setting. Hospitals with an NRP must provide administrative support for space, resources, and personnel. Hospitals with an NRP should develop a policy for who is required to obtain/maintain provider or instructor status and delineate how this is accomplished.

4. Discuss your proposed agendas for an NRP Provider Course and an NRP Hospital-based Instructor Course.	The NRP allows flexibility with NRP course curriculum. The regional trainer creates the course to meet learning objectives of the course participants. Uses Experience Survey for NRP Provider Course development. The regional trainer candidate can identify what a Provider Course and Instructor Course covers and where to find resources for creating an agenda.
5. Identify strategies for how the regional trainer can oversee implementation of NRP within a region (if applicable).	The regional trainer should know which hospitals in the region are included in the trainer's scope of responsibility. The regional trainer should assess the stage of NRP development (if any) attained by each hospital in the region. In addition, the regional trainer should create strategies for enhancing existing programs without duplicating activities in tertiary care centers. The regional trainer serves as a resource for hospitals initiating a Neonatal Resuscitation Program. Activities may include assisting hospitals to • Define resuscitation responsibilities of staff. • Identify resuscitation training needs. • Implement initial NRP courses. • Develop a process for evaluation and selection of resuscitation equipment for the hospital.
6. List the most important elements of a Regional Trainer Course.	A regional trainer may be called upon to train a fellow regional trainer; therefore, the Regional Trainer Course should include the following: • Criteria for being a regional trainer • Reasons to train additional regional trainers • Regional trainer role and responsibilities • Course documentation procedures • Acquisition procedures for course materials and equipment
7. Identify strategies for providing ongoing support of hospital-based instructors.	Implement a plan for interacting with hospital-based instructors at hospitals for which the regional trainer is responsible. Activities may include the following: • Responding to NRP and resuscitation-related questions from hospital-based instructors • Assisting hospital-based instructors with NRP-related problem solving • Identifying strategies to help hospital-based instructors meet teaching requirements for renewal • Developing a process for recognition and reinforcement of hospital-based instructor efforts Discuss ways of assisting hospital-based instructors in interacting with their administration. Activities may include the following: • Determining benefits to hospital of NRP training • Identifying strategies to encourage physician involvement
8. Describe the liaison role between AAP Life Support staff and hospital-based instructors.	Discuss how to access the *NRP Instructor Update* to familiarize participants with the mechanism for learning about changes in policy and procedure. Give the AAP Life Support e-mail address and phone number to participants. Discuss mechanism for distributing changes in policy and procedure to hospital-based instructors.

SAMPLE LETTER "Registration Confirmation in Regional Trainer Course"

Hospital letterhead or logo

Thank you for registering for the Neonatal Resuscitation Program™ (NRP™) Regional Trainer Course. To complete your registration, send:

- Evidence of current licensure as an RN, MD (or DO), Respiratory Care Practitioner, or Physician Assistant
- Photocopy of both sides of your current NRP Hospital-based Instructor Card

We are expecting you: **Date:**   **Time:**   **Location:**

See the attached information for driving directions and parking information.

Lunch on your own (brown bag encouraged due to short time for lunch; a microwave is available).

These course prerequisites must be complete by the course date:

- Self-study the *Textbook of Neonatal Resuscitation, 6th Edition.*
- Take and pass the NRP online examination, Lessons 1 through 9, *during the 30 days before* the Regional Trainer Course.
- View the *NRP Instructor DVD*. Review the DVD if you already viewed it and completed the education activity as a hospital-based instructor.
- Self-study the *Instructor Manual for Neonatal Resuscitation, 5th Edition.*
- Take the NRP Instructor Self-assessment (page 187 of the *Instructor Manual for Neonatal Resuscitation*).

To gain admittance to the course, you must bring your

- Examination verification for NRP Online Examination, Lessons 1 through 9
- Certificate of Completion for the *NRP Instructor DVD (you may bring your certificate from the first time you completed this requirement as a hospital-based instructor)*
- Copy of the completed NRP Instructor Self-assessment Answer Sheet

This is a hands-on interactive course. You successfully pass the course after you

- Can identify and discuss the role as conceptualized by the American Academy of Pediatrics.
- Demonstrate developing abilities to plan and implement all levels of NRP instruction.
- Demonstrate knowledge of NRP in the region and explain expectations of the role.
- Demonstrate excellent interpersonal skills and the ability to facilitate learning to diverse groups.
- Demonstrate excellent NRP cognitive, technical, and communication skills.
- Demonstrate developing abilities at simulation and debriefing skills.

If you have questions about this NRP course, contact: _____

Neonatal Resuscitation Program

Neonatal Resuscitation Program™ Regional Trainer Course

SAMPLE Individual Recording Sheet

Name: _____ Credentials: RN MD DO RT PA

Work Phone: _____ Home Phone (optional): _____

Address (American Academy of Pediatrics [AAP] will use this address to correspond with you and mail Neonatal Resuscitation Program [NRP™] Provider Course Completion Cards):

_____

E-mail address: _____

Institution: _____ Department: _____

```
For Regional Trainer Use:

_____ Evidence of current NRP hospital-based instructor status (required)

_____ Examination verification for NRP online examination, Lessons 1 through 9 (required)

_____ Certificate of Completion for the NRP Instructor DVD (may be from a previous viewing)

_____ NRP Instructor Self-assessment Answer Sheet (strongly recommended)
```

_____ Learner can identify and discuss the role as conceptualized by the AAP.

_____ Learner demonstrates abilities (or developing abilities) to plan and implement all levels of NRP instruction, if this is a region-specific expectation of the role.

_____ Learner demonstrates knowledge of NRP in the region and can explain the expectations of the role.

_____ Learner demonstrates excellent interpersonal skills and ability to facilitate learning to a diverse group of learners with different learning styles and abilities, and is ready to represent the region's NRP as an expert resource and respected leader.

The regional trainer should be able to demonstrate

_____ Technical skills at all Performance Stations and at the Integrated Skills Station

_____ Excellent communication skills and ability to facilitate the trainee's learning

_____ Developing skills at creating and conducting a scenario and facilitating a debriefing

Course Participant Roster Information: American Academy of Pediatrics Online Roster for Instructor Courses

This is what the regional trainer needs to know about each person in an instructor course to complete the online roster for the AAP following the course. The regional trainer may request that each course participant complete this form during the Hospital-based Instructor Course.

First Name:	
Last Name:	
Title	
Temporary ID Number (8 Digits)	8 Digit Temporary ID printed on NRP Instructor DVD Completion Certificate

Applicant Information

Business Address: (Required)

Address:

City:

State/Zip:

Country: United States

Phone:

Fax:

Email:

Home Address:

Address:

City:

State/Zip:

Country: United States

Phone:

Fax:

Preferred Mailing Address:

☐ Business

☐ Home

☐ Another address below

Other Mailing Address:

Address:

City:

State/Zip:

Country: United States

Medical Education:

Available credentials [R8]

AA
APRN
ARNP
BA
BSN
CCE
CFP

Selected credentials

Course Documentation

Neonatal Resuscitation Program™ (NRP™) instructors not only facilitate learning for their course participants, they have administrative duties. The lead instructor for each course is responsible for completing the online Course Roster and submitting it to the American Academy of Pediatrics (AAP). This is how NRP instructors receive credit for teaching a course and register course participants as NRP providers.

In Chapter 10 you will learn about

- **How to complete an online Provider Course Roster**

- **Things to know about completing an Instructor Course Roster**

- **Common errors when submitting a Course Roster**

- **Completion and distribution of the NRP Course Completion Cards**

- **Record Keeping**

"Instructor Self-assessment" for Chapter 10 starts on page 198.

After studying this chapter, complete the Chapter 10 questions, using the answer sheets that begin on page 188. Your regional trainer may ask you to bring the answer sheets to your NRP Instructor Course.

> The NRP Course Roster is submitted *online* within 30 days after completion of the program. Submission of a hard-copy Course Roster is not permitted.

When is the Course Roster submitted?

Instructors must submit completed NRP Course Rosters to the AAP within 30 days after completion of the program. If your Course Roster is not submitted in a reasonable time, the Life Support staff is not obligated to provide Course Completion Cards for learners or give credit to instructors for teaching a course.

Participants must complete the NRP course within 30 days of completing the online examination, and the instructor must submit Course Rosters within 30 days of course completion.

- Course Rosters for several participants, each with different course completion dates within the same month, may be submitted on the same roster, if desired. For example, 6 learners who completed the course on different dates in the same month may be listed on the same roster. The instructor may decide if it is more beneficial to "batch" completed courses and submit them on the same roster, or count them as separate courses and submit them on separate rosters. If employing this method, use the most recent course date when submitting the roster.

- Each form should include only those students who were taught at the same course level (Provider, Hospital-based Instructor, or Regional Trainer). If more than one type of course is taught on the same day, separate NRP Course Rosters must be submitted.

How do I complete the Neonatal Resuscitation Program Course Roster?

The NRP Course Roster is designed to provide instructors with the information necessary to ensure that instructors and students receive credit. Rosters must be submitted online.

💻www Find the online roster at **www.aap.org/nrp.**

Screen shots on page 175 and 176 illustrate the steps to roster completion.

The Roster List view defaults to the current period. The current period is defined as the time from the instructor's last renewal to the present.

To view past rosters, select the "Current Period" menu, and choose from 5 years, 10 years, or All.

Neonatal Resuscitation Program Course Roster

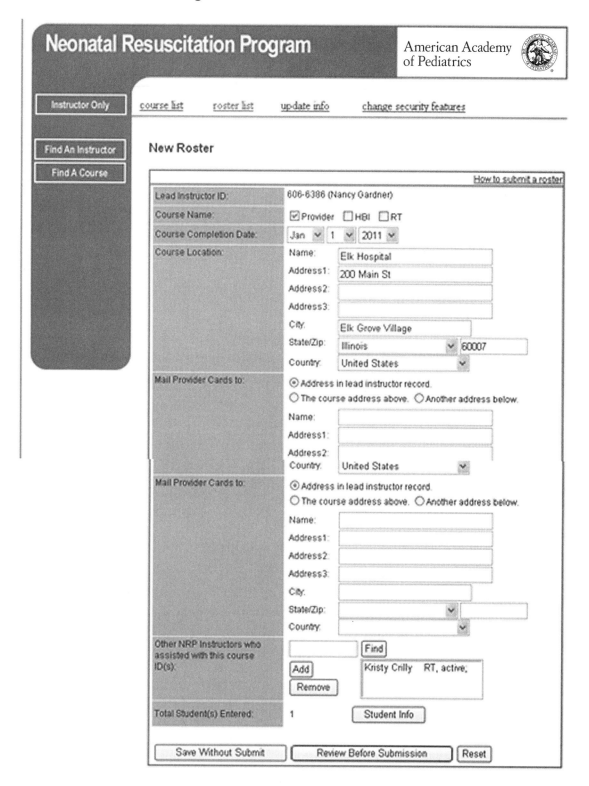

Neonatal Resuscitation Program

American Academy
of Pediatrics

Instructor Only

course list   roster list   update info   change security features

Find An Instructor

Find A Course

Student Information

*First Name		*Last Name	
Address		City	
State	[▼]	Zip	
*Credential	[▼] Or another:	Phone	

Lessons Learned   ☐ 1-4, 9 ☐ 5 ☐ 6 ☐ 7 ☐ 8

[Add] [Update] [Delete] [Clear]   * are required fields.

Name	Address	City	State	Zip	Credential
○ Kim Kelly					RN

[OK]

Instructions for Completing the Online Course Roster

If necessary, update your listed address, e-mail address, and security question by clicking on "Update Info".

A. Course Information

1. Date of Course: Please use the drop-down box to select the exact date on which the course was taught.
2. Neonatal Resuscitation Program Course Taught: Check type of course(s) being reported (Provider Course, Hospital-based Instructor Course, or Regional Trainer Course).

B. Lead Instructor Information

3. Lead Instructor's NRP Identification Number: Automatically populates the field.
4. Lead Instructor's Name: Automatically populates the field. Only one lead instructor may be designated per course. All others must be listed as assistant instructors. The lead instructor will receive the Provider Course Completion Cards, unless otherwise

indicated. Serving as either a lead instructor or an assistant instructor counts toward renewal of NRP instructor status.

5. Lead Instructor's NRP Level (hospital-based instructor or regional trainer): Automatically populates the field.

6. Neonatal Resuscitation Program Provider Cards Mailed to: Indicate the address where you would like the cards sent. Also, indicate if NRP Course Completion Cards are to be sent to someone other than the lead instructor. The AAP will not send Course Completion Cards directly to a student in the course. If the student is designated as the recipient, the roster will be rejected.

C. Assistant Instructor Information

7. Assistant Instructors: Type in each instructor's ID number and click "Add", or select "Find" and enter the assistant instructor(s) name. For best results, use only the first few letters of the first and last names and leave other fields blank.

8. Neonatal Resuscitation Program staff will not provide information regarding the status of NRP providers or instructors to third parties; therefore, you cannot call the Life Support Division and ask for an instructor's number or ask if an individual is currently an instructor or an NRP provider.

D. Submitting Student Information

9. Student Name: List the student's full name (no initials) as it should appear on the Course Completion Card.

10. Credentials: Select the student's current credentials. Please specify credentials if different than options listed.

11. Address and E-mail Address: These are required for NRP Instructor Courses because the AAP mails instructor cards directly to instructors. Enter complete home address, including zip code, for each student. If using a work address, a Department name must be specified. Enter complete e-mail address. See page 172 for roster information required for an Instructor Course.

12. Telephone: Business and home telephone numbers are required for each participant listed on the Instructor Course roster; optional for Provider Course.

Common Errors

Course Rosters that are incomplete or incorrect will be rejected. Cards will not be issued until an approved roster is on file. The most common errors include the following:

- **Forgetting to enter assistant instructors.** Sometimes when instructors submit rosters online, they do not include the other instructors who assisted in teaching the course. If the assistant instructors are not listed on the roster, they will not receive credit for teaching the course.

- **Accessing the database with alternative Web browsers** (eg, Netscape, Mozilla, Firefox, or Safari) is not recommended. The NRP database functions best when accessed with Internet Explorer (IE). In non-IE browsers, assistant instructors cannot be added to a Provider Roster, nor can Instructor Rosters be completed properly.

- **Not entering valid credentials for all students.** Credentials must be listed for all students on the roster. Options are available in the drop-down box, or they can be typed in if the desired credential is not listed in the "Other" field. Examples of unacceptable entries are "student" or a license number.

- **Entering students' names incorrectly.** The names of the students on the rosters should be entered as the first name, then last name. Instructors sometimes switch the names, include "Dr" in front of first names, enter only initials, or simply misspell the names. This makes it difficult or impossible to look up these students by name to verify participation in a Provider Course.

- **Submitting the same roster more than once.** This happens if instructors make mistakes on rosters and are unable to change them because they have already submitted the roster. If a mistake is identified on a submitted roster, contact the Life Support staff to make the changes. Instructors also sometimes inadvertently submit duplicates. Please notify Life Support staff of a duplication.

- **Saving, but not submitting, a roster.** When a roster is completed, sometimes instructors click on the "Save without submit" button. This saves the roster only in the instructor's window, and does not send it to Life Support staff. To submit the roster, instructors must click on the button that says, "Review before submission." A summary screen appears for the instructor to review. If the summary is accurate, he or she can scroll down and click on "Submit roster".

- **Indicating on the roster to mail cards to a student.** After a roster is processed, Course Completion Cards are sent to the address indicated on the roster. The cards must be filled out by the instructor before being given to students; therefore, the cards must be mailed to the instructor or to a third party as directed by the instructor, and not directly to students.

- **Roster missing from Roster List.** To avoid losing the information entered into a roster, be sure to submit or save the roster before exiting your browser. Please be aware that instructors are able to delete rosters from the Roster List if the roster has been rejected or not submitted.

What does the Life Support staff send to me after I submit the Course Roster?

An explanatory e-mail is sent if the roster is rejected. A verification e-mail is sent to the lead instructor upon submission and upon approval of the roster. Course Completion Cards and a letter of receipt will be mailed via regular mail to the lead instructor. You have the option of using a printer to print (instead of hand write) the students' name, course completion date, and renewal date directly onto the cards that will be mailed to you from the Life Support office. A print template is available on line at **www.aap.org.**   ⬛www

What should I do with the blank Course Completion Cards?

Instructors are responsible for writing (or printing, using the online template) the name, indicating lessons completed, signing the cards, filling out expiration dates, and distributing the cards to participants. As an instructor, you must ensure that learners receive their NRP Provider Cards within 30 days of the course. The recommended renewal date is 2 years from the date the course was completed. Correctly completed Course Completion Cards are shown in Figure 10.1 A and B.

Instructor tip: If you are conducting a course that will include participants from another institution, consider asking the participants to bring or fill out a self-addressed return envelope for the mailing of their Provider Cards.

A   B

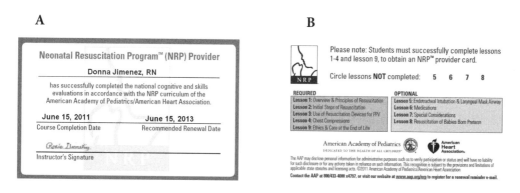

Figure 10.1. Correctly completed Course Completion Cards

Should providers keep their old Course Completion Cards or throw them away after expiration?

Some hospital risk managers advise NRP providers and instructors to keep all of their own expired cards as a personal record of NRP education. The Life Support staff keeps records for the current time frame. If a health care professional is asked to provide evidence of past education in neonatal resuscitation, old NRP Course Completion Cards could be helpful.

I taught a Hospital-based Instructor Course and never received Course Completion Cards for my participants. What happened?

After the Life Support staff receives the Course Roster for new instructors, the cards are mailed directly to participants, not to the instructor. That is why it is crucial to include new instructors' correct mailing addresses on the Course Roster form.

Sometimes former class participants come to me and want to replace a lost Course Completion Card. Can I refer them to the Life Support staff for this?

Life Support staff cannot always verify a person's provider status by the provider's name alone. The course participant needs the city and state where the course was held, and the instructor's name. The Life Support staff can find the participant's name as long as the course instructor correctly submitted the Course Roster after the course. A letter of verification can be sent to the course participant verifying course participation; however, because the Life Support staff cannot always determine which lessons were included in the course, the Life Support staff cannot provide a new Course Completion Card. Your own records should provide this information, enabling you to provide a replacement Course Completion Card.

How can I verify that someone has attained NRP provider status?

Due to privacy concerns, the NRP does not provide third-party verification of NRP provider status. The provider may contact the NRP office directly to request a letter of verification; however, the letter will not provide vertification of lessons completed.

Our hospital requires that staff go through a Provider Course every year. Do I send in my Course Roster every year, or should I wait and send it every 2 years as recommended?

You are encouraged to submit a Course Roster for every NRP course that you teach.

How should I keep track of old Course Rosters and class documents?

If you have arranged for continuing education credits for your course, the accrediting body may have requirements for record keeping. As a minimum, and to fulfill record keeping requirements for the AAP, course instructors need to maintain the following records for at least 3 years after the date of the course:

- A completed Course Roster. Although your electronically submitted Course Rosters are available online, they are protected by the instructor's password. It may be helpful to file them electronically in a shared drive and/or print a copy of each roster and store them in a file so that others can access this information.

- A copy of each student's Individual Recording Sheet for each course. This sheet lists the name of each course participant along with activities successfully completed.

Your hospital risk manager may advise keeping these records for a longer time period. Ask about your hospital's policy or recommendation for record retention.

How can I streamline my documentation? For example, staff on my unit are separated into groups and I run a Provider Course a few times a month. If the Course Roster allows only one course completion date, how can I avoid submitting a separate Course Roster each time a group completes a Provider Course?

The Course Roster supports only one course completion date because of the capabilities of the current electronic filing system. It is allowable to "batch" Provider Courses done in the same month and submit the roster under one course date. Because the instructor should submit the Course Roster within 30 days of course completion, a large discrepancy should not occur between the date the instructor chooses to record for AAP use and the dates that the learners actually completed their courses within the month. Try to limit the dates on the Roster to 1 calendar month and record the date of the last course on the Course Roster. This facilitates choosing the month of expiration.

The Master Recording Sheet (Appendix D) is a good place to record each learner's completed course components and actual course completion date. The instructor or facility protocol for renewal can decide if the learner needs to renew by the exact day and month of expiration, or within the calendar month of expiration.

- The instructor should write the actual course completion date on the NRP Course Completion Card when it is received from the AAP.

How does the AAP maintain records?

- Each Course Roster submitted is kept in an electronic file. Neonatal Resuscitation Program provider status verification can only be provided within the current period. However, you do have the option of viewing rosters in other time periods.

- The AAP maintains a database of instructors by NRP instructor level. The database includes basic identifying information plus a record of the courses taught by each instructor.

Instructor Q & A

Why is it important to submit the Course Roster?
If the lead instructor does not submit the Course Roster, the Life Support staff cannot verify participation by instructors or participants. If a class participant calls the AAP to verify his or her provider status, no such record will exist. Instructors, who need to teach 2 courses in 2 years to maintain their instructor status, will not receive credit for teaching an unreported course and will lose their instructor status.

Why do I need to write in every Instructor Course participant's address and e-mail address?
When you teach an Instructor Course, it is important to record both the home and business address of each new instructor. The Life Support staff mails Instructor Cards directly to participants of these classes. The business address must include Department Name, Hospital Name, and Address.

New instructors also receive the *NRP Instructor Update* periodically throughout the year, and additional mailings with information about the NRP. The e-mail address is required to receive verification of roster submissions and approvals, and other important notices.

Instructors must distribute the Course Completion Card to each Provider Course participant after receiving the cards from the AAP. Therefore, it is helpful for the instructor to have an address for each Provider Course participant.

Students want to leave the NRP Provider Course with their Course Completion Card. I would like to have a stack of Course Completion Cards sent to me when I become an NRP instructor so I can distribute cards as my participants leave the course.
Because many instructors never act as the lead, and some never even teach, it would be wasteful and expensive to mail out Course Completion Cards in advance.

Appendices

Introduction

Appendix A: Neonatal Resuscitation Program™ Instructor Self-assessment

Answer Sheets for Chapters 2 Through 10

Questions for Chapters 2 Through 10

Answers for Chapters 2 Through 10

Appendix B: Roster Samples

Completed Course Roster Sample

Neonatal Resuscitation Program Course Roster Sample

Information Needed to Complete the Instructor Course Roster

Appendix C: Planning a Course

Basic Equipment and Supplies Needed for Most Neonatal Resuscitation Program Courses

Experience Survey

Create a Medication Performance Skills Station

Make a Medication Performance Skills Station Doll

How to Prepare Umbilical Cords for Skills Stations

Sample Timeline and Details for a Neonatal Resuscitation Program Provider Course

Sample Projected Budget Worksheet

Appendix D: Neonatal Resuscitation Program Provider Course

Registration Confirmation: Sample Letter

Course Agenda: Sample 1

Course Agenda: Sample 2

Diagram for Neonatal Resuscitation Program Course Setup

Provider Course Individual Recording Sheet: Sample

Master Recording Sheet

Provider Course Evaluation: Sample 1

Provider Course Evaluation: Sample 2

Neonatal Resuscitation Program Provider Card Mailing: Sample Letter

Appendix E: Performance Skills Checklists and Textbook Key Points

Equipment Check

Initial Steps

Positive-Pressure Ventilation

Chest Compressions

Endotracheal Intubation and Laryngeal Mask Airway Placement

Medication Administration via Endotracheal Tube and Emergency Umbilical Venous Catheter

Integrated Skills Station Performance Checklist (basic)

Integrated Skills Station Performance Checklist (advanced)

List of Neonatal Resuscitation Program Resuscitation Skills Videos

Key Points: Lessons 1 Through 9

Appendix F: Scenario and Debriefing Tools

Neonatal Resuscitation Program Key Behavioral Skills

NRP Key Behavioral Skills in Action

Ground Rules for Simulation and Debriefing: Sample

CAPE Confidentiality Agreement: Sample

Scenario Template (blank and completed)

Instructions for Using the Sample Scenario Template

Scenario Building Tool

Simulation Preparation, Tips, and Sample Debriefing Questions

CAPE Debriefing Evaluation Tool® and Instructions for Use

Ready, Set, Go: Neonatal Resuscitation Program Instructor Prep Sheet for Simulation and Debriefing

NRP Instructor Simulation and Debriefing Checklist

The Art of Moulage: Guidelines, Recipes, and Easy Techniques

    Guidelines for Moulage

    Recipes for Blood, Vernix, Meconium

    Acrocyanosis

    Abdominal Defect

    Myelomeningocele

    Chest "Glow" With Transillumination

Make a Pulse Oximeter Out of a Box

Make a Pulse Oximeter From a Desktop Card File

The Neonatal Mock Code

Appendix G: Instructor Courses
Hospital-based Instructor Course

Hospital-based Instructor Course Sample Curriculum

Sample Letter: Eligibility Confirmation

Sample: Letter of Support From Hospital-based Instructor Applicant's Manager/Supervisor/Hospital Administrator

Sample Letter: Registration Confirmation in Instructor Course

Hospital-based Instructor Course: Sample Individual Recording Sheet

Sample Letter: Neonatal Resuscitation Program Resources

Sample Hospital-based Instructor Course Evaluation

Regional Trainer Course

Registration Confirmation in Regional Trainer Course: Sample Letter

Regional Trainer Course: Individual Recording Sheet: Sample

Regional Trainer Course Evaluation: Sample

Managing Challenging Classroom Situations

Appendix H: Neonatal Code Forms and Documentation

Neonatal Code Documentation Form: Sample 1

Neonatal Code Documentation Form: Sample 2

Neonatal Code Documentation Form: Sample 3

Sample Narrative Note to Accompany Code Documentation Form

Medications for Neonatal Resuscitation

How to Administer Dopamine Hydrochloride

American Academy of Pediatrics Policy Statement: The Apgar Score (includes expanded Apgar form)

American College of Obstetricians and Gynecologists Practice Bulletin: Intrapartum Fetal Heart Rate Monitoring: Nomenclature, Interpretation, and General Management Principles

Appendix I: Resuscitation Supplies and Equipment

Neonatal Resuscitation Supplies and Equipment

Neonatal Resuscitation Program Quick Pre-resuscitation Checklist

Organizing Resuscitation Supplies and Equipment

Introduction

These Appendices contain Neonatal Resuscitation Program™ (NRP™) standard forms as well as samples of correspondence, course schedules, course evaluations, and other information the instructor may find useful for implementing the NRP and optional activities. Many of these samples were contributed by NRP instructors across the United States and updated to concur with the revised program. These sample materials should be adapted to fit the specifications of your NRP course and the requirements of your institution.

🖥 **www** Many of the forms contained within these Appendices are available in an electronic form on the NRP Web site at **www.aap.org/nrp** for easy downloading and customization.

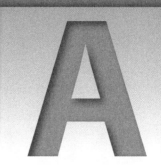

Neonatal Resuscitation Program™ Instructor Self-assessment

The Instructor Self-assessment is an optional tool that may be used to help ensure that current Neonatal Resuscitation Program (NRP™) instructors and NRP instructor candidates understand important concepts in the *Instructor Manual for Neonatal Resuscitation.* There is no pass/fail scoring stipulated by the American Academy of Pediatrics (AAP) and there are no documents to submit to the AAP related to this self-assessment tool. Because the regional trainer should not spend course time reviewing material from the *Instructor Manual* that the instructor candidate can learn through self-study, the regional trainer may require the instructor candidate to bring a copy of the completed answer sheets (Chapters 2 through 10) to the Instructor Course. This mirrors the requirement of learners who must pass the NRP online examination and bring their online examination verification to the NRP Provider Course.

Instructor Self-assessment Answer Sheets

Questions Begin on Page 191

Your regional trainer may ask you to bring a copy of your Answer Sheets to your Instructor Course

Chapter 2: Core Elements and Course Requirements

1. A.   B.   C.
2. A.   B.   C.
3. A.   B.   C.
4. A.   B.   C.
5. A.   B.   C.   D.   E.

Chapter 3: Course Planning: Who Learns What and How

1. A.   B.   C.   D.
2. Pass the _____, complete the _____ Station, and participate in _____ and
   _____ .
3. One instructor for every _____ to _____ learners
4. Minimum requirement for the NRP Provider Course is Lessons _____
   and Lesson _____.
5. _____
6. A.   B.   C.   D.

Chapter 4: The Online Examination

1. True   False
2. _____, _____ and
   _____
3. A. Institution already is a HealthStream customer _____
   B. Institution uses a different system than HealthStream _____
   C. Learners pay for their own examination _____
4. A.   B.   C.   D.
5. A.   B.   C.   D.
6. _____ and
   _____

Chapter 5: Organizing Supplies and Arranging the Classroom

1. Describe your current or proposed system for organizing Neonatal Resuscitation Program (NRP) course supplies.

2. How will you set up practice stations prior to your Provider Course? Who will ensure that supplies and equipment are maintained and functioning? How will learners access an NRP instructor, if necessary?

3. Using one of the sample Provider Course agendas in Chapter 3 or your own Provider Course agenda, make a room diagram as shown on page 244 and show how your course components are arranged for student check-in and checkout; Performance Skills Stations, if used; Integrated Skills Stations; optional learning stations, if used; and Simulation and Debriefing. Will you organize your learners into teams, with

one instructor who stays at a complete learning station with his or her team and conducts all course components from there, or will your learners "travel" from station to station to complete course requirements? After you have finished, show your diagram to a colleague and ask if that person could use the diagram and successfully set up an NRP Provider Course if you could not be there.

4. Make a standard NRP Provider Course packet for learners. List what is included in your packet. Are your packets standardized so that every course uses the same materials and you do not need to type in revisions or make new copies for each course?

Your standardized course packet items

1. _____
2. _____
3. _____
4. _____
5. _____

Chapter 6: Administering Performance Skills Stations

1. Your response: _____
2. _____
3. True   False
4. True   False
5. Main points of your introduction for learners to the Performance Skills Stations and Integrated Skills Station _____

Chapter 7: Simulation

1. _____
2. _____ _____
3. True   False
4. _____
_____
_____
5. A.   B.   C.
6. Write your own ground rule: _____
7. _____
8. A.   B.   C.

Chapter 8: Debriefing

1. Three important goals for debriefing
_____
_____
_____
2. A.   B.   C.   D.   E.
3. A.   B.   C.   D.

4. True   False
5. True   False
6. _____ and _____

Chapter 9: Instructor Courses

1. Eligible health care professionals: _____, _____,
   _____ and _____

2. Instructor maintenance requirements
   1. (teaching requirement): _____
   2. (examination requirement): _____
   3. (DVD requirement) _____
   4. (instructor candidates' DVD requirement) _____

3. Three items to ensure eligibility prior to acceptance into an Instructor Course

   _____

   _____

   _____

4. Five Instructor Course prerequisites

   _____

   _____

   _____

   _____

   _____

5. Three eligibility requirements of a regional trainer

   _____

   _____

   _____

6. A.   B.   C.
7. A.   B.   C.   D.   E.
8. A.   B.   C.

Chapter 10: Course Documentation

1. Submit roster within _____ days of course completion
2. A.   B.   C.
3. A. Web site: _____
   B. Click on: _____
   C. Enter your: _____
   D. Click on: _____
   E. Click on: _____
4. True   False
5. To replace a lost Provider Card: _____

Instructor Self-assessment Questions

Chapter 2: Core Elements and Course Requirements
Questions

1. Neonatal Resuscitation Program (NRP) education materials, such as the *Textbook of Neonatal Resuscitation, 6th Edition,* are based on evidence from

   A. The International Liaison Committee on Resuscitation (ILCOR) process that results in international resuscitation treatment recommendations

   B. The experiences and opinions of the NRP Steering Committee members

   C. The American Heart Association Board of Directors annual report

2. Neonatal Resuscitation Program instructors should know that

   A. Simulation-based training must include the use of a sophisticated electronic simulator.

   B. Learners who pass the NRP Provider Course are NRP certified for 2 years.

   C. Debriefing is not instructor feedback. The instructor's role is to ask reflective questions and enable the team to discover what went well and how team performance could be improved.

3. The NRP Provider Course curriculum has 3 primary components.

   A. Provider Course, Renewal Course, and Instructor Course

   B. Knowledge, Skills, and Teamwork/Communication

   C. Initial steps, Chest Compressions, and Medications

4. Which of the following statements reflect the new philosophy of NRP learning?

   A. The majority of instructor-participant interaction is now focused on hands-on learning, immersive simulations, and constructive debriefings.

   B. Simulation-based learning allows learners to make mistakes and learn from them in a safe and supportive training environment.

   C. The instructor is less of a "teacher" and more of a "learning facilitator" because the learner now takes responsibility for much of his or her own learning.

5. Which of the following are core elements of the NRP Provider Course?

   A. Self-study and online examination prior to the Provider Course

B. Lecture about resuscitation concepts and skills (preferably a review of each Lesson's Key Points), from an NRP instructor at the Provider Course

C. Performance Skills Stations

D. Integrated Skills Station

E. Simulation and Debriefing

Instructor Self-assessment

Chapter 3: Course Planning: Who Learns What, and How?
Questions

1. Which of the following groups may receive a Neonatal Resuscitation Program (NRP) Provider Course Completion Card?

   A. Nurses, physicians, respiratory therapists and medical students who complete the course requirements

   B. Paramedics and other emergency medical services workers who complete the course requirements

   C. Social workers, physical therapists, or chaplains who observe the course

   D. Participants who complete your course requirements in a course you teach outside of the United States (for example, in Mongolia)

2. Successful completion of the NRP Provider Course requires that the learner pass the _____, complete the _____ _____ Station, and participate in _____ and _____ _____.

3. The recommended instructor:learner ratio for a Provider Course is one instructor for every _____ to _____ learners.

4. The minimum requirement for the NRP Provider Course is Lessons _____ and Lesson _____.

5. What is the difference between the Performance Skills Stations and the Integrated Skills Station?

6. Select the activities for which the American Academy of Pediatrics (AAP) and American Heart Association (AHA) offer continuing education credits.

   A. The NRP Provider Course

   B. The *NRP Instructor DVD: An Interactive Tool for Facilitation of Simulation-based Learning*.

   C. The NRP online examination

   D. The NRP Hospital-based Instructor Course

Instructor Self-assessment

Chapter 4: The Online Examination
Questions

1. True or False? The hard-copy format of the 6th edition Neonatal Resuscitation Program (NRP) examination is available by ordering online from the Division of Life Support.

2. Who is required to take the NRP online examination?

   _____, _____, and

   _____

3. The 3 potential scenarios for NRP learners who need to access the online examination are listed below. What should you tell the learner who has questions about how to access the online examination, depending on which situation fits the learner?

   A. My institution is a HealthStream customer and gets online courses through HealthStream.

   B. My facility uses a different Learning Management System (LMS) than HealthStream.

   C. I have to pay for it myself.

4. Which of the following statements are true?

   A. The learner may skip questions within a lesson and come back to them. The learner also may change answers on any question until the lesson is submitted for grading.

   B. The online examination program ends the testing session as soon as Lessons 1 through 4 and 9 are completed. This is why it is a good idea to save Lesson 9 for last if the learner is testing on more than Lessons 1 through 4 and 9.

   C. Lessons can be retaken immediately, or a lesson can be retaken on a different day, within 14 days of the original purchase date. After 14 days, the unfinished online examination becomes invalid, and the learner needs to pay the fee and begin again. The original examination fee is not refunded.

   D. If the learner fails a second time, the learner needs to pay the examination fee again and retake the entire examination. The original examination charge is not refunded.

5. Advantages of online testing include

   A. The learner can take the online examination anywhere and at his or her own convenience within 30 days prior to the scheduled NRP Provider Course.

   B. Continuing education credits for physicians, nurses, and respiratory therapists are offered for online testing.

C. The online examination is financially advantageous for the institution.

D. Learners who pass the examination for each leasson will be able to see and print which questions they missed.

6. List 2 reasons why instructors are now required to take the online examination every 2 years.

Instructor Self-assessment

Chapter 5: Organizing Supplies and Arranging the Classroom
Questions

1. Describe your current or proposed system for organizing Neonatal Resuscitation Program (NRP) course supplies.

2. How will you set up practice stations prior to your Provider Course? Who will ensure that supplies and equipment are maintained and functioning? How will learners access an NRP instructor, if necessary?

3. Using one of the sample Provider Course agendas in Chapter 3 or your own Provider Course agenda, make a room diagram as shown on page 244 and show how your course components are arranged for student check-in and checkout; Performance Skills Stations, if used; Integrated Skills Stations; optional learning stations, if used; and Simulation and Debriefing. Will you organize your learners into teams, with one instructor who stays at a complete learning station with his or her team and conducts all course components from there, or will your learners "travel" from station to station to complete course requirements? After you have finished, show your diagram to a colleague and ask if that person could use the diagram and successfully set up an NRP Provider Course if you could not be there.

4. Make a standard NRP Provider Course packet for learners. List the items included in your packet. Are your packets standardized so that every course uses the same materials and you do not need to type in revisions or make new copies for each course?

Instructor Self-assessment

Chapter 6: Administering Performance Skills Stations
Questions

1. What is your response to this comment from a participant at your Neonatal Resuscitation Program (NRP) Provider Course?

"Thank goodness we're allowed to learn how to intubate at this course. Sometimes I have to go to high-risk deliveries and the doctor can't get there in time for the birth. Now I can intubate the baby myself."

2. What is the difference between a Performance Skills Station and the Integrated Skills Station?

3. True or False: The Performance Skills Stations and use of the Performance Checklists to assist learners with resuscitation techniques are an optional part of the NRP Provider Course.

4. True or False: The Integrated Skills Station must be done perfectly according to the Integrated Skills Station Checklist. If any errors are made, the participant fails the NRP course.

5. Describe your step-by-step strategies for introducing Performance Skills Stations to learners and facilitating performance at the Integrated Skills Station.

Instructor Self-assessment

Chapter 7: Simulation
Questions

1. West Cupcake Regional Medical Center encourages the use of simulation and debriefing to improve skills and teamwork. Its Neonatal Resuscitation Program (NRP) instructors created "Scenario Challenge," in which 3 teams are given the same scenario, then scored by observers according to how well they performed resuscitation interventions, how quickly they resuscitated the newborn, and how many Key Behavioral Skills were used during the scenario. The highest scoring team is declared the winner. Does this activity match the intentions of simulation-based learning? Why or why not?

2. A scenario is always based on _____ _____.

3. True or False: The main focus of a resuscitation scenario is practice and refinement of hands-on resuscitation skills.

4. Name at least 3 visual cues that are important for helping the learner "suspend disbelief."

5. You are facilitating a scenario with a traditional manikin on a radiant warmer in a birthing room. You have already oriented the 3 learners to the supplies and equipment, and how they will know the manikin's vital signs such as breathing, heart rate, pulse oximetry, tone, etc. The scenario begins, and you place the manikin on the radiant warmer. The leader is drying the baby and suctioning the mouth and nose as he asks you, "What's the baby's heart rate?" What is your response?

   A. Announce the heart rate or give him an auditory heart rate (metronome or tapping heart rate) then discuss this problem during debriefing.

   B. Stop the scenario, tell him what he did wrong, and start over from the beginning.

C. Do not respond to the question immediately. Wait for him to listen with the stethoscope or palpate the umbilicus. If he still does not understand what to do, and does not get help from his team, ask, "How do you assess heart rate?" and wait for him to listen or palpate before you reveal an auditory heart rate.

6. Create a ground rule for simulation and debriefing for learners or instructors that is not on the sample list on page 121 but is important to you.

7. Your NRP Provider Course participants are arriving and checking in. One of your students approaches you and states that she refuses to sign the Confidentiality Agreement. What should you do?

8. Filming a scenario is valuable to the learning experience and assists with debriefing because

A. Videotaping provides an objective record of who said and did what, and when it occurred.

B. Videotaping saves a lot of time during debriefing, because learners do not need to recount each event out loud.

C. The learner's manager can use the videotape at a performance evaluation to counsel or congratulate the learner on his or her resuscitation skills.

Instructor Self-assessment
Chapter 8: Debriefing
Questions

1. List at least 3 important goals a Neonatal Resuscitation Program (NRP) instructor has for a debriefing.

2. Which of these are the debriefer's responsibility?

A. Help the learners identify topics and facilitate discussion as necessary.

B. Give immediate feedback about what went well and what skills need improvement.

C. Act as a resource for teamwork/communication and NRP issues.

D. Keep the discussion learner-centered rather than instructor-centered.

E. Ensure that the scenario objectives are met.

3. You are debriefing a group and you notice that one learner is very quiet and not engaged in the discussion. Which of these questions may help draw the learner into the debriefing and help the team meet its learning objectives?

A. "Kathy, what happened next?"

B. "Kathy, what else might have Steve done to help you in this situation?"

C. "Kathy, how did you feel about that scenario?"

D. "Kathy, you are very quiet. Do you have anything to add to the discussion?"

4. True or False: A team who does everything well during a scenario does not really benefit from debriefing.

5. True or False: The best way to use film during a debriefing is to let the film run from start to finish, which encourages learners to watch closely and make comments quickly.

6. An effective debriefing focuses on _____ and _____.

Instructor Self-assessment

Chapter 9: Instructor Courses
Questions

1. Who is eligible to become a hospital-based instructor or a regional trainer?

2. What are the 4 things a Neonatal Resuscitation Program (NRP) instructor should know about requirements for maintaining instructor status?

3. List the 3 documents the regional trainer receives from the instructor candidate to verify eligibility for the course.

4. Name the 5 course prerequisites for the Hospital-based Instructor Course.

5. List 3 eligibility requirements of an NRP regional trainer.

6. Which of these duties describe those of an NRP regional trainer?

   A. Facilitating regional implementation of the NRP

   B. Training hospital-based instructors and regional trainers

   C. Providing a crucial link between local programs and the NRP Steering Committee

7. What are the requirements for successful completion of a Regional Trainer Course?

   A. Learner meets American Academy of Pediatrics (AAP) eligibility and training requirements.

   B. Learner can identify and discuss the role as conceptualized by the AAP.

   C. Learner demonstrates abilities (or developing abilities) to plan and implement all levels of NRP instruction, if this is a region-specific expectation of the role.

    D. Learner demonstrates knowledge of NRP in his or her region and can explain the expectations of the role.

    E. Learner demonstrates excellent interpersonal skills, ability to facilitate learning to a diverse group of learners with different learning styles and abilities, and is ready to represent his or her region's NRP as an expert resource and respected leader.

8. You are a regional trainer who just taught a Provider Course, followed the next day by a different group of learners in a Hospital-based Instructor Course. Which cards should you expect to receive in the mail?

    A. NRP Provider Course Completion Cards

    B. NRP Hospital-based Instructor Cards

    C. Both sets should be mailed to your address

Instructor Self-assessment

Chapter 10: Course Documentation
Questions

1. The Course Roster must be submitted to the American Academy of Pediatrics (AAP) within _____ days of course completion.

2. The Course Roster may be submitted

    A. Online

    B. Hard copy sent by mail (hard copy requires a fee)

    C. Either online or hard copy

3. Where do I go to submit my Course Roster? How do I begin?

4. True or False: Neonatal Resuscitation Program (NRP) Instructor Cards are sent to the regional trainer to distribute to course participants.

5. How does an NRP provider replace a lost Provider Card?

Instructor Self-assessment Answers

Chapter 2 Answers

1. A

2. C (Note re option B: NRP learners are not "certified" to do anything. Learners obtain provider status.)

3. B (Note re option A: All NRP learners take a Provider Course. There is no Renewal Course.)

4. A, B, C

5. A, C, D, E

Chapter 3 Answers

1. A, B (Note re options C and D: Observers in your course may not receive a Course Completion Card. Neonatal Resuscitation Program Course Completion Cards cannot be issued by the AAP for courses given internationally.)

2. Pass the *NRP online examination,* complete the *Integrated Skills* Station, and participate in *Simulation* and *Debriefing.*

3. One instructor for every 3 to 4 learners

4. Lessons 1 through 4 and Lesson 9

5. *Performance Skills Station* (optional activity): This is a learning activity where learners have the opportunity to work with an NRP instructor who will discuss the cognitive aspects of the intervention (why and when to use the intervention) and help the learner practice and improve technique (technical component). When the learner and instructor agree that the learner can perform the intervention smoothly and without assistance, the learner incorporates the intervention into a clinical scenario. Each Performance Skills Station scenario builds on the one that came before it. The learner and instructor use a Performance Skills Checklist as a reference.

   Integrated Skills Station (required activity): This is an evaluation activity where the learner integrates the "what, when, and how" of the resuscitation interventions appropriate to his or her NRP learning objectives. One or more clinical scenarios may be used to evaluate the learner. The instructor does not interrupt, coach, or assist the learner. For major deficiencies in knowledge or skill, the learner is sent back to the appropriate Performance Skills Station for additional review and practice. This evaluation precedes the Simulation and Debriefing component of the course.

6. B and C

Chapter 4 Answers

1. False. The hard copy of the examination is no longer available with the 6th Edition materials.

2. Required to take the NRP online examination:

   • Neonatal Resuscitation Program Provider Course participants are required to self-study the *Textbook of Neonatal Resuscitation, 6th Edition,* and take the online examination during the 30 days before their scheduled NRP Provider Course.

   • Hospital-based instructors and regional trainers are required to complete the NRP online examination every 2 years, beginning in 2013, based on their renewal date. For example, an instructor with a renewal date of March 1, 2011, must complete the online examination by March 1, 2013, and every 2 years thereafter. The examination will be provided at no charge to instructors.

   • Neonatal Resuscitation Program providers who are applicants for any NRP Instructor Course must have taken and passed Lessons 1 through 9 of the online examination during the 30 days before the Instructor Course or Regional Trainer Course.

3. Three potential scenarios for accessing the online examination:

   • My institution is a HealthStream customer and gets online courses through HealthStream: Your facility's HealthStream administrator will purchase and deliver the course to your students in the same way as other online courses currently delivered to your HealthStream system. Although your facility must purchase the examination from HealthStream for online use, there is no additional setup fee and no additional per-student fee.

   • My facility uses a different learning management system (LMS) than HealthStream: In this case, your facility may have the NRP examination delivered via your current LMS, or your facility may purchase "batches" of examinations for NRP learners to access at an Express Web site HealthStream will set up for your institution.

   • *I have to pay for it myself.* If you are an individual purchaser of one NRP examination (paying for the examination with a credit card), access the online test at **www.aap.org/nrp** and click on the "Online Examination" symbol.

   ⌨www

4. A, B, C, D

5. A, B, C, D

6. Instructors take the NRP online examination every 2 years, which

   • Helps ensure that instructors and regional trainers have current knowledge for teaching their courses

   • Helps ensure the quality of NRP instruction

Chapter 5 Answers

(Your responses are best assessed by you and your colleagues.)

Chapter 6 Answers

1. Remind participants that the NRP Provider Course does not certify or authorize them to perform any resuscitation technique, and course participants should not exceed their scope of practice defined by their professional governing body and institutional job description. This comment also prompts a discussion about the goal of having one person at each birth who is capable of initiating resuscitation, and one person who is immediately available who has skills required to perform a complete resuscitation, including intubation, line placement, and medication administration.

2. The Performance Skills Stations for individual skills such as Equipment Check, Initial Steps, Positive-Pressure Ventilation, Chest Compressions, and Intubation are for the purpose of learning. The Integrated Skills Station is for evaluation.

3. True. Most NRP courses will include all Performance Skills Stations, but this is not required. The NRP instructor assesses the learning needs of the participants prior to the NRP course and determines which elements of the NRP course would best meet their learning objectives. (See Table 3-1 on page 39.) Even experienced learners, whose course includes all 9 textbook lessons, benefit from review and discussion of all Performance Skills Stations; however, the instructor who knows and works with the course participants who perform frequent complex resuscitation may choose to include only the unfamiliar or rarely practiced skills, such as laryngeal mask airway placement or the medication station. If the instructor determines that all participants are experts at neonatal resuscitation, it would be permissible to begin with the Integrated Skills Station.

4. False. If the learner makes significant mistakes in the sequence, timing, or technique of the individual skills, he or she should return to the appropriate Performance Skills Station for additional practice before repeating the Integrated Skills Station Checklist. The learner then may proceed to the Simulation and Debriefing component of the course. While technical skills can be refined during the simulation, significant problems with hands-on skills interfere with the intended focus of simulation and debriefing, which is teamwork and communication. If a reasonable amount of time and effort working both independently and with instructor assistance does not improve performance, the learner and instructor should agree on a remediation plan.

5. Suggested strategies:

Introduction: Consider a group orientation by the NRP lead instructor that introduces the purpose of the Performance Skills Stations and a demonstration of the Integrated Skills Station checklist.

Performance Skills Station: Remind learners that Skills Stations are for learning. Ask about cognitive aspects of the skill. Provide a demonstration, and model behaviors such as talking aloud and directing assistants as needed. Orient learners to how they know about the manikin's breathing, heart rate, pulse oximetry, tone, or other physiologic signs that influence interventions. Encourage hands-on practice and discussion and refine the learner's technique. When the skill can be performed smoothly and without instructor assistance, ask the learner to demonstrate the skill within the context of a scenario. Use the Performance Checklist as your reference. Request that the learner begin with the Equipment Check and move forward in real time through the skills up to and including the skill that is the focus of the Performance Checklist. Assess performance using Reflective Questions.

Integrated Skills Station: Remind learners that the Integrated Skills Station is for evaluation, and clarify expectations of performance. Know what skills are to be included in the learner's scenario. Use one or more scenarios to allow the learner to demonstrate all relevant skills in proper sequence and with correct technique. Do not coach or assist the learner during the scenario. Assess performance with the learner using Reflective Questions. Significant deficiencies in performance require that the learner return to the Performance Skills Stations for additional practice. After the learner successfully completes the Integrated Skills Station, the learner may proceed to the Simulation and Debriefing component of the course.

Chapter 7 Answers

1. Although this activity is well-intentioned and entertaining for observers, it does not match the aims or purpose of simulation-based learning because

   - A competition with scorekeepers is not a safe environment in which to make errors. The goal of simulation training is learning, not perfection, and the best learning often occurs through making mistakes.

   - It uses a score-sheet approach to evaluate the activity, instead of a team-centered discussion that enables self-discovery about what went well and what needs improvement.

- The responsibilities for an effective or ineffective simulation-based learning experience are shared among the instructor and the learners. In this game, all the responsibilities for being "best" lie with the learners.

2. A scenario is always based on *learning objectives*.

3. False. The main focus of simulation-based learning is teamwork and communication.

4. Visual cues include: Radiant warmer, simulated blood, meconium, or vernix, people wearing scrubs or cover gowns and gloves, and hospital linen and blankets.

5. Do not respond to the question immediately. Wait for him to listen with the stethoscope or palpate the umbilicus. If he still does not understand what to do, and he does not get help from his team, ask, "How do you assess heart rate?" and wait for him to listen or palpate before you reveal an auditory heart rate.

   A. If you announce the heart rate and discuss this during debriefing, the learner has missed multiple opportunities to assess his ability to count the heart rate correctly. The instructor has missed the opportunity to correct the behavior and help the learner understand how simulation-based learning works.

   B. Stopping the scenario is disruptive and punitive. Telling him what he did wrong is providing feedback, and this feedback does not pertain to hands-on skills or teamwork behaviors. Feedback is not the same as enabling the learner to self-assess and determine what went well and what needs improvement.

6. Write your own ground rule.

7. If a course participant refuses to sign the confidentiality agreement, find a private place to have a short conversation and ask why. Be polite and nonjudgmental during this conversation. Perhaps the participant does not understand that the agreement is for her protection and to ensure that future participants have the same opportunities for a powerful learning experience. If this is not the problem, allow the participant to make changes, with a pen, on her agreement before signing it. If the changes do not adversely affect the intent of confidentiality, allow the learner to participate in the simulation-based training.

8. A and B. The film should be erased immediately after debriefing unless the learner has given written permission to use the film for another stated purpose, such as educating others about simulation-based learning. The film should never be used for disciplinary or evaluative purposes by a manager or supervisor.

Chapter 8 Answers

1. List at least 3 important goals for debriefing. The NRP instructor aims to

    A. Facilitate a discussion where learners talk mostly with one another—not to the instructor.

    B. Ask open-ended questions that enable learners to analyze the situations that confronted them during the scenario, and evaluate how well they managed those situations.

    C. Guide the learners to relate the events of the scenario to real life. It is hoped that they will draw upon this information in the future and perform effectively when faced with the real-life situations they encountered in the scenarios.

2. A, C, D, E. The debriefer holds his own opinion and feedback until the team has finished its discussion. When the team has finished its analysis, you can reinforce the positive points of the performance. If necessary, fill in any important points the team has missed, make sure the learning objectives have been met.

3. A and B may help draw Kathy into the debriefing. Asking Kathy to talk about her feelings (C) distracts Kathy and the team from assessing performance. Asking Kathy a yes/no question (D) may result in her answering "no," and you will not have made any progress guiding Kathy into the discussion.

4. False. The team who performed well benefits from analyzing its scenario and figuring out why it went so well. Which Key Behavioral Skills were used that resulted in a positive performance? The team that knows why it works well together can transfer these skills to other scenarios where teamwork is more challenging.

5. False. The instructor does not show long video segments that will not be discussed. The debriefer introduces each video segment that is to be shown. Set the scene and tell viewers what you want them to analyze: "This segment begins as the team decides to begin chest compressions. Watch your performance and think about what went well here, and what could be improved." Pause the tape when asking a question, or when someone is making a point.

6. An effective debriefing focuses on teamwork and communication. The debriefer guides learners into discussing which Key Behavioral Skills helped them manage, or could have helped them manage, the events during the scenario.

Chapter 9 Answers

1. Eligibility: Neonatal Resuscitation Program hospital-based instructors and regional trainers are *physicians (and DOs), registered nurses, respiratory care practitioners, and physician assistants* who have experience in the hospital care of newborns in the delivery room, newborn nursery, or newborn intensive care

setting. Ideally, the NRP instructor has ongoing delivery room experience and current educational or clinical responsibility within a hospital setting. Instructors are selected for their experience in newborn care, good interpersonal skills and self-confidence working with all levels of professionals, and ability to implement and maintain the NRP enthusiastically in their institution.

2. Maintenance requirements:

   A. Teach or assist with at least 2 NRP courses during the 2 years for which his or her Instructor Card is valid. For a regional trainer, at least one course during the 2-year period must include a Provider Course. Instructors do not need to maintain a separate NRP Provider Card.

   B. Beginning in 2013, instructors will be required to complete and pass all 9 lessons of the NRP online examination every 2 years, based on their renewal date. For example, an instructor with a renewal date of March 1, 2011, must complete the online examination by March 1, 2013, and every 2 years thereafter. The examination will be provided at no charge to instructors renewing their instructor status.

   C. Every instructor who has attained hospital-based instructor status or regional trainer status before January 1, 2012, must watch the *NRP Instructor DVD: An Interactive Tool for Facilitation of Simulation-based Learning* by January 1, 2012.

   D. Instructors who attain instructor status after January 1, 2012, are required to watch the *NRP Instructor DVD: An Interactive Tool for Facilitation of Simulation-based Learning* as a prerequisite for attending the Hospital-based Instructor or Regional Trainer Course.

3. The following 3 items ensure eligibility prior to acceptance into a Hospital-based Instructor Course:

   • Evidence of current licensure as an RN, MD, Respiratory Care Practitioner, or Physician Assistant

   • Evidence of current NRP Provider Card (Lessons 1 through 9)

   • Evidence that the instructor candidate is supported and recommended by his or her institution as a person who has the necessary skills and abilities to be a hospital-based instructor (letter of recommendation)

4. Five course prerequisites

   • Self-study the *Textbook of Neonatal Resuscitation, 6th Edition*.

   • Take and pass the NRP online examination, Lessons 1 through 9, during the 30 days before the Instructor Course.

   • View the *NRP Instructor DVD: An Interactive Tool for Facilitation of Simulation-based Learning* during the 30 days *before* the Instructor Course date.

- Study the *Instructor Manual for Neonatal Resuscitation*.
- Take the NRP Instructor Self-assessment (Appendix A) prior to the Instructor Course (strongly recommended).

5. Three eligibility requirements of a regional trainer:
   - Have current licensure as a physician (or DO), registered nurse, respiratory care practitioner, or physician assistant with current newborn training or experience.
   - Have a current Hospital-based Instructor Course Completion Card. If the regional trainer candidate is not an experienced hospital-based instructor, he or she must complete an NRP Instructor Course prior to becoming a regional trainer.
   - Be available to assume leadership responsibilities at the request of the NRP Steering Committee.

6. A, B, C

7. All choices are correct.

8. A. Only NRP Provider Course Completion Cards are mailed to the instructor for distribution to course participants. The AAP will mail instructor cards directly to the new instructors.

Chapter 10 Answers

1. The Course Roster must be submitted to the AAP within 30 days of course completion.

2. The Course Roster must be submitted
   A. Online

3. To submit Course Rosters online,
   - www
   A. Go to **http://www.aap.org/nrp/nrpmain.html.**
   B. Click on "Instructor Log In Only".
   C. Enter your ID number (this is your instructor ID number on your Instructor card) and password.
   D. Click on "Roster List".
   E. Click on "New Roster" and fill out the roster form.

4. False. Instructor Cards are sent directly to the new instructors at the mailing address indicated by the regional trainer who submitted the Instructor Course Roster.

5. To replace a Provider Card, the provider contacts the instructor of the course he or she took. By looking at the records in his or her file, the instructor should be able to verify the course date and the lessons completed, and issue the provider a replacement card. If the provider is unable to locate his or her course instructor, he or she can contact the Life Support staff for a letter of verification. Life Support staff cannot verify lessons completed.

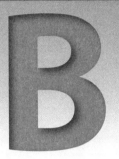
Roster Samples

Completed Course Roster Sample

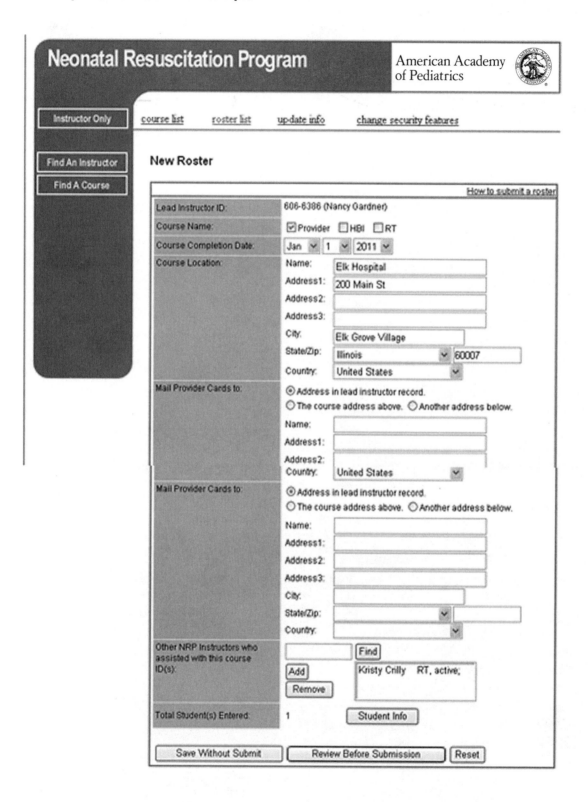

Neonatal Resuscitation Program Course Roster Sample

Neonatal Resuscitation Program

American Academy of Pediatrics

Instructor Only

course list   roster list   update info   change security features

Find An Instructor

Find A Course

Student Information

*First Name [____] *Last Name [____]

Address [____] City [____]

State [____ ▾] Zip [____]

*Credential [____ ▾] Or another: [____] Phone [____]

Lessons Learned ☐ 1-4, 9 ☐ 5 ☐ 6 ☐ 7 ☐ 8

[Add] [Update] [Delete] [Clear] * are required fields.

	Name	Address	City	State	Zip	Credential
○	Kim Kelly					RN

[OK]

Information Needed to Complete the Instructor Course Roster

This is what the regional trainer needs to know about each person in an Instructor Course to complete the AAP online roster after the course. The Regional Trainer may want to print a hard copy of this form and request that each course participant complete this form during the Hospital-based Instructor Course.

First Name:	
Last Name:	
Title	
Temporary ID Number (8 Digits)	8-Digit Temporary ID printed on NRP Instructor DVD Completion Certificate

Applicant Information

Business Address: (Required)	Address:			
	City:	
	State/Zip:	
	Country:	United States
	Phone:	
	Fax:	
	Email:	
Home Address:	Address:			
	City:	
	State/Zip:	
	Country:	United States
	Phone:	
	Fax:	

Preferred Mailing Address:
- ☐ Business
- ☐ Home
- ☐ Another address below

Other Mailing Address:	Address:			
	City:	
	State/Zip:	
	Country:	United States

Medical Education:

Available credentials [R8]
- AA
- APRN
- ARNP
- BA
- BSN
- CCE
- CFP

Selected credentials

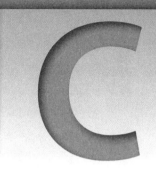

Planning a Course

Basic Equipment and Supplies Needed for Most Neonatal Resuscitation Program Courses

• **Newborn manikin** • **Neonatal intubation head or full-body intubation manikin** • **Gloves**
• **Cover gowns or size-XL scrub tops to cover street clothing**

Optional: Simply NRP **kit control board to simulate radiant warmer power switch, wall suction, oxygen and blender, pulse oximetry, and "Help" button**

Warm	• Radiant warmer or simulation (tabletop) with surface area to hold equipment • Towels or blankets, including small towel or cloth diaper for optional shoulder roll For resuscitation of preterm newborn <29 weeks • Food-grade polyethylene bag (1-gallon size) or plastic wrap • Chemically activated warming pad (or simulated pad)
Suction	• Bulb syringe • Mechanical suction (or simulation) and suction tubing with 10F or 12F suction catheter • Meconium aspirator
Auscultate	• Stethoscope(s)
Oxygenate	• Oxygen tubing, mask, or flow-inflating bag and mask to deliver free-flow oxygen • Oxygen or air source with flowmeter and nipple adapter (required for use with flow-inflating bag or T-piece resuscitator) • Pulse oximeter probe for newborn use • Pulse oximeter device, such as on the *Simply NRP* control board, or simulated
Ventilate	• Self-inflating bag, flow-inflating bag, or T-piece resuscitator • Oxygen tubing • Face masks (preterm and term sizes) • Oxygen or air source with flowmeter and nipple adapter (required for flow-inflating bag and T-piece resuscitator) • 8F feeding tube and 20-mL syringe • Oral airways (various sizes)
Intubate	• Intubation head or full-body intubation manikin • Laryngoscope with straight blades, size 0 (preterm), size 1 (term), and size 00 (optional) • Endotracheal (ET) tubes sizes 2.5, 3.0, 3.5, and 4.0 • Stylets • Scissors • Tape or securing device for ET tube • End-tidal CO_2 detector • Size-1 laryngeal mask airway with 5-mL syringe

Medicate	• Equipment for emergency umbilical venous catheter (UVC) placement
	   – Umbilical catheters, 3.5F or 5F (preferred)
	   – 10-cc and 20-cc syringes (may be prefilled with non-bacteriostatic normal saline or simulate with water)
	   – Volume expander of choice (such as 100-mL bag of normal saline or prefilled syringes)
	   – Needle or puncture device to access volume expander, if needed
	   – Curved forceps or instrument to stabilize umbilical cord or catheter
	   – Three-way stopcocks and/or Luer lock connectors
	   – Antiseptic prep solution (may simulate with cotton-tipped applicators)
	   – Umbilical tape (may simulate with narrow, white cloth ribbon)

Basic Equipment and Supplies Needed for Most Neonatal Resuscitation Program Courses—*continued*

Medicate—*continued*	– Scalpel blade and handle – Securing device for UVC (optional) • Epinephrine 1:10,000 in 3-mL or 10-mL ampules (or substitute water in ampules) • 1-mL syringes, 5- or 6-mL syringes • Three-way stopcocks or Luer lock syringe connectors • Volume expander: normal saline (preferred), Ringer's lactate (or substitute water) • Assorted syringes, needles, or puncture devices/needleless system supplies • Medication labels and waterproof pen
Available for each course	• Silicone spray for use with some types of intubation heads • Extra balloons and rubber bands for intubation head "lungs" • Extra bulbs and batteries for laryngoscope • Oxygen regulator and key or wrench for oxygen or air tank, if used • Clock with second hand • Apgar timer or stopwatch to assess newborn's age in minutes
Simulate	• Metronome to simulate various newborn heart rates • Flash cards or dry-erase board to give learners physiologic feedback (optional for breathing, color, tone, oximetry) • Supplies for simulated blood, meconium, vernix – Small cups for mixing, and coffee stirrer, spoons, and sections of drinking straws for stirring fluids – Purchased simulated blood or red finger paint/green finger paint, OR ingredients for alternate recipe – Baby oil or mineral oil – Blue dishwashing liquid – Meconium: Pureed baby food green beans or peas OR split pea soup OR ingredients for alternate recipe – Vernix: unscented heavy hand cream, instant potato flakes OR ingredients for alternate recipe • Disposable wipes or alternate method for manikin cleanup • Spray bottle of simulated blood for towels and manikin, if needed • Camcorder • Tripod • Method for showing filmed scenario to viewers (TV monitor, computer screen, LCD projector)
Instructor Resources	Scenario template for creating scenarios Table of Pre-ductal Oxygen Saturation Targets (from NRP flow diagram) List of NRP Key Behaviors to post for reference during debriefing NRP Instructor Simulation and Debriefing Checklist and/or CAPE Debriefing Evaluation Tool® Simulation Preparation, Tips, and Sample Debriefing Questions Ready, Set, Go: NRP Instructor Prep Sheet for Simulation and Debriefing Institution's Neonatal Code Documentation form
Optional	• Cardiac monitor/leads/alcohol sponges • Umbilical cord model for UVC placement (page 217) • Medication doll (page 218)

Experience Survey

Complete and submit to instructor prior to course.

Name _____

E-mail address _____

Contact number _____

Institution _____

Credentials:

MD _____ RN _____ LPN _____ Respiratory Therapist _____

Advanced practice RN (specify type: CRNP, NNP, PNP, CNM, etc) _____

Prehospital professional (specify) _____

Other (specify) _____

Current position

MD: Obstetrics/Gynecology _____ Neonatology _____ General Pediatrics _____

Family Medicine _____ Emergency Medicine _____ Anesthesiology _____

Other (specify) _____

RN/LPN: Labor and Delivery _____ Newborn Nursery _____

Special Care Nursery/NICU _____

Nursing Education _____ Operating Room _____ Emergency Department _____

Other (specify) _____

Other health care professional (specify) _____

Is this your first NRP course? Yes _____ No _____

What is your role at a newborn resuscitation?

_____ I have primary responsibility for all aspects of resuscitation, including airway management, umbilical line placement, and administration of medications.

_____ I have primary responsibility for providing initial steps, positive-pressure ventilation (PPV), and chest compressions until help arrives.

_____ I have primary responsibility for providing initial steps, and PPV, assisting with airway management, drawing up and administering medications, and assisting with umbilical line placement.

_____ I have a different role than any described above. My role is: _____

In the past 6 months, how many times have you participated in the resuscitation of a newborn?

None _____   1-4 _____   5-9 _____   10-20 _____   More than 20 _____

During those resuscitations, how many times have you performed the following:

Initial steps _____   Bag-and-mask ventilation _____   Ventilation with T-piece resuscitator _____

Chest compressions _____   Endotracheal intubation _____   Laryngeal mask airway _____

Preparation and/or administration of epinephrine _____

Preparation and/or insertion of emergency umbilical venous catheter _____

In the next 6 months, how many times do you anticipate participating in newborn resuscitation?

None _____   1-4 _____   5-9 _____   10-20 _____   More than 20 _____

What specific goals do you have for the course?

Improve team communication _____

Participate in simulation-based training _____

Improve skills performance:

Ventilation with bag and mask _____   Ventilation with T-piece resuscitator _____

Chest compressions _____

Endotracheal intubation (assist or perform) _____

Laryngeal mask airway placement _____

Epinephrine and volume administration _____

Emergency umbilical venous catheter placement (assist or perform) _____

Other personal objective for attending this course: _____

Have you participated in simulated neonatal resuscitations, mock codes, or similar exercises in the past 2 years?

Yes _____   No _____

Please add any other comments you think would help the instructor in meeting your educational goals:

_____

_____

_____

_____

_____

Create a Medication Performance Skills Station

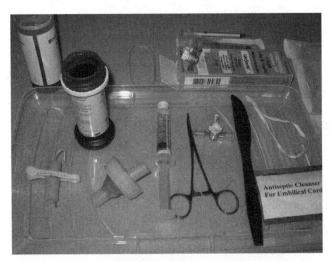

If you do not have a commercial umbilical vessel insertion kit, you can easily assemble essential supplies and create the Medication Station pictured here. This station allows the learner to simulate preparation of the umbilical catheter (in wrapper on right), insertion of the catheter, drawing up epinephrine, and administering epinephrine and volume.

Most newborns who need resuscitation respond quickly to positive-pressure ventilation. Medications are rarely required. The medication skills station provides hands-on practice for these rarely used lifesaving procedures.

It is optimal to use the supplies and equipment that are used in your birth setting to prepare and insert an emergency UVC. If your unit uses a commercial kit, purchase one or obtain one that is clean but would otherwise be discarded. Add missing items, such as pre-filled normal saline syringes (refill with water if necessary) and the size 5F umbilical catheter, which can be reused many times.

If you must simulate the setup with essential items instead of using a commercial kit, your Medication Station may look similar to the photo above. All the supplies for this setup are kept in a clear plastic box. (See page 76.) When in use, the umbilical catheter setup is positioned in the box lid to contain spills.

Supplies for creating a Medication Performance Skills Station
Simulated blood (purchase or make your own)
Bottle filled to top with simulated blood
Bottle nipple with simulated reusable umbilical cord (see directions that
    follow)
Size 5F umbilical catheter
3-way stopcock

Labeled syringe(s) filled with normal saline (or simulated with water)
Antiseptic prep with swab
Umbilical tie (tape)
"Scalpel" (plastic knife or other simulated scalpel)
Forceps
(sterile) Gloves
Sterile drape (desirable)

Create a reusable umbilical cord.

The "umbilicus" can be "cut" and reused many times. Create a reusable umbilicus using the following steps:

- Obtain a plastic bottle that fits a commercial bottle nipple, as pictured.

- Cut the tip off the nipple.

- Obtain a simulated umbilical segment approximately 5- to 6-cm long (available commercially).

- Cut the umbilicus with sharp scissors straight across, leaving the lower umbilical segment approximately 5-cm long.

- Thread this segment through the bottle nipple and screw-on ring.

- Insert the plastic zip tie (cable tie) through an arterial vessel in the other umbilical segment. The plastic tie should protrude through the bottom of the umbilical segment.

- Clamp the plastic cord clamp about one-third from the top of this umbilical segment. This holds the plastic tie in place and simulates the portion of the umbilical cord that is cut and discarded.

- When the umbilicus is set up for practice, insert the plastic tie into the arterial vessel of the lower umbilical setup. This allows the learner to "cut" the umbilicus and discard the upper portion of the umbilical cord, and use the lower portion of the umbilical cord for umbilical catheter insertion.

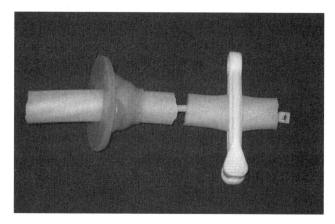

Reusable umbilical segment for practicing emergency umbilical venous catheter placement. The nipple ring goes around the nipple and screws onto the baby bottle. The learner "cuts" the umbilicus in the precut area and separates the top segment from the bottom segment of the cord. The upper segment maintains the plastic zip tie so that the umbilical segment can be reattached to the lower segment for the next learner.

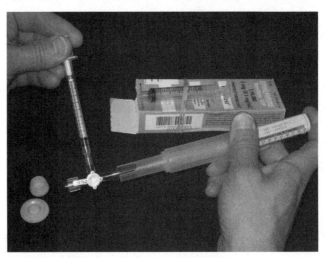

Using a 3-way stopcock to draw up epinephrine

Supplies for Drawing Up Epinephrine

1:10,000 epinephrine

1-mL syringe for intravenous administration

5-mL syringe for intratracheal administration

3-way stopcock or Luer Lock syringe connector

Make a Medication Performance Skills Station Doll

You can create a "manikin" with an endotracheal tube for administration of intratracheal epinephrine and an "umbilicus" for placing an emergency umbilical venous catheter (UVC) and administering epinephrine and volume per the UVC.

Create a Medication/UVC doll by following these steps:

1. Poke a small hole in the lips of the plastic doll and insert an endotracheal tube. Make the hole small enough to make a tight fit. This allows epinephrine administration via the endotracheal tube and also allows practice securing the endotracheal (ET) tube with tape or the tube-securing device used by your hospital.

2. Cut a hole in the back of the doll's head to allow for air circulation and drying of any fluids that enter the doll's head through the ET tube. This helps prevent mold and mildew from forming inside the doll's head.

3. Find a small container, as tall as the anterior-posterior diameter of the doll's chest, to hold the simulated blood. This container will fit into a hole cut into the doll's back, directly across from the doll's

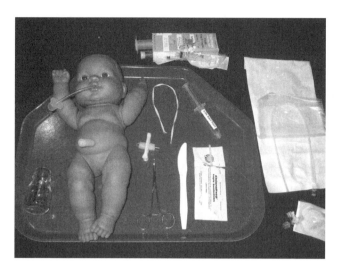

The photograph illustrates a medication station that uses an inexpensive newborn baby doll purchased from a toy store. When ready for use, the glass bottle on the left is filled with simulated blood and sits on the tray and fits in a hole in the doll's back. The simulated umbilicus protrudes into the doll's abdominal cavity and lies in the simulated blood container. The doll is on a plastic cafeteria tray to contain supplies and spills.

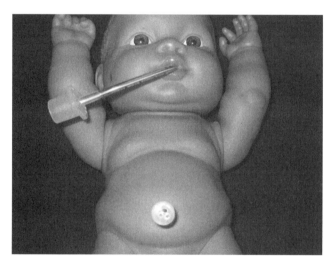

The medication doll has a hole cut in the mouth to hold an endotracheal tube and a hole cut in the location of the umbilicus to hold the umbilical segment. See page 217 for instructions to create a reusable umbilicus for emergency umbilical venous catheter placement.

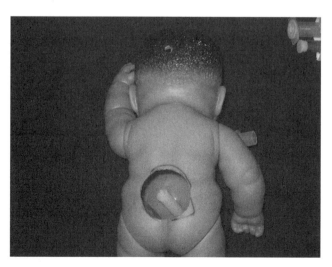

This photo illustrates the small hole cut in the back of the doll's head to allow moisture to evaporate, if necessary, and a hole cut in the doll's back to hold the container of simulated blood. Place the doll carefully over the blood container and ensure that the end of the umbilicus is inside the container of blood.

umbilicus. The doll fits over the top of the container of simulated blood. The glass container pictured on the tray is a small ketchup bottle from a restaurant. If the container is too short, the umbilical segment inserted through the doll's abdomen will need to be too long to realistically simulate insertion of an emergency UVC. The total insertion length of the umbilical catheter, through the umbilicus at the doll's abdomen and into the simulated blood container, should be approximately 5 cm—the depth of insertion for an emergency UVC in a term newborn.

4. Cut a small hole, slightly smaller than the umbilical cord segment in the place where the doll would have an umbilicus. The "umbilicus" fits snugly through this hole and lies just inside the small container of simulated blood. See page 217 for directions about creating a reusable umbilical cord segment for practicing emergency UVC insertion.

5. See page 216 for the supply list to complete your Medication Station.

How to Prepare Umbilical Cords for Skill Stations

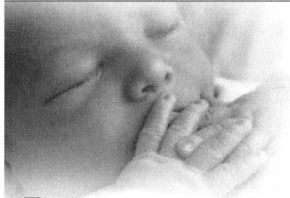

The umbilical vein is the most quickly accessible direct intravenous route in a newborn and may be used in the administration of epinephrine or other medications during resuscitation. Hands-on training on the proper use and handling of umbilical cords is an important skill that can be incorporated into an NRP course.

The Children's Hospital and the University of Colorado Health Sciences Center, Denver, have for some time incorporated skills training with the use of human umbilical cord segments within their NRP courses. "We had, in the past, used human umbilical cord segments and felt in order to continue to use them, we really needed to have a statement that set forth safeguards for the students and recognized, to some extent, the patients who allowed us to do this for training purposes," explained Susan Niermeyer, MD, FAAP, of the University of Colorado Health Sciences Center, Division of Neonatology, in Denver.

"WE HAD, IN THE PAST, USED HUMAN UMBILICAL CORD SEGMENTS AND FELT IN ORDER TO CONTINUE TO USE THEM, WE REALLY NEEDED TO HAVE A STATEMENT THAT SET FORTH SAFEGUARDS FOR THE STUDENTS AND RECOGNIZED, TO SOME EXTENT, THE PATIENTS WHO ALLOWED US TO DO THIS FOR TRAINING PURPOSES."

Based on this need, the institution's policy statement on the proper use and handling of umbilical cords for training was developed several years ago by Sharon Glass, RNC, MS, NNP, Coordinator of Neonatal Nurse Practitioners at The Children's Hospital, Denver, the University of Colorado Hospital, and a network of regional hospitals in Colorado. According to the policy, umbilical cords are provided by donors who sign

an informed consent agreement supplied by hospital personnel. The agreement explains the purpose of the donation, how the baby's umbilical cord will be used for teaching purposes, and that proper handling precautions will be followed at all times. The instructor's signature also appears on the consent agreement.

In order to set up similar training exercises in your institution, various types of equipment are recommended, including, but not limited to, the following:

- Specimen containers
- Label with donor's name and hospital medical records number*
- Normal saline
- 3cc syringes
- Gloves
- Scalpel
- Hemostat
- Baby bottles (glass, if possible)
- Nipples
- Scissors
- Artificial blood
- Umbilical catheter kit

Some helpful hints for teaching the procedure:

Universal precautions in handling human tissue must be used at all times. After obtaining a donor's consent, try to acquire enough umbilical cord from one source (at least 2 inches of cord for each skill station) for use by the entire class. Cords can be stored in the refrigerator, in saline in a covered specimen container, for up to 48 hours. Be sure to label the container with the donor's identification.

Use baby bottles to hold saline colored with the artificial blood. Cut a hole large enough to snugly hold the cord and gently pull a 2-inch piece of cord through the bottle's nipple using the hemostat. There should be about half an inch of cord protruding from the top of the nipple.

This is a good time to practice proper sterile techniques and how to prepare the catheter for insertion into the cord by attaching a stopcock and flushing with a saline-filled syringe. Other hands-on opportunities include flushing the artificial blood from the catheter, moving the stopcock handle back to the closed position, changing syringes and injecting medication, and flushing between medications. At the end of training, be sure to dispose of tissue samples and supplies in the appropriate biohazard containers.

"We incorporate skills training with umbilical cord segments and follow the institution's umbilical cord statement in every NRP instructor course we teach. This is important so instructors can then share the knowledge and hands-on training they've received at the course with their own hospital or institution," Dr. Niermeyer said.

*This information should be available in case of accidental exposure to blood or body fluid, but should not be disclosed to the participants in the training exercise.

(From *NRP Instructor Update.* Vol 16 No 1. spring/summer 2007; p 14.)

Sample Timeline and Details for a Neonatal Resuscitation Program Provider Course

Each of these steps is described in detail beginning on page 224. The timeline is created for use in planning a Neonatal Resuscitation Program Provider Course for community participants. Choose the steps most applicable to your planning needs and make your own course-planning timeline.

Sample Timeline for Neonatal Resuscitation Program Course Preparation*

Choose the tasks applicable to your course.

Setting a date for a course

- ❏ Determine need for course and what type of course (Provider, Hospital-based Instructor, or Regional Trainer Course).
- ❏ Determine need to jointly sponsor or desire to cosponsor with another institution or organization.
- ❏ Select potential participants.
- ❏ Determine date(s) of course.
- ❏ Research continuing education application(s).
  - — Submission deadlines vary from 6 weeks to 12 months prior to offering.

Three to 12 months before the course

- ❏ Prepare mailing list.
- ❏ Arrange and reserve space for practice, if necessary.
- ❏ Select course location.
- ❏ Choose faculty and verify instructor status.
- ❏ Have faculty planning meeting.
- ❏ Notify person who is responsible for staffing/scheduling of the course date to facilitate course attendance.
- ❏ Determine how learners will access the online examination.
- ❏ Prepare budget.
- ❏ Prepare course flyer or announcement.
- ❏ Submit continuing education application(s), if not already done.

Six to 8 weeks before the course

- ❏ Advertise course and mail flyer to participants outside your institution.
- ❏ Order textbooks for participants if you supply them.
- ❏ Order additional Neonatal Resuscitation Program (NRP) supplies if needed.

Four to 6 weeks before the course

- ❏ Begin registration list of participants' names, addresses, and phone numbers.
- ❏ Distribute textbooks (if applicable to your course procedure) with instructions to read and study the textbook and/or accompanying DVD and pass the online examination prior to course.
- ❏ Send confirmation letter and attachments (map, study aids, Experience Survey) as registrations are received.
- ❏ Arrange for food and beverages, if applicable.
- ❏ Order additional course supplies.
- ❏ Inventory equipment and make arrangements to borrow supplies, if necessary.
- ❏ Plan time for faculty planning meeting; plan site visit if teaching at an unfamiliar institution.
- ❏ Arrange opportunity for practice periods, if necessary for your course.

Two weeks before the course

- ❏ Write or request checks for honoraria and other expenses due, if applicable.
- ❏ Review responses to Experience Survey for NRP Provider Course.
- ❏ Prepare written handouts.
- ❏ Prepare administrative handouts and directional signs.
- ❏ Have faculty planning meeting periods, if necessary for your course.
- ❏ Continue opportunities for learners to practice, if necessary for your course.
- ❏ Confirm course date(s) and expectations of instructors.
- ❏ Remind participants of the requirement to study the material and pass the online examination before the course.

One week before the course

- ❏ Collate written handouts for learners.
- ❏ Organize resuscitation supplies to take to classroom.
- ❏ Confirm room reservation, catering arrangements, and audiovisual equipment.

Day of the course

- ❏ Arrive early.
- ❏ Post directional signs.
- ❏ Check classroom and, if necessary, refreshment setup.
- ❏ Set up Performance Skills Stations, Integrated Skills Stations, and area for simulation and debriefing.
- ❏ Test audiovisual equipment.
- ❏ Ensure that you have or can access instructor information for the Course Roster (full name and instructor ID number).

After the course

- ❏ Clean up, restock, and reorganize NRP equipment. Replace and repair equipment, if necessary.
- ❏ Return borrowed equipment.
- ❏ Complete American Academy of Pediatrics (AAP) Course Roster electronically at www.aap.org/nrp, make a copy for your file, and submit to the AAP.
- ❏ Summarize evaluations and distribute to faculty and continuing education provider, if applicable.
- ❏ Make personal notes of what worked well and what to do differently next time.
- ❏ Notify students' supervisors of students' attendance, if necessary.
- ❏ Make copies for your file, then send continuing education forms, evaluation summary, and budget to appropriate parties.
- ❏ Send thank-you notes as appropriate.
- ❏ Complete and distribute NRP Course Completion Cards when received from the AAP.

*The timeline is created for use in planning a comprehensive NRP Provider Course for community participants. Choose the steps most applicable to your planning needs and make your own course-planning timeline.

Sample Timeline Details

Scheduling a Course
What should I know about scheduling my course(s)?

The date you choose for your course(s) plays a major part in its success or failure. Do NOT schedule your course

- The day before or after a holiday weekend

- In close proximity to a major religious holiday

- During a major school holiday, such as spring break

- On the same day as another previously planned educational event or meeting for the same audience of learners

- Near the same day as another course that requires the same group of learners to study ahead of time, such as an Advanced Cardiac Life Support (ACLS) course or a Pediatric Advanced Life Support (PALS) course

Following are other considerations when you choose your course date(s):

- Physicians and certified nurse midwives may prefer a weekend or evening class to a weekday class. This prevents loss of time and income from an office practice.

- Learners are more likely to attend an educational opportunity in the spring and fall months. Learners tend to be busy and less interested in attending class during the winter holiday season and during summer vacation times.

Three to 12 Months Before the Course
What are some ways to prepare my mailing list?

Who is interested in attending your course? If you can accommodate only a small group, do not advertise extensively or use a large mailing list. Target only those people who have expressed an interest in the course or those who have top priority learning needs.

You must have enough instructors to support your learners. *The recommended ratio is one instructor for every 3 to 4 learners.*

To develop a mailing list for learners in your institution only,

- Ask your medical staff support office if you can access its mailing list of potential learners by specialty (eg, the list of pediatricians, obstetricians, nurse practitioners, family practitioners, and nurse midwives who have practice privileges in your institution).

- Ask your hospital education department if you can access mailing lists of learners who have previously attended or expressed interest in pediatric learning opportunities (such as PALS).

- Use your institution's phone directory and medical staff directory as a resource to develop your own mailing list.

- Access the registration list of attendees from a Neonatal Resuscitation Program (NRP) course held about 2 years ago. These people may be interested in renewing their NRP provider status now.

To reach learners outside your institution,

- Use the process of cosponsorship to access learners from more than 1 institution.

- Use your local telephone directory to develop your own mailing list.

- Contact professional nursing or medical associations for a list of members.

- Contact NRP regional trainers who may be aware of persons seeking courses.

- Develop a separate mailing list if some of your NRP Provider Courses target prehospital professionals, such as law enforcement and emergency medical services personnel.

What do I need to know about choosing a location for my NRP course?

Sometimes you will not have much choice about where your NRP course is held. As an NRP instructor, you may need to be flexible and creative under challenging conditions.

If you have some choices of location within your institution, find out about the

- Availability of room(s) on your selected date(s). Ideally, one room is available for the Performance Skills Stations and simulation and another is available for debriefing.

- Size of room(s) and choices for classroom setup.

- Availability of audiovisual equipment (DVD player, laptop, LCD projector).

- Food and beverage policy—Can you bring in your own refreshments from outside sources, such as grocery stores and bakeries; can you hire catering services from outside the institution, or must you use on-site catering facilities?

- Classroom setup, takedown, and cleaning services.

If you are holding your course outside the institution, ensure that

- The proposed area of town is familiar to your audience or an easy-to-read map or directions are available.

- Room size is adequate.

- More than one room is available, if necessary.

- Parking is adequate or public transportation is available.

- Restroom facilities are sufficient for the number of people in your course.

- Setup and takedown services are available.

- Catering is available and affordable, or outside catering is permissible.

- Audiovisual equipment and support are adequate and affordable. This includes
  - Adequate size and location of a wall or screen for projection, including a screen larger than 21 inches for visibility for large groups.
  - Adequate number of electrical outlets and extension cords.
  - Ability to support electronic media presentations.

- Location does not preclude transportation of equipment to the site.

- Location does not preclude receiving deliveries (eg, air or oxygen tanks) at the site.

- Cancellation policy is clearly stated and meets your needs.

- Total cost to use this facility is within your budget.

What should I know about choosing faculty for my course?

Instructors for NRP courses must meet the training requirements outlined in the following table.

Course Level	Instructor Must Be
Provider Course	Hospital-based instructor or regional trainer.
Hospital-based Instructor Course	Regional trainer. (Hospital-based instructors may assist, if needed.)
Regional Trainer Course	Regional trainer. (Hospital-based instructors may assist, if needed.)

In addition, instructors should have a grasp of adult learning principles. They should be enthusiastic and supportive of all learning styles. Instructors should be confident of their resuscitation skills and their teaching skills and be able to convey their knowledge in an engaging and supportive manner.

What happens at the first course-planning meeting?

Request that all faculty bring the following:

- Neonatal Resuscitation Program instructor number.

- Curriculum vitae.

- Name, credentials, and institutional affiliation as they wish to see it printed on the course flyer. These items will help you get started on continuing education applications and the course flyer.

- Personal and professional calendars for scheduling future meetings.

You and your course faculty should discuss and answer the following questions:

- Do the course date(s) and time(s) work for faculty members?

- Who are your targeted learners?

- What are the course objectives?

- If this course involves joint sponsorship, are both institutions/ organizations adequately represented?

- Who will supply or arrange for NRP course equipment and supplies?

- What is the schedule for the day?

- Are guest lecturers who are not NRP instructors needed to present supplementary content, such as pharmacology or sequelae of perinatal asphyxia? (These lecturers are not listed on the NRP Course Roster.)

- Who is available for supervised practice before the course?

- Are all instructors staying for the full length of the course?

- Who requires an honorarium? What amount? What is the payment process?

- How do others charge for their time?

- Are faculty disclosure statements needed? This is a form signed by faculty to disclose any conflict of interest or financial involvement or gain from the course information or recommended equipment (often necessary when your course has been approved for continuing education credit). Who is responsible for distributing and submitting these forms?

How do I prepare a budget?

Most educational programs are required to submit a budget to some type of authoritative body. Requirements for budgetary components will vary. Your NRP may be a service provided at no charge for participants within your region. Your NRP may be a planned expense for your department's fiscal budget. In any case, a projected budget will help you plan expenses and calculate costs. A sample budget worksheet is located on page 238 of this Appendix.

What is important to know about flyer development?

Your program announcement gives the learner his or her first impression of your course. It is important that your flyer is attractive and easy to read, and that it presents a clear picture of the course you are offering. Your organization may have specific requirements for flyer design and components. If not, collect different types of flyers from other offerings and analyze their strong and weak points, and then design a flyer of your own.

Your course announcement should answer the following questions:

- What is your course about?

- What are the course objectives?

- What are the responsibilities of the learners?

- What are the requirements for successful completion of the course?

- What is the day of the week, date, and time of the course?

- What is the course agenda?

- Where will it be held? (Include a map if offered to learners outside your institution.)

- Who should attend?

- Why should learners attend?

- Who is teaching and what qualifies the main speakers as experts?

- What is the cost, if any?

- Are there cost variations (eg, program free of charge to institution employees, reduced cost to students)?

- What does registration include (textbook, online examination, lunch)?

- Is registration limited to a certain number of registrants?

- Are continuing education credits granted (or is the application pending approval)? What types of credits are offered? (Inquire about specific wording that may be required in the flyer by the organization granting the continuing education credits.)

- How will the learner obtain the *Textbook of Neonatal Resuscitation, 6th Edition,* and/or the *Instructor Manual for Neonatal Resuscitation* and other required materials? If learners are required to obtain their own textbooks, include information on how to best do that and how long it takes to receive the books.

- When and where are skills practice sessions held? If supervised, when are instructors available?

- What is the cancellation policy?

- How do participants register and pay (fax, e-mail, check, credit card)?

- What is the registration mailing address?

- What is the registration cutoff date?

- Who is the contact person in case the registrant has questions about the course?

Components of an attractive course announcement include the following:

- Correct spelling and punctuation.

- Correct month, date, and year of offering.

- Organization for fast and easy comprehension.

- Attractive font.
  - Simple and easy to read, not overcrowded with multiple fonts and graphics.

- Adequate "white space."

- If photos or graphics are used, they are clear and appropriate images for the subject matter. (Copyrighted materials, such as the American Academy of Pediatrics [AAP] and American Heart Association [AHA] logo or the NRP logo, cannot be used on course announcements.)

- Designed so that important information, such as the date, time, place, or map, is not cut off or lost when the participant mails in the registration form.

Six to 8 Weeks Before the Course
What are possible ways to advertise my course?

Within your institution,

- Post the course announcement on major bulletin boards, in staff elevators, and in the cafeteria.

- Use interdepartmental mail and institutional e-mail to deliver course announcements to people and departments other than your own.

- Ask department managers and the medical staff support office about the possibility of delivering a course announcement to staff mailboxes.

- Talk about your course at unit staff meetings.

- Submit a course announcement to the editor of your hospital newsletter.

To hospitals and other institutions within your area,

- Mail a packet of announcements to neonatal nursing units and medical clinic practices that may be interested in your course.

- Use the process of cosponsorship to deliver brochures to more than one institution.

- Send course announcements to medical schools, residency programs, and schools of nursing.

- Send course announcements to the newsletter editors of local nursing and medical associations in your area.

🖥**www** • Post your course on the NRP Web site at **www.aap.org/nrp.**

A few additional points to consider:

- Have you included the faculty members on the mailing list?

- Do you want the flyer mailed to your administrators as a way to promote your work?

- Have you met any special requirements for mail that is sent from your organization or institution?

- Have you saved several flyers for your own files? You also will need a few extra to include in your continuing education applications.

I'm still working on the application(s) for continuing education credits. Am I running out of time?

Time is running short for approval of your application. It may come back to you for corrections before approval is given. Do not delay this step any longer or you risk the ability to grant continuing education credits at all.

How do I order the *Textbook of Neonatal Resuscitation, 6th Edition,* and other NRP supplies?

Each learner is required to have access to a copy of the *Textbook of Neonatal Resuscitation, 6th Edition.* It can be provided by the hospital or purchased by the participant. Because the NRP requires self-study, the participant will need to have the book about a month before the beginning of a course or evaluation. Each textbook includes a DVD that presents the content of the textbook in an expandable, interactive multimedia format.

Anyone can order the *Textbook of Neonatal Resuscitation, 6th Edition,* and the *Instructor Manual for Neonatal Resuscitation,* from the AAP.

Call the AAP Publications Division at 888/227-1770 (847/434-4000 outside the United States) for more information, or order from the
🖥**www** AAP Web site (**www.aap.org/bookstorepubs.html**).

Instructors can order these items from the AAP by

Phone
888/227-1770 (847/434-4000 outside the United States)

Mail
AAP Publications
PO Box 747
Elk Grove Village, IL 60009-0747

Fax
847/228-1281

Internet
www.aap.org/bookstorepubs.html   🖥www

Other ways instructors and students can obtain the textbook:

- The institution purchases the textbook for each employee who requires it.

- The institution has a loaner program.

- Students purchase a personal copy of the textbook.

- A regional outreach education program may have a stock of books for sale.

- A regional outreach education program may have a book loan program.

- A university bookstore may carry the textbook, especially if the university offers health care studies.

- Students purchase the textbook from an online bookstore.

Optional supplies available from the AAP:

- *Textbook of Neonatal Resuscitation, 6th Edition, Spanish Version*

- NRP Wall Chart

- NRP Key Behavioral Skills poster

- NRP Code Cart Cards

- NRP Pocket Cards

- NRP Provider Pins

- NRP Instructor Pins

What other supplies do I need to order now?

Think about

- Name tags

- Folders for class materials

- Pens

Four to 6 Weeks Before the Course
Registrations are beginning to come in. What should I do now?

Elicit administrative support, if possible. It is helpful to have one central phone number where a person is available during business hours to answer questions about the course or to take a message for a course coordinator or lead instructor. As registrations are received,

- Log the registrant's name, address, phone number, and professional discipline (MD, RN, RT, etc). This is important for completing the NRP Course Roster. You also will use this information for sending each registrant a confirmation letter, creating an attendance sign-in sheet, and mailing the participant an NRP Course Completion Card after the course. You also may need an identifying number for continuing education credit. This may be the registrant's professional license number, or some other identifier as required by the accrediting organization.

- Do not throw away anyone's registration form. File it in a folder specified for this purpose.

- If applicable, log the amount of money received and method of payment.

- If applicable, follow your institution's protocol for depositing registration moneys.

Send a confirmation letter and attachments as registrations are received. This letter (sample on page 240) serves to

- Confirm receipt of the registration and fee. This may seem obvious, but, if the registration was sent by the learner's supervisor or by someone from another department in the institution, the confirmation letter might be the only way the participant knows that the registration process is complete.

- Remind registrants of the class date, time, and location.

- Reiterate important information, such as what NRP material needs to be completed prior to the course.

- Inform students what to bring to class.

- Provide a way to mail additional attachments to the learner, such as the following:
    - Schedule of supervised or independent practice periods
    - *Textbook of Neonatal Resuscitation, 6th Edition*
    - Study aids, such as a list of Key Points from each lesson in the *Textbook of Neonatal Resuscitation, 6th Edition* (see Appendix E)
    - Experience Survey (see page 214)

- Provide a contact person's name and telephone number for additional information, if needed by the registrant.

What if I need to borrow equipment for my course?

It is smart to inventory your equipment well before your course date. This is the time to make sure you have enough equipment in good working order to run a course of the expected size. If you need to borrow equipment, check with

- The regional education outreach program in your area
- Neighboring hospitals
- The fire department or law enforcement agencies who conduct cardiopulmonary resuscitation training
- Schools of medicine and nursing
- Local nursing and medical associations

What are the objectives of the planning meeting I arrange now?

This meeting (in person or by telephone) is usually necessary to

- Confirm delegated responsibilities.
- Review progress of registration.
- Review the detailed plan for the day of the course.
  - Responsibilities of the lead instructor
  - Responsibilities of assistant instructors
  - Time allotted to each section of the course
  - Assignments for Performance Skills Stations, Integrated Skills Stations, and Simulation and Debriefing.
- Plan a site visit or telephone assessment if you will be teaching in an institution unfamiliar to you. Learn who resuscitates newborns and how responsibilities are delegated, what kind of equipment is used, and what the participants hope to gain from the NRP course.
- Schedule supervised practice sessions, if necessary for your course format. Consider the following:
  - A sign-up sheet for participants. Ask that participants sign up in advance. This prevents instructors from waiting for learners who never show up.
  - Various times of the day and various days of the week. Participants are more likely to come to a practice session before or after their shift.
  - Participants will be more likely to come to practice sessions as the day of the course grows near.

How can I best use the lunch break for continued learning?

The lunch break offers time to network and an opportunity to gain insight into how participants view resuscitation, barriers to performing effectively, and participants' level of self-efficacy. If learners leave the site to have lunch, encourage groups to mingle and include others. Lunch options include the following:

- On your own. (Allow 90 minutes for lunch if people must use transportation to find lunch.)

- On-site box lunch catered by your institution or an outside source.

Two Weeks Before the Course

Is it time to pay the bills?

If you have not already done so, write or request checks for honoraria, facilities, or miscellaneous expenses.

I know every instructor's set of course materials will be a little different. What are the typical course handouts?

- Schedule for the day (see page 245)

- Neonatal Resuscitation Program Individual Recording Sheet (see page 245)

- Course evaluation form (see pages 247-248)

- Envelope for participants to self-address so that the instructor can easily mail successful participants the NRP Course Completion Card after it is received from the AAP Life Support office

What other written materials are needed for the administrative portions of the course?

- Attendance sheet or some type of sign-in sheet to document attendance.

- Certificate of attendance—usually not necessary if NRP Course Completion Card or continuing education certificate is distributed.

- Course evaluation form. (See pages 247-248.)
  - Every institution has its own format for course evaluation. In addition, find out if the accrediting agency has specific requirements for wording on the evaluation form. If your evaluation form fails to meet the requirements of the accrediting agency, you may lose the ability to grant continuing education credits.
  - A course evaluation form should include space for comments and suggestions and some sort of evaluative scoring for assessing the following:
    - If course objectives were met
    - If personal objectives were met

How the learner will utilize what was learned

- Quality of speaker(s) and instructor(s)

- Quality of presentation, such as audiovisual material, class handouts, and textbooks

- Quality of learning environment

Do I need another faculty meeting now?

Some lead instructors need a final meeting to iron out last-minute details. Instructors should know the following:

- Where and when to come on the day of the course

- How to account for their time or method of payment for services

- Time schedule for the course

- Who is attending the course (skill level, professional level)

- Any accommodations for registrants with special needs

People are beginning to attend the supervised practice periods. Is there anything else I need to know?

Attendance may climb as the course date gets closer. You may need to schedule extra time or instructors to staff the practice site this week.

One Week Before the Course

What are my last-minute preparations for written handouts, resuscitation supplies, and practice periods?

Do not save all your course preparation until a day or 2 before class. Things can come up that will prevent you from having time to adequately prepare. Absence from work, missing equipment, and broken copy machines are only a few examples of unexpected problems that cause stressful pre-course emergencies.

- Collate written handouts for learners and place the attendance sheet on top of the stack. Place handouts in folders or put them together with a rubber band in a box. On the course day, simply unload your box and arrange your written materials on your tables.

- Organize resuscitation supplies to take to the classroom.

- Collect all your supplies. Gather posters, DVDs, and other materials.

- Continue supervised practice periods for your course, if necessary.

- Confirm your room reservation, food or catering provisions, and audiovisual equipment. Know whom to contact if things are not as expected on course day.

One Day Before the Course

Can you set up your classroom today and lock the room? This will save you a lot of time and stress on course day. If not, how will you transport your equipment to the classroom? Do you need carts? Do you need extra help to transport equipment to the site? Do you need to load your car today?

Day of the Course

- Arrive early.

- Post directional signs if your course location is unfamiliar to registrants. Signs should be printer processed, not handwritten. A sign written in felt marker and hung crooked with a ragged piece of masking tape will not make a good first impression or promote confidence in the day.

- Notify the hosting facility's information desk and switchboard of the exact location of the course, in case participants ask for directions.

- Ensure that the classroom is set up correctly. Avoid theater or classroom style for the interactive portion of the day. If necessary, rearrange tables and chairs or call your facilities contact to correct the room setup.

- Locate restrooms, telephones, emergency exits, and the closest fire alarm pull station.

- Set up refreshments or, if catered, ensure that your order is correct and well presented.

- Put out attendance sheet, student handout materials, name tags, and pens.

- Ask that assistant instructors fill out a sign-in form with their correct name, address, and instructor identification number.

- Set up practice stations, if necessary.

- Familiarize yourself with the classroom audiovisual equipment, if necessary.

Learn how to operate heating/ventilation/air-conditioning or whom to contact for adjustments.

- − Familiarize yourself with room lights and dimmers.
- − Practice using the microphone or lavalier microphone.

- When course participants arrive,
  - − Introduce yourself and assistant instructors.
  - − Tell learners about locations of restrooms, telephones, and snack/beverage machines.

- Discuss the objectives of the course and how you plan to meet those objectives.
- Discuss guidelines for the day (schedule, organization of practice/performance stations, lunch plan, if applicable).
- Go over written handout material.
- Clarify instructions for attendance sheets and continuing education credits.
- Be friendly, supportive, and professional.
- Stay on schedule.
- Encourage learner participation. If your course is a small- or medium-sized group of learners from different settings, have participants introduce themselves to the group.

After the Course

- Make a remedial plan for learners who did not meet the performance objectives.

- Clean up, restock, and reorganize course materials and equipment. Clean and return borrowed equipment. Replace or repair damaged equipment, if necessary.

- Complete the online NRP Course Roster form, make a copy for your own files, and submit the Roster to the AAP. (Instructions for administrative responsibilities are in Chapter 10.)

- Summarize course evaluations. Make personal notes of what worked well and what to do differently next time.

- Distribute evaluation summary to interested parties (your manager, participating instructors, sponsoring parties).

- Notify learners' supervisors of learners' attendance at class, if necessary.

- Pay bills as necessary. Ensure that instructors and lecturers receive payment as arranged.

- File continuing education paperwork, pay fees, and complete any processes as designated by the accrediting agency.

- Complete and distribute NRP Course Completion Cards when received from the AAP. Remember that the AAP sends Instructor Cards directly to the course participants, not to the regional trainer who taught the course.

- Send thank-you notes to guest lecturers and others who made your course possible.

Sample Projected Budget Worksheet

Customize this worksheet to include your projected expenses.

Expenses	Subtotal	Total
Staff expenses		
Conference coordinator	____ hours of preparation time at $____ per hour ____ hours of teaching time at $____ per hour	
Neonatal Resuscitation Program (NRP) instructor 1	____ hours of preparation time at $____ per hour ____ hours of teaching time at $____ per hour	
NRP instructor 2	____ hours of preparation time at $____ per hour ____ hours of teaching time at $____ per hour	
Administrative support	____ hours at $____ per hour	
Faculty honorarium	____ faculty at $____ each	
	Total staff expenses	

Supply expenses		
Brochure/flyer printing	____ brochures/flyers at $____	
Textbook of Neonatal Resuscitation *Instructor Manual for Neonatal Resuscitation*	____ textbooks at $____ (including shipping) ____ manuals at $____ (including shipping)	
Fee for online NRP examinations, if necessary	____ online examinations at $____	
NRP optional supplies (wall charts, pocket cards, etc)		
Miscellaneous course supplies (name tags, folders, pencils, written handouts)	____ name tags at $____ ____ folders at $____ ____ pencils at $____	
	Total supply expenses	

Facility expenses		
General meeting room and breakout room	$____ + $____	
Audiovisual support	$____	
Catering	Service per registrant	
Morning: coffee, tea, light refreshment	$____ x ____ registrants	
Afternoon: beverages, light refreshment	$____ x ____ registrants	
	Total facility expenses	

Miscellaneous expenses		
Mailing, correspondence		
Parking lot passes for faculty/participants	$____ x ____ faculty members	
	Total miscellaneous expenses	
	Total expenses	
Registration fee	$____ per participant (including text) $____ per participant (not including text)	

Divide course expenses by proposed number of registrants to establish the registration fee.

Course requires _____ registrants at $_____ per person to maintain a neutral budget.

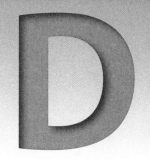

Neonatal Resuscitation Program™ Provider Course

SAMPLE LETTER FOR NEONATAL RESUSCITATION PROGRAM COURSE PARTICIPANTS

Hospital logo

Welcome to the American Academy of Pediatrics/American Heart Association Neonatal Resuscitation Program™ (NRP™) course. While this course does not guarantee proficiency during an actual resuscitation, it lays the foundation of knowledge, technical skills, and teamwork and communication skills that enable participants to continue development of neonatal resuscitation skills. Successful completion earns the participant an NRP Provider Card. Neonatal Resuscitation Program provider status should be renewed every 2 years.

Prior to the course, you must read the *Textbook of Neonatal Resuscitation, 6ᵗʰ Edition* (or view the DVD that accompanies the textbook) and **pass the NRP online examination.** You may find it helpful to go to **www.aap.org/nrp** and read the resources under the Online Examination tab.

We are expecting you

Date: _____

Time: _____

Location: _____

This is a hands-on interactive course. You successfully pass the course after you

- Produce your online examination verification from the NRP online examination on course day. You are assigned

_____ *Lessons 1-4* and *Lesson 9*

_____ *Lessons 1-9*

_____ *Lessons 1-4,* _____, _____, _____, _____, and *Lesson 9*

- Demonstrate the above assigned neonatal resuscitation lessons within the context of a clinical scenario in correct sequence according to the NRP flow diagram, with correct timing and proper technique. Use the Integrated Skills Assessment Checklist (Basic or Advanced) in the textbook as your guide.

- Participate in simulation training and debriefing exercises.

Information About NRP Online Examination

Bring your online examination verification to your NRP Course.

To access the NRP online examination *(instructor fills in information appropriate to the institutional process),* _____

You must take the online examination at your convenience on any computer prior to your NRP course, during the **30 days before the course. You must finish testing within 14 days of your original start date. If you complete the examination more than 30 days before your scheduled course, the examination is invalid and you must pay to take it again.**

This test covers the material in Lessons 1 through 9 the *Textbook of Neonatal Resuscitation, 6ᵗʰ Edition.* The test is not difficult for learners who focus on each lesson's Key Points and know the correct answers to each lesson's Review section (practice test). Most new learners require several hours of study time. You may not agree with the NRP approach to every clinical scenario. We will allow discussion time at the course for these differences in opinion.

Please note: Lessons 1 through 4 and Lesson 9 are required Lessons. Once you complete the final required lesson, the examination is considered complete, and you will not have the opportunity to test on additional lessons. To prevent being shut out of the examination prior to taking all the required lesson examinations for your course, take the Lesson 9 examination last.

The average time to complete the full examination (all 9 lessons) is 55 minutes. The online test is arranged by lesson, in the same order as in the textbook. You may skip questions and come back to them. You may change your answers on any question until you submit the lesson for grading. The computer scores each lesson as you submit answers. You may stop testing after a lesson, and resume testing later.

If you do not attain a passing score (80%) for a lesson, you may retake that section immediately, or on a different day, **within 14 days** of the original testing date. After 14 days, the online testing becomes invalid and requires payment to begin again.

You may retake sections ONE time. If you fail a second time, contact _____ at _____ to make a new plan. If you do not finish testing or cannot pass the test prior to the course start time, you may practice hands-on skills at the course with other learners, but you will not receive your NRP provider status on this course day.

The registration for online examination will ask if you have designated an NRP instructor for the in-person components of the NRP Provider Course. The answer is YES. You do not need to name the instructor.

After completing the examination, you will receive online examination verification. **Bring this with you to the NRP course** and give it to the instructor. If you cannot produce online examination verification, you cannot receive NRP provider status at this course.

If you have questions about this NRP course or online examination process, contact

_____ at _____ (phone) or

_____ (e-mail).

Sample NRP Provider Course Agenda #1

Learners: Community Hospital Physicians, Special Care Nursery RNs, and Labor and Delivery RNs

Time	Activity	Notes
8:00-8:15 am	Introductions, paperwork.	Ensure that all learners have online examination verification. Orient learners to written materials, such as confidentiality agreement.
8:15-8:20 am	What NRP is, what it is not.	The NRP is not a certification course. Learners may practice all skills, but must stay within the designated scope of practice during actual resuscitation. Learners renew provider status every 2 years.
8:20-8:30 am	How the day works.	Course requirements: What do learners need to do? This may vary depending on learners' needs. See Table 3-1 for examples. (See sample script on page 86.)
8:30-8:45 am	"What's the Baby Doing Now?"	Orientation to breathing, heart rate, oximetry. Allow learners to see, hear, and touch manikin and methods of physiologic feedback, such as metronome. Orient to supplies and equipment.
8:45-8:55 am	Demonstrate simulation and debriefing using short scenario.	Allow learners to see how learners prepare for resuscitation, talk through actions as they perform them (no pretending), receive physiologic feedback from the manikin, and observe instructor/learner roles during debriefing.
8:55-9:00 am	Divide into teams based on learning needs.	Each team of 3 or 4 learners is assigned an instructor who is aware of the group's learning objectives.
9:00-11:50 am Instructor manages time for each component based on learners' needs	Each instructor has a complete resuscitation setup and manikin, and takes the team of 3 or 4 learners through Performance Skills Stations in place. Rotate to Laryngeal Mask Airway Performance Skills Station. Rotate to Medication Performance Skills Station.	Each team progresses at its own pace. In this course, the Laryngeal Mask Airway and Medication Performance Skills Stations are separate stations so that each learner can have a setup and practice/review the procedure simultaneously. If each team has one setup for laryngeal mask airway placement and one setup for umbilical venous catheter line placement and medications, learners must practice one person at a time.
	Integrated Skills Stations in progress.	The NRP instructor decides when each learner is ready for the Integrated Skills Station.
	Simulation and Debriefing in progress.	The NRP instructor may conduct Simulation and Debriefing at the same station where practice and learning occurred, or at a different station with additional instructor assistance.
11:50 am-12:00 noon	Evaluation and adjournment.	Learners turn in their Individual Recording Sheet, online examination verification, and course evaluation.

Sample NRP Course Agenda #2

Learners: Neonatal nurse practitioners, neonatal intensive care unit (NICU) RNs, and respiratory therapists who are the Delivery Room Resuscitation Team in a Busy Level III setting. *Prior to the course, instructors and the NICU Resuscitation Team collaborated on what to include at a "Delivery Room Management of the ELBW Infant" Performance Skills Station (based on the Resuscitation Skills Video of the same name in the textbook DVD) to meet this team's learning needs.*

Time	Activity	Notes
8:00-8:15 am	Introductions, paperwork.	Ensure that all learners have online examination verification. Orient learners to written materials such as confidentiality agreement.
8:15-8:20 am	What NRP is, what it is not.	The NRP is not a certification course. Learners may practice all skills but must stay within designated scope of practice during actual resuscitation. Learners renew provider status every 2 years.
8:20-8:30 am	How the day works.	Course requirements: What do learners need to do? (NRP instructors assessed the group's needs and selected specific Performance Skills Stations.)
8:30-8:45 am	"What's the Baby Doing Now?"	Orientation to breathing, heart rate, oximetry. Allow learners to see, hear, and touch manikin and methods of physiologic feedback, such as metronome. Orient to supplies and equipment.
8:45-8:55 am	Demonstrate simulation and debriefing using short scenario.	Allow learners to see how learners prepare for resuscitation, talk through actions as they perform them (no pretending), receive physiologic feedback from the manikin, and observe instructor/learner roles during debriefing.
8:55-9:00 am	Divide into teams composed of typical resuscitation team (NNP, 2 RNs, RT for this course).	Each team of 3 or 4 learners is assigned an instructor who is aware of the group's learning objectives.
9:00-10:00 am	Four teams rotate to 4 stations. (Instructors added Station 4 to this course based on learners' needs and followed recommendations in the *NRP Instructor DVD* Resuscitation Skills videos of the same title.)	Station 1: Intubation Performance Skills Station (including meconium management) Station 2: Medication Performance Skills Station Station 3: Laryngeal Mask Airway Performance Skills Station Station 4: The ELBW: Aspects of Delivery Room Management (additional station created by NRP instructors)
10:00-10:30 am	Integrated Skills Stations in Progress.	The NRP instructor decides when each learner is ready for the Integrated Skills Station.
10:30-11:50 am	Simulation and Debriefing in Progress.	The NRP instructor may conduct Simulation and Debriefing at the same station where practice and learning occurred, or at a different station with additional instructor assistance.
11:50 am-noon	Evaluation and adjournment.	Learners turn in their Individual Recording Sheet, online examination verification, and course evaluation.

Diagram for Sample Neonatal Resuscitation Program Course Setup

Neonatal Resuscitation Program™ Provider Course Individual Recording Sheet: Sample
(hospital name)

RETURN THIS SHEET TO ANY INSTRUCTOR AT THE END OF THE COURSE

Provider Course Date: _____

Name: _____

Credentials: RN MSN NNP RT MD DO PA Other _____

Mailing Address (your NRP™ Provider Card will be *mailed in an envelope* to you at this address, if necessary): _____

Phone or e-mail: _____ Hospital: _____

_____ NRP online examination verification received

_____ **Lessons 1-9** _____ **Lessons 1-4 and Lesson 9** _____ **Lessons 1-4, 9 and** _____

Performance Skills Stations

Instructor Initials

_____ Equipment Check

_____ Initial Steps

_____ Positive-Pressure Ventilation

_____ Chest Compressions

_____ Intubation (perform or assist)

_____ Laryngeal Mask Airway

_____ Draw up epinephrine

_____ Administer epinephrine via endotracheal tube

_____ Administer epinephrine via emergency umbilical venous catheter (UVC)

_____ Prepare emergency UVC for placement

_____ Place or assist with placement of emergency UVC

_____ **Integrated Skills Station** _____ **Basic** _____ **Advanced**

_____ **Simulation and Debriefing**

INSTRUCTOR INITIALS/SIGNATURES

_____ _____ _____ _____

_____ _____ _____ _____

Instructor Reminder: Participant must pass all components of the course within 1 month of beginning the NRP online examination.

_____ Participant's name recorded on AAP Course Roster

_____ Instructors' names recorded on AAP Course Roster

Master Recording Sheet

American Academy of Pediatrics/American Heart Association Neonatal Resuscitation Program™ Provider Course

Date of course _____ Course location _____

Lead instructor _____ Asst. instructor _____

Asst. instructor _____ Asst. instructor _____

Continuing education credit awarded _____ _____ _____

Place a check in the appropriate box of each completed course component.

Student Name	Online examination verification received	Lessons 1-4 and Lesson 9	Lessons 1 through 9	Lessons 1-4, 9 and _____ (additional)	Performance Skills Stations Lessons 1-4, 5, 6	Integrated Skills Station BASIC or ADVANCED	Simulation and Debriefing	Date completed (if different than course date)

Neonatal Resuscitation Program™ Provider Course Evaluation: Sample 1

(hospital name)

Date: _____

Course Title: Neonatal Resuscitation Program (NRP™) Provider Course

Course Objectives

1. Demonstrate understanding of neonatal resuscitation key concepts by successfully completing the NRP online examination.

2. Name the most important and effective action in neonatal resuscitation.

3. Demonstrate appropriate resuscitation procedures in proper sequence for a compromised newborn.

4. Through simulation-based training, identify neonatal resuscitation skills and aspects of teamwork that are well-developed, and those that require continuing improvement.

1. Did the course meet the written objectives? ❏ Yes ❏ No

2. Did the course meet your personal objectives? ❏ Yes ❏ No

Please rate the following with 1=lowest/5=highest. Low High

3. Course expectations and requirements were clear. 1 2 3 4 5

4. The textbook or textbook DVD was useful. 1 2 3 4 5

5. My NRP instructor(s) was knowledgeable, supportive, and facilitated my learning. 1 2 3 4 5

6. The Performance Skills Stations were useful. 1 2 3 4 5

7. The environment was conducive to learning. 1 2 3 4 5

8. The information was useful to your work setting. 1 2 3 4 5

9. What was the best part of this course?

10. What needs improvement?

Neonatal Resuscitation Program™ Provider Course Evaluation: Sample 2

(hospital name)

Date: _____

Course Title: Neonatal Resuscitation Program (NRP™) Provider Course

Please rate the following:	Very Satisfied 5	4	3	2	Very Dissatisfied 1
1. Overall rating of this offering	❏	❏	❏	❏	❏
2. Your expectations/objectives were met	❏	❏	❏	❏	❏
3. Applicability of course to your practice	❏	❏	❏	❏	❏
4. Registration procedure	❏	❏	❏	❏	❏
5. Ease of accessing NRP online examination	❏	❏	❏	❏	❏
6. Simulation and debriefing experience	❏	❏	❏	❏	❏

Instructor's Name _____

Mastery of NRP knowledge and skills	❏	❏	❏	❏	❏
Ability to listen, communicate well	❏	❏	❏	❏	❏
Ability to create a safe supportive learning environment	❏	❏	❏	❏	❏

Instructor's Name _____

Mastery of NRP knowledge and skills	❏	❏	❏	❏	❏
Audience to listen, communicate well	❏	❏	❏	❏	❏
Ability to create a safe supportive learning environment	❏	❏	❏	❏	❏

What did you like most about this program?

What could we improve about this program?

How did you learn about this program?

Additional comments:

Neonatal Resuscitation Program™ Provider Card Mailing: Sample Letter

(hospital logo)

Thank you for participating in a Neonatal Resuscitation Program (NRP™) course at

_____ Hospital. Please find your enclosed NRP Provider Course Completion Card.

Your NRP instructor will register you online as an NRP provider with the American Academy of Pediatrics and report the course date. Your NRP provider status is current for 2 years.

To comply with our hospital requirements, you need to take your next NRP Provider

Course by _____(month) _____(day) _____(year).

Or (instructor modifies letter to meet learners' needs)

Find out when your organization expects you to take another NRP Provider Course. Although the American Academy of Pediatrics (AAP) expects you to take your next NRP Provider Course 2 years from now, by the end of the month in which you took your course, some hospitals have different requirements.

The AAP will remind you of your need to take your next Provider Course if you register for a renewal reminder e-mail. Go to www.aap.org/nrp and click on Provider Resources.

Thank you again for participating in our NRP course. Please let me know if you have questions or if I can be of any assistance with your Neonatal Resuscitation Program.

Sincerely,

(Name)

NRP Regional Trainer

(Contact information)

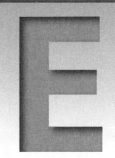

Performance Skills Checklists and Textbook Key Points

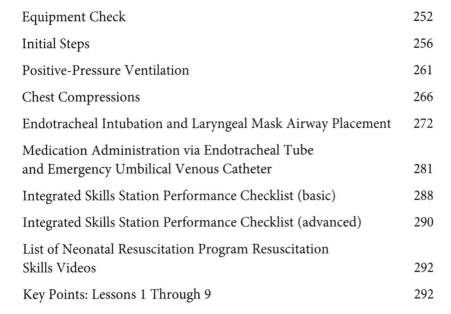

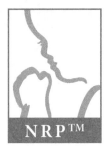

Lesson 1: Equipment Check Performance Checklist

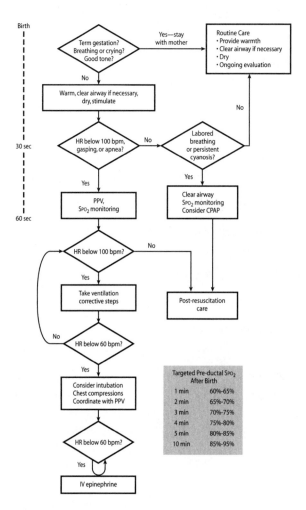

The Performance Checklist Is a Learning Tool

The learner uses the checklist as a reference during independent practice, or as a guide for discussion and practice with a Neonatal Resuscitation Program™ (NRP™) instructor. When the learner and instructor agree that the learner can perform the skills correctly and smoothly without coaching and within the context of a scenario, the learner may move on to the next lesson's Performance Checklist.

This Equipment Check Performance Checklist includes only the most essential supplies and equipment for neonatal resuscitation. You may wish to add supplies or additional safety checks to meet your unit's standards or protocols. When the learner knows the routine and supplies are present and functioning, the Equipment Check should take approximately 1 minute to complete.

Knowledge Check

- Why is it important to have an organized routine for checking the presence and function of resuscitation supplies and equipment prior to every birth?

- Besides checking presence and function of equipment, what other resources should be assembled prior to a birth identified as high-risk?

Learning Objectives

1. Demonstrate an organized routine for checking presence and function of supplies and equipment necessary for newborn resuscitation, using the NRP flow diagram interventions as your guide.

2. Identify any additional preparatory routines for high-risk birth specific to this birth setting.

3. Locate the Quick Pre-resuscitation Checklist on page 380.

"You are notified that a woman has been admitted to the hospital in active labor. Check your supplies and equipment to prepare for the birth. As you work, say your thoughts and actions aloud so I will know what you are thinking and doing."

Instructor should check boxes as the learner responds correctly. The learner may refer to this checklist or the Quick Pre-resuscitation Checklist that follows it to ensure the availability and function of essential supplies and equipment.

Performance Steps	Details
Warm: ☐ Preheat warmer ☐ Lay out towels or blankets	Learner begins with equipment needed for initial steps of resuscitation and ends with equipment needed for complex resuscitation.
Clear the airway 3 ways: ☐ Bulb syringe ☐ 10F or 12F suction catheter attached to wall suction, set at 80-100 mm Hg ☐ Meconium aspirator	Turns on wall suction to "continuous" and occludes suction tubing; adjusts suction to 80-100 mm Hg.
Auscultate ☐ Stethoscope	Picks up stethoscope, places in ears, and taps on diaphragm to ensure function.

Performance Steps	Details
Oxygenate ☐ Turn on oxygen flowmeter to 5-10 L/min	If birth is imminent, suction and air/oxygen should be turned on and ready for use.
☐ Adjust blender to hospital standard for initiation of resuscitation	Are air/O_2 tanks full, if used in your setting?
☐ Pulse oximeter probe ☐ Pulse oximeter	Safety Check: Even if beginning resuscitation with 21% oxygen, the air/oxygen flow should be turned on in the event that supplemental oxygen is needed. A self-inflating bag will work even without gas flow; therefore, turn on air/oxygen so that gas is flowing if blender is turned up to administer supplemental oxygen.
Ventilate ☐ Check presence and function of positive-pressure ventilation (PPV) device ☐ Check presence of term- and preterm-size masks ☐ 8F feeding tube and 20-mL syringe	It is most important to check that safety features are working to prevent over-inflation of lungs with PPV. Manometers present and functioning? Connected to oxygen/air? Self-inflating bag: Pop-off valve working? Flow-inflating bag: Does it inflate properly (no rips or missing attachments)? T-piece: Maximum circuit pressure set appropriately? Peak inspiratory pressure and positive end-expiratory pressure set appropriately?
Intubate ☐ Laryngoscope ☐ Size 0 and 1 blades with bright light ☐ Stylet (optional) ☐ Endotracheal (ET) tubes (2.5, 3.0, 3.5, 4.0) ☐ End tidal CO_2 detector ☐ Laryngeal mask airway and 5-mL syringe	Learner should know how to attach and detach blade from laryngoscope; check laryngoscope light. If setting up for intubation, ET tube should stay clean inside its package even if package is open and stylet is inserted.
Medicate Access to ☐ 1:10,000 epinephrine ☐ Supplies for administering medications and placing emergency umbilical venous catheter ☐ Documentation supplies	Location and protocol for checking emergency medications and supplies for vascular access are specific to each birth unit.

Performance Steps	Details
Thermoregulate For very preterm newborns ☐ Plastic wrap or bag ☐ Chemically activated warming pad ☐ Transport incubator	
Other Unit-specific items ☐ ☐ ☐ ☐	These items may be specific to your unit. Tailor the Equipment Checklist to meet facility requirements.

Instructor asks the learner Reflective Questions to enable self-assessment, such as:

1. Tell me how using this organized approach to checking resuscitation equipment works for you.

2. If all equipment and supplies were present, how long would it take you to confirm readiness for a birth?

3. Did you notice anything in this Equipment Checklist that is missing, specific to our birth setting? What would you change about this checklist?

Neonatal Resuscitation Program Key Behavioral Skills

Know your environment.
Anticipate and plan.
Assume the leadership role.
Communicate effectively.
Delegate workload optimally.

Allocate attention wisely.
Use all available information.
Use all available resources.
Call for help when needed.
Maintain professional behavior.

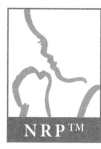

Lesson 2: Initial Steps
Performance Checklist

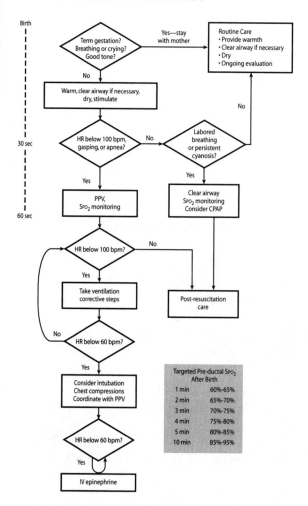

The Performance Checklist Is a Learning Tool

The learner uses the checklist as a reference during independent practice or as a guide for discussion and practice with a Neonatal Resuscitation Program™ (NRP™) instructor. When the learner and instructor agree that the learner can perform the skills correctly and smoothly without coaching and within the context of a scenario, the learner may move on to the next lesson's Performance Checklist.

Knowledge Check

- How do you determine if a newborn requires resuscitation?

- How do you manage the baby who is born with meconium-stained amniotic fluid?

- How does pulse oximetry work and what is its function?

Learning Objectives

1 Identify the newborn who requires initial steps of resuscitation.

2 Demonstrate correct technique for performing initial steps, including decision making for a baby born with meconium-stained amniotic fluid.

3 Demonstrate correct placement of oximeter probe and interpretation of pulse oximetry.

"You are called to attend a cesarean birth due to breech presentation. How would you prepare for the birth of this baby? As you work, say your thoughts and actions aloud so your assistant and I will know what you are thinking and doing."

Instructor should check boxes as the learner responds correctly.

Participant Name:		
	☐ Obtains relevant perinatal history	Gestational age? Fluid clear? How many babies? Other risk factors?
	Performs equipment check ☐ If obstetric provider indicates that meconium is present in amniotic fluid, prepares for intubation and meconium aspiration	**Warmer** on and towels to dry, **Clear airway** (bulb syringe, wall suction set at 80-100 mm Hg, meconium aspirator), **Auscultate** (stethoscope), **Oxygenate** (checks oxygen, blender, pulse oximeter and probe), **Ventilate** (checks positive-pressure ventilation [PPV] device), **Intubate** (laryngoscope and blades, endotracheal tubes, stylets, end-tidal CO_2 detector), **Medicate** (code cart accessible), **Thermoregulate**
Option 1: Meconium-stained amniotic fluid, vigorous newborn.		
"The baby has been born."		

Sample Vital Signs	Performance Steps	Details
Appears term Respiratory rate (RR)-crying Tone-flexed	Completes initial assessment when baby is born. ☐ Learner asks 3 questions: • Term? • Breathing or crying? • Good tone?	Initial assessment determines whether or not baby will receive initial steps of resuscitation at the radiant warmer.
	☐ Allows baby to stay with his mother for routine care: Warm, clear airway if necessary, dry, stimulate if necessary, continue evaluation	"Vigorous" meconium-stained baby is defined by • Strong respiratory efforts • Good muscle tone • Heart rate (HR) >100 beats per minute (bpm) Assume that a crying baby with good tone has HR >100 bpm.

Option 2: Meconium-stained amniotic fluid; non-vigorous newborn		
"The baby has been born."		
Sample Vital Signs	**Performance Steps**	**Details**
Appears term Not breathing Limp	Completes initial assessment when baby is born. ☐ Learner asks 3 questions: • Term? • Breathing or crying? • Good tone?	This baby requires initial steps, even without the additional risk factor of meconium-stained amniotic fluid.
RR-apneic HR-70 bpm Tone-limp	☐ Receives at radiant warmer. Does not dry or stimulate to breathe. ☐ Assesses breathing, heart rate, tone. ☐ Indicates tracheal suctioning would be required.	This is a "non-vigorous" meconium-stained baby. Intubation and tracheal suctioning procedure discussed in Lesson 5.
Baby has been intubated and suctioned. Continue with any option below and begin with "Receives baby at radiant warmer."		
Option 3: Clear fluid, newborn requires initial steps		
"The baby has been born."		
Term-yes RR-weak Tone-limp	Completes initial assessment when baby is born ☐ Learner asks 3 questions: • Term? • Breathing or crying? • Good tone?	Instructor may tailor scenario to meet learner needs; any or all of the assessment questions may prompt initiation of initial steps.
	☐ **Receives baby at radiant warmer** • Positions airway • Suctions mouth and nose • Dries with towel or blanket • Removes wet linen • Stimulates by flicking soles or rubbing back	Learner should move quickly through these steps.
RR-cry HR-120 bpm Tone–fair Color-cyanotic	☐ Assesses breathing and heart rate	If learner believes baby is cyanotic and requires supplemental oxygen, learner should administer free-flow oxygen and immediately connect pulse oximeter to confirm the perception of cyanosis.
"The baby is now 3 minutes old and appears cyanotic"		
Breathing HR-140 bpm Appears cyanotic	☐ Begins supplemental oxygen ☐ Places oximeter probe on right hand or wrist, then connects oximeter ☐ Confirms reliable signal by ensuring audio/pulsing light correlates with baby's actual heart rate	Free-flow oxygen may be given by oxygen mask, flow-inflating bag and mask, T-piece resuscitator, or oxygen tubing. It may not be given through the mask of a self-inflating bag.

SpO$_2$-65%	☐ Continues free-flow oxygen and weans per oximetry target range for age	Target range for 3 minutes of age = 70%-75%.
SpO$_2$-72%	☐ Does not begin supplemental oxygen and continues to monitor baby's transition	

Option 4: Clear fluid, newborn requires initial steps.

"The baby has been born."

Sample Vital Signs	Performance Steps	Details
Appears term Weak cry Limp	Completes initial assessment when baby is born ☐ Learner asks 3 questions: • Term? • Breathing or crying? • Good tone? ☐ Receives baby at radiant warmer • Positions airway • Suctions mouth and nose • Dries with towel or blanket • Removes wet linen • Stimulates by flicking soles or rubbing back	Learner should move through these steps quickly; handle baby gently, do not use bulb syringe aggressively, do not waste time continuing to stimulate baby if unresponsive.
RR-labored HR-110 bpm Tone-fair Color-cyanotic	☐ Assesses breathing, heart rate	Visual perception of cyanosis is unreliable. If newborn seems persistently cyanotic, start supplemental oxygen and confirm cyanosis with pulse oximetry.
	☐ Begins free-flow oxygen ☐ Attaches oximeter probe to right hand or wrist; then attaches to oximeter ☐ Considers continuous positive airway pressure (CPAP)	Free-flow oxygen may be given by oxygen mask, flow-inflating bag and mask, T-piece resuscitator, or oxygen tubing. It may not be given through the mask of a self-inflating bag. CPAP is possible with flow-inflating bag or T-piece resuscitator.
RR-40 breaths per minute HR-120 bpm SpO$_2$-74%	☐ Evaluates oximetry reading in relation to age.	Refers to table of pre-ductal oxygen saturation targets on Neonatal Resuscitation Program flow diagram.
RR-40 breaths per minute and unlabored HR-140 bpm SpO$_2$-97% or SpO$_2$-65%	At 3 minutes of age: ☐ Weans supplemental oxygen ☐ Indicates need for PPV	 Increases free-flow oxygen concentration and/or indicates need for trial of PPV.

Instructor asks the learner Reflective Questions to enable self-assessment, such as:

1. How did you know if the newborn required
   A. Initial steps at the radiant warmer?
   B. Intubation and suction of meconium from the trachea?
   C. Routine care and could stay with his mother?
   D. Supplemental oxygen?

2. Tell us about how you used pulse oximetry to guide your actions.

3. At what point would you need to call for more help?

4. What went well during this resuscitation?

5. Would you do anything differently when faced with this scenario (indicate which scenario) again?

Neonatal Resuscitation Program Key Behavioral Skills

Know your environment.	Allocate attention wisely.
Anticipate and plan.	Use all available information.
Assume the leadership role.	Use all available resources.
Communicate effectively.	Call for help when needed.
Delegate workload optimally.	Maintain professional behavior.

Lesson 3: Positive-Pressure Ventilation Performance Checklist

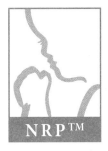

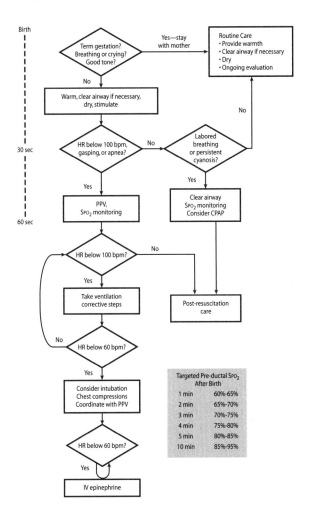

Targeted Pre-ductal SpO$_2$ After Birth	
1 min	60%-65%
2 min	65%-70%
3 min	70%-75%
4 min	75%-80%
5 min	80%-85%
10 min	85%-95%

The Performance Checklist Is a Learning Tool

The learner uses the checklist as a reference during independent practice, or as a guide for discussion and practice with a Neonatal Resuscitation Program™ (NRP™) instructor. When the learner and instructor agree that the learner can perform the skills correctly and smoothly without coaching and within the context of a scenario, the learner may move on to the next lesson's Performance Checklist.

If the institution policy is that a T-piece resuscitator normally is used in the delivery room, the learner should demonstrate proficiency with that device. However, he or she also should demonstrate ability to use a bag and mask.

Knowledge Check

- How will you check the function of the positive-pressure ventilation (PPV) device you will use?

- What are the indicators for beginning PPV?

- What is the correct ventilation rate?

- Which 2 indicators are evaluated when you first begin PPV? If those 2 indicators are not improving, what 2 indicators are next in evaluating effective ventilation?

- How is pulse oximetry used during PPV?

- What are the ventilation corrective steps (MR SOPA)?

- What is the purpose of an orogastric tube and when is it placed?

- What are the indications for stopping PPV?

Learning Objectives

1. Identify the newborn who requires PPV.

2. Demonstrate correct technique for PPV, including placement of mask on the newborn's face, rate and pressure, and corrective steps (MR SOPA).

3. Demonstrate correct placement and interpretation of pulse oximetry.

4. Recognize improvement during PPV by first assessing for increasing heart rate and oxygen saturation; if those are not improving, recognize the need to perform ventilation corrective steps and achieve audible breath sounds and chest movement with ventilation.

5. Identify signs that PPV may be discontinued.

6. Demonstrate pertinent key behavioral skills to optimize team performance.

"You are called to attend the birth of a baby because of failure to progress and maternal fever. How would you prepare for the resuscitation of this baby? As you work, say your thoughts and actions aloud so your assistant and I will know what you are thinking and doing."

Instructor should check boxes as the learner responds correctly.

Participant Name:		
	☐ Obtains relevant perinatal history	Gestational age? Fluid clear? How many babies? Other risk factors?
	☐ Performs equipment check ☐ Ensures correct size mask, and depending on device, checks function and inspiratory pressure, turns on gas flow 5-10 L/min, sets oxygen blender setting per hospital protocol ☐ If obstetric (OB) provider indicates that meconium is present in amniotic fluid, prepares for intubation and tracheal suctioning	**Warm, Clear airway, Auscultate, Oxygenate, Ventilate** (check PPV device), **Intubate, Medicate, Thermoregulate**

"The baby has been born."		
Sample Vital Signs	**Performance Steps**	**Details**
Gestational age as indicated Apneic Limp	Completes initial assessment when baby is born ☐ Learner asks 3 questions • Term? • Breathing or crying? • Good tone?	Initial assessment determines whether or not baby will receive initial steps of resuscitation at the radiant warmer.
	☐ Receives newborn at radiant warmer	
	☐ Meconium management (optional)	Intubation and suction indicated if meconium-stained and not vigorous.
	☐ Performs initial steps	Warm, position airway, suction mouth and nose, dry, remove wet linen, stimulate.
Respiratory Rate (RR)-apneic Heart Rate (HR)-40 beats per minute (bpm)	☐ Evaluates breathing and heart rate	Auscultate or palpate umbilical pulse.
	☐ Applies mask correctly and starts PPV at 20 cm H_2O; rate 40-60 bpm	Begin PPV with ____% oxygen per hospital protocol.
	☐ Calls for additional help	PPV requires 2 resuscitators.
	☐ Requests pulse oximetry	Assistant places probe on right hand or wrist, then plugs into oximeter. Oximeter has no signal.
HR-40 bpm SPO_2 - - - -	☐ Requests HR and saturation response within 5-10 breaths	Assistant auscultates chest and monitors oximetry.
Poor breath sounds; no chest movement	☐ Assesses bilateral breath sounds and chest movement	

Sample Vital Signs	Performance Steps	Details
	Ventilation Corrective Steps	Instructor may indicate chest movement and breath sounds at any step along sequence.
	Mask adjustment **R**eposition head **S**uction mouth and nose **O**pen mouth Increase **P**ressure	Do **M, R** first and reattempt PPV If no breath sounds or chest movement, do **S and O** and reattempt PPV. If no breath sounds or chest movement, gradually increase **P**ressure every few breaths, until there are bilateral breath sounds and chest movement with each breath, up to maximum of 40 cm H_2O pressure.
	Consider **A**lternative airway	If no breath sounds or chest movement, consider endotracheal intubation or laryngeal mask airway. (Lesson 5 notes limitations of the laryngeal mask airway.)
	After achieving breath sounds and chest movement ☐ Administers effective PPV for 30 seconds	Monitor for overinflation of lungs as functional residual capacity is established with first effective breaths.
	☐ Assesses HR and Sp_{O_2}	Instructor chooses from options below.
Option 1		
HR-70 bpm RR-4 breaths per minute (gasping) Sp_{O_2}-67%	☐ Continues effective PPV as long as HR is rising ☐ If HR not rising, repeats all ventilation corrective steps (MR SOPA) to ensure effective ventilation ☐ Adjusts oxygen per oximetry ☐ Considers intubation if HR continues >60 bpm and <100 bpm	If HR rises >100 bpm, proceed to Option 2. Learner demonstrates continuous assessment of HR and Sp_{O_2} and ability to problem solve based on newborn's response.
Option 2		
HR-120 bpm RR-10 breaths per minute (weak cry) Sp_{O_2}-74%	☐ Stimulates newborn to breathe spontaneously and slows PPV rate as breathing becomes effective ☐ Adjusts oxygen per oximetry	
HR-140 bpm RR-60 breaths per minute (grunting) Sp_{O_2}-97%	☐ Monitors newborn's respiratory effort, HR, and Sp_{O_2} ☐ Gradually withdraws PPV and adjusts oxygen as Sp_{O_2} rises and then discontinues free-flow oxygen	
	☐ Updates family ☐ Directs post-resuscitation care	

Sample Vital Signs	Performance Steps	Details
Option 3		
HR-40 bpm RR-apneic SpO$_2$ - - -	☐ Quickly assesses reasons why baby may not be responding ☐ If no apparent reason for poor response, indicate need to intubate and begin chest compressions	Consider equipment malfunction, oxygen concentration, need for orogastric tube, or other problem (pneumothorax, hypovolemia). Oximeter—no signal.

Instructor asks the learner reflective questions to enable self-assessment, such as,

1. How did you know the newborn required
   a. Initial steps at the radiant warmer?
   b. Positive-pressure ventilation?
   c. Corrective steps (MR SOPA)?
   d. Supplemental oxygen?

2. Tell me about how you used pulse oximetry to guide your actions.

3. At what point would you need to call for more help?

4. What are some examples of the Key Behavioral Skills you used to communicate clearly with your assistant?

5. What went well during this resuscitation?

6. Would you do anything differently when faced with this scenario (indicate which scenario) again?

Neonatal Resuscitation Program Key Behavioral Skills

Know your environment.
Anticipate and plan.
Assume the leadership role.
Communicate effectively.
Delegate workload optimally.

Allocate attention wisely.
Use all available information.
Use all available resources.
Call for help when needed.
Maintain professional behavior.

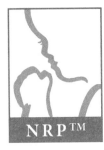

NRP™

Lesson 4: Chest Compressions Performance Checklist

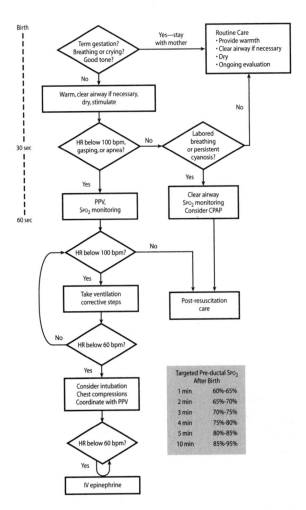

Birth

Term gestation?
Breathing or crying?
Good tone? → Yes—stay with mother → Routine Care
• Provide warmth
• Clear airway if necessary
• Dry
• Ongoing evaluation

No ↓

Warm, clear airway if necessary, dry, stimulate

30 sec

HR below 100 bpm, gasping, or apnea? → No → Labored breathing or persistent cyanosis? → No

Yes ↓   Yes ↓

PPV, SpO₂ monitoring   Clear airway
                                  SpO₂ monitoring
                                  Consider CPAP

60 sec

HR below 100 bpm? → No

Yes ↓

Take ventilation corrective steps   Post-resuscitation care

HR below 60 bpm? → No

Yes ↓

Consider intubation
Chest compressions
Coordinate with PPV

Targeted Pre-ductal SpO₂ After Birth	
1 min	60%-65%
2 min	65%-70%
3 min	70%-75%
4 min	75%-80%
5 min	80%-85%
10 min	85%-95%

HR below 60 bpm?

Yes ↓

IV epinephrine

The Performance Checklist Is a Learning Tool

The learner uses the checklist as a reference during independent practice or as a guide for discussion and practice with a Neonatal Resuscitation Program™ (NRP™) instructor. When the learner and instructor agree that the learner can perform the skills correctly and smoothly without coaching and within the context of a scenario, the learner may move on to the next lesson's Performance Checklist.

Knowledge Check

- What are the indications for beginning chest compressions?

- Which method is preferred: 2-finger or thumb technique? Why?

- What is the indication for discontinuing chest compressions?

Learning Objectives

1 Identify the newborn who requires chest compressions.

2 Demonstrate correct technique for performing chest compressions.

3 Identify the sign that indicates chest compressions should be discontinued.

4 Demonstrate behavioral skills to ensure clear communication and teamwork during this critical component of newborn resuscitation.

"You are called to attend an emergency cesarean birth due to fetal bradycardia. How would you prepare for the resuscitation of this baby? As you work, say your thoughts and actions aloud so your assistant and I will know what you are thinking and doing."

Instructor should check boxes as the learner responds correctly.

Note: This scenario takes the learner from Lesson 1 through Lesson 4. The instructor who finds the "Details" column helpful for assessing performance may use this Performance Checklist as the Basic Integrated Skills Station Checklist (Lessons 1 through 4) instead of the more abbreviated Basic Integrated Skills Performance Checklist.

Participant Name:		
	☐ Obtains relevant perinatal history	Gestational age? Fluid clear? How many babies? Other risk factors?
	☐ Performs equipment check ☐ Assembles resuscitation team (at least one other person) and discusses plan and roles ☐ If obstetric provider indicates that meconium is present in amniotic fluid, prepares for intubation and suctioning meconium	Warm, Clear airway, Auscultate, Oxygenate, Ventilate, Intubate, Medicate, Thermoregulate
	"The baby has just been born."	
Sample Vital Signs	**Performance Steps**	**Details**
Gestational age as indicated Apneic Limp	☐ Completes initial assessment ☐ Receives baby at radiant warmer	Asks 3 questions: Term? Breathing or crying? Good tone?

Sample Vital Signs	Performance Steps	Details
	Meconium management (optional)	
	☐ Performs initial steps	Warm, position airway, suction mouth and nose, dry, remove wet linen, stimulate.
Respiratory rate (RR)-apneic Heart rate (HR)-40 beats per minute (bpm)	☐ Evaluates respirations and heart rate	Auscultates apical pulse or palpates umbilicus.
	☐ Initiates positive-pressure ventilation (PPV)	Begins with ___% oxygen per hospital protocol at about 20 cm H_2O pressure. Rate = 40-60/min
	☐ Calls for additional help if necessary	A minimum of 2 resuscitators are necessary if PPV required. Team should be assembled before birth.
	☐ Requests pulse oximetry	Assistant places probe on right hand or wrist before plugging into monitor.
RR-apneic HR-40 bpm Sp_{O_2} — — - - No breath sounds or chest movement	☐ Requests assessment of heart rate, pulse oximetry ☐ If not rising, requests assessment of bilateral breath sounds and chest movement	Pulse oximetry not functioning at low HR.
	☐ Takes ventilation corrective steps (MR SOPA)	**M**ask adjustment and **R**eposition airway (reattempt 5-10 breaths). **S**uction mouth and nose and **o**pen mouth (reattempt 5-10 breaths). Gradually increase the pressure every few breaths until there are bilateral breath sounds and visible chest movement with each breath, up to a maximum of 40 cm H_2O pressure, if necessary.
+ chest movement + breath sounds	☐ Requests evaluation of chest rise and breath sounds	If all corrective steps done but still no chest movement, breath sounds, or rising heart rate, learner indicates need for **a**lternative airway, such as intubation.
+ chest movement + breath sounds	☐ Performs 30 seconds of PPV; notes breath sounds and chest movement	Assistant notes bilateral breath sounds and chest movement.
HR-50 bpm Sp_{O_2} — — —	☐ Evaluates heart rate and Sp_{O_2}	Assistant auscultates or palpates HR (oximetry not yet functioning due to low heart rate).
	☐ Calls for additional help ☐ Initiates chest compressions ☐ Increases oxygen to 100%	Team may already be present. Do not forget someone needs to document events on the code sheet. Leader delegates PPV and other tasks as necessary.
	☐ Locates appropriate position on lower third of sternum	

Sample Vital Signs	Performance Steps	Details
	☐ 2-finger technique: • Uses fingertips of middle and index or ring fingers ☐ Thumb technique: • Uses distal portion of both thumbs (one thumb over the other if baby is small)	Thumb technique is preferred because you can control the depth of compression better than with 2-finger technique. Thumb technique generates superior peak systolic and coronary arterial perfusion pressure.
	☐ Compresses sternum one-third of anterior-posterior diameter of chest, straight up and down. ☐ Keeps fingertips/thumbs on sternum during release. Allows chest expansion between compressions, but does not lift thumbs or fingers from chest.	Duration of downward stroke should be somewhat shorter than the duration of the release for generation of maximum cardiac output. During thumb technique, beware of tight grip around thorax that impedes ventilation.
	☐ Compressor counts cadence: "One-and-Two-and-Three-and-Breathe-and" ☐ Ventilates during pause at "Breathe-and"	One cycle of 3 compressions and 1 breath takes 2 seconds.
	☐ Provides 45-60 seconds of chest compressions and coordinated ventilations Assesses heart rate: ☐ Palpates umbilicus and continues ventilation Or, if no pulsations felt, ☐ Auscultates apical pulse and pauses ventilation	Heart rate assessment is a good place to ask learner and assistant to change places so learner can demonstrate roles of compressor and ventilator. Instructor chooses **Option 1:** Recovery to free-flow oxygen. **Option 2:** Indicate need to proceed to umbilical venous catheter (UVC) placement and administration of epinephrine.
Option 1		
HR-70 bpm SpO_2-67% Apneic + breath sounds + chest movement	☐ Discontinues compressions ☐ Continues ventilations ☐ Adjusts oxygen based on oximetry and newborn's age	Discontinue compressions when HR >60 bpm. Continue to monitor HR and SpO_2.

Sample Vital Signs	Performance Steps	Details
HR-120 bpm SpO₂-74% RR-10 breaths per minute HR-140 bpm SpO₂-97% RR-weak cry	☐ Provides additional 30 seconds of effective ventilation *without* chest compressions. ☐ Assesses newborn's respiratory effort, HR, pulse oximetry. ☐ Slows PPV rate as newborn breathes spontaneously. ☐ Gradually withdraws PPV and adjusts free-flow oxygen based on oximetry. Eventually discontinues free-flow oxygen based on oximetry.	Team should be noting newborn's improving vital signs and discussing next steps together.
	☐ Updates family ☐ Directs appropriate post-resuscitation care	
Option 2		
HR-40 bpm SpO₂ - - - (Oximeter—no signal)	☐ Provides additional 45-60 seconds of chest compressions and coordinated ventilations and considers reasons for poor response	Consider reasons for poor response: • Ineffective ventilation? • Dislodged endotracheal tube (or need to intubate now)? • Supplemental oxygen being given? • Appropriate compression technique (location, depth, rate)? • Coordinated compressions and ventilations?
HR-50 bpm SpO₂ - - - (Oximeter—no signal)	☐ Requests HR assessment after completing more than 45-60 seconds of coordinated compressions and PPV ☐ Communicates plan for next steps • Intubate if not yet done • Insert emergency UVC and give epinephrine	Team may need additional help to place emergency UVC and administer epinephrine and intubate newborn.

Instructor asks the learner Reflective Questions to enable self-assessment, such as:

1. What went well during this resuscitation?

2. Who assumed the leadership role in this scenario?

3. Did you (leader) get what you needed from your assistant(s)? What behavioral skills did you use to ensure good teamwork? Give me an example of what you did or said that used that behavioral skill.

4. When the baby did not respond to chest compressions and coordinated, effective ventilation, what did team members do to support (or not support) each other?

5. What would you do differently when faced with this scenario again?

Neonatal Resuscitation Program Key Behavioral Skills

Know your environment.	Allocate attention wisely.
Anticipate and plan.	Use all available information.
Assume the leadership role.	Use all available resources.
Communicate effectively.	Call for help when needed.
Delegate workload optimally.	Maintain professional behavior.

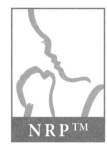

Lesson 5: Endotracheal Intubation and Laryngeal Mask Airway Placement

Performance Checklist

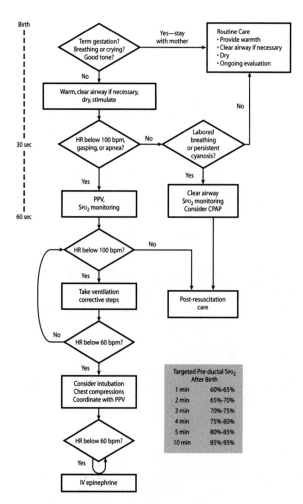

The Performance Checklist Is a Learning Tool

The learner uses the checklist as a reference during independent practice, or as a guide for discussion and practice with a Neonatal Resuscitation Program™ (NRP™) instructor. When the learner and instructor agree that the learner can perform the skills correctly and smoothly without coaching and within the context of a scenario, the learner may move on to the next lesson's Performance Checklist.

Knowledge Check

- What are the indications for endotracheal intubation during resuscitation?

- How do you determine if a baby born with meconium-stained amniotic fluid requires tracheal suction?

- What are the signs of correct placement of the endotracheal tube in the trachea?

- What are the indications for placing a laryngeal mask airway?

- What are the limitations of a laryngeal mask airway?

Learning Objectives

1 Identify the newborn who requires endotracheal intubation during resuscitation.

2 Demonstrate correct technique for performing/assisting with endotracheal intubation and administering positive-pressure ventilation (PPV).

3 Demonstrate correct technique for suctioning meconium from the trachea of a non-vigorous newborn.

4 Identify when placement of a laryngeal mask airway is indicated.

5 List the limitations of a laryngeal mask airway.

6 Demonstrate correct technique in placing and removing a laryngeal mask airway.

7 Demonstrate behavioral skills to ensure clear communication and teamwork during this critical component of newborn resuscitation.

"You are called to attend the birth of a full-term newborn because of meconium in the amniotic fluid. How would you prepare for the resuscitation of this baby? As you work, say your thoughts and actions aloud so your assistant and I will know what you are thinking and doing."

Instructor should check boxes as the learner responds correctly.

Participant Name:		
	☐ Obtains relevant perinatal history	Gestational age? (confirms information) Fluid clear? (confirms information) How many babies? Other risk factors?
	☐ Performs equipment check ☐ Assembles resuscitation team (at least one other person) and discusses plan and roles	**Warm**er on, Towels to **dry**, **Clear airway** (bulb syringe, wall suction set at 80-100 mm Hg, meconium aspirator), **Auscultate** (stethoscope), **Oxygenate** (checks oxygen, blender, pulse oximeter, and probe), **Ventilate** (checks positive-pressure ventilation [PPV] device), **Intubate** (laryngoscope and blades, endotracheal tubes, stylets, end-tidal CO_2 detector) **Medicate** (code cart accessible), **Thermoregulate.**
	Prepares for intubation • Selects correct-sized tube • Inserts stylet correctly (stylet optional) • Checks light on blade (size 1 for full-term newborn) • Ensures that suction functions at 80-100 mm Hg and ensures connection to 10F or 12F catheter • Obtains meconium aspiration device • Obtains end-tidal CO_2 detector • Prepares tape or obtains endotracheal tube securing device	The team prepares for a non-vigorous newborn who will require intubation and tracheal suction with a meconium aspiration device. Due to the high-risk scenario, the team also prepares to intubate and ventilate with an endotracheal tube and PPV device.

"The baby has been born."		
Sample Vital Signs	**Performance Steps**	**Details**
Appears term Apneic Limp	Completes initial assessment when baby is born. ☐ Asks 3 questions: Term? Breathing or crying? Good tone?	
	☐ Indicates tracheal suctioning is required	Newborn is meconium stained and not vigorous (apneic, and poor muscle tone).
Respiratory Rate (RR)-apneic Heart rate (HR)-<100 beats per minute (bpm) Tone-limp	☐ Receives baby at radiant warmer, does not dry or stimulate	Vigorous meconium-stained newborn may stay with his mother and receive routine care.

During the intubation procedure, the role of the intubator is in the left column and the role of the assistant is in the right column. Some actions and decisions can be made by either or both the intubator and assistant (merged columns).

Performing Intubation	Assisting With Intubation
☐ Holds laryngoscope correctly in left hand	☐ Positions newborn's head.
☐ Inserts blade carefully to base of tongue	☐ Monitors 30-second time frame for intubation.
☐ Requests suction if needed for visualization	☐ Places suction catheter in intubator's hand and provides suction if needed. Intubator should not have to look away from landmarks.
☐ Lifts using correct motion (no rocking back)	☐ Taps out heart rate (HR) (if no audio HR from pulse oximeter) where intubator can view with peripheral vision.
☐ Requests cricoid pressure if needed	☐ Applies cricoid pressure if requested.
☐ Identifies landmarks seen	
☐ Takes corrective action to visualize glottis if needed	
☐ Inserts tube from right side, does not insert tube down center of laryngoscope blade	
☐ Aligns vocal cord guide with vocal cords	☐ Attaches meconium aspiration device to suction tubing.
☐ Removes laryngoscope (and stylet) while firmly holding tube against baby's palate	☐ Attaches meconium aspiration device to endotracheal tube.
☐ Holds endotracheal tube in place and applies suction to meconium aspiration device; slowly withdraws endotracheal tube from trachea	
☐ Assesses the need to repeat procedure with a clean endotracheal tube (decision is based on amount of meconium recovered and baby's status) **OR** ☐ Proceeds with Initial Steps	

Proceeds With Initial Steps		
Sample Vital Signs	**Performance Steps**	**Details**
	☐ Performs initial steps	Position airway, dry, stimulate, remove wet linen.
RR-apneic HR-40 bpm	☐ Evaluates respirations and heart rate	Auscultates apical pulse or palpates umbilicus.
	☐ Initiates PPV	Begins with ___% oxygen per hospital protocol at about 20 cm H_2O pressure. Rate = 40-60/min
	☐ Calls for additional help if necessary	A minimum of 2 resuscitators are necessary if PPV required. Team should already be assembled.
	☐ Requests pulse oximetry	Places probe on right hand or wrist before plugging into monitor.
RR-apneic HR-40 bpm S_{PO_2} - - - No breath sounds or chest movement	☐ Requests assessment of heart rate, pulse oximetry ☐ If not rising, requests assessment of bilateral breath sounds and chest movement	Pulse oximetry not functioning at low HR.
	☐ Takes ventilation corrective steps (MR SOPA)	**M**ask adjustment, **R**eposition airway (re-attempt PPV). **S**uction mouth and nose and **o**pen mouth (re-attempt PPV). If no breath sounds or chest movement, gradually increase **p**ressure every few breaths until there are bilateral breath sounds and chest movement with each breath. Move to next step if reaching 40 cm H_2O.
No chest movement No breath sounds HR-50 bpm S_{PO_2} - - -	☐ Requests evaluation of chest movement and breath sounds ☐ Evaluates heart rate and pulse oximetry	If all corrective steps are done but there still is no chest movement, breath sounds, or rising heart rate, learner indicates need for intubation.
	☐ Indicates need for intubation	Ventilation of the newborn is the highest priority; chest compressions will be ineffective until ventilation is established by mask or endotracheal tube.
	☐ Directs assistant to continue monitoring HR and oxygen saturation (S_{PO_2}) ☐ Turns up oxygen to 100% in preparation for chest compressions ☐ Assistant may continue to try corrective steps to improve PPV	Assistant monitors HR and S_{PO_2} (if possible) throughout procedure.

Performing Intubation	Assisting With Intubation
☐ **Prepares for intubation** (Most of these steps were done in preparation for the birth.) • Selects correct-sized tube • Inserts stylet correctly (stylet optional) • Checks light on blade (size 1 for full-term newborn) • Ensures that suction functions at 80-100 mm Hg and ensures connection to 10F or 12F catheter • Obtains end-tidal CO_2 detector • Prepares tape or obtains endotracheal tube securing device	
☐ Holds laryngoscope correctly in left hand	☐ Positions newborn's head.
☐ Inserts blade carefully to base of tongue	☐ Monitors 30-second time frame for intubation.
☐ Requests suction if needed for visualization	☐ Places suction catheter in intubator's hand and provides suction if needed. Intubator should not have to look away from landmarks.
☐ Lifts using correct motion (no rocking back)	☐ Taps out heart rate (HR) (if no audio HR from pulse oximeter) where intubator can view with peripheral vision.
☐ Requests cricoid pressure if needed	☐ Applies cricoid pressure if requested.
☐ Identifies landmarks seen	
☐ Takes corrective action to visualize glottis if needed	
☐ Inserts tube from right side, does not insert tube down center of laryngoscope blade	
☐ Aligns vocal cord guide with vocal cords	
☐ Removes laryngoscope (and stylet) while firmly holding tube against baby's palate	☐ Removes mask from positive-pressure ventilation (PPV) device. Attaches CO_2 detector to endotracheal tube and attaches PPV device to CO_2 detector.
☐ Holds tube against baby's palate with one hand and PPV device with other hand and resumes ventilation	☐ Assistant hands off PPV device to intubator so that intubator is holding both the endotracheal tube and the PPV device.
☐ Ensures correct depth of insertion: Estimate weight of newborn in kg + 6 Example: 3 kg + 6 = 9 cm marking at upper lip ☐ Looks and listens for signs to confirm correct tube placement. • Mist in tube during exhalation • CO_2 detector confirmation (may not function if newborn has very poor cardiac perfusion) • Rising heart rate • Rising oxygen saturation • Bilateral breath sounds • Symmetrical chest movement (do not over inflate)	

If correct placement cannot be confirmed, assistant and intubator discuss and take necessary corrective action.
☐ Repeat confirmation steps.
☐ Reassess correct tip-to-lip measurement.
☐ Reinsert laryngoscope and visualize placement of stripe at vocal cords.
and/or
☐ Remove endotracheal tube, ventilate with mask and PPV device, and repeat intubation.
  Or
☐ Consider rescue airway (laryngeal mask airway). GO TO ALTERNATIVE AIRWAY.

Chest compressions resume after successful intubation

Sample Vital Signs	Performance Steps	Details
HR-50 bpm	☐ Assesses respiratory effort, HR, and SPO₂ as PPV resumes	
	☐ Chest compressions resume	Assistant resumes chest compressions and calls out cadence. Now that baby is intubated, compressor may move to head of bed to allow access to umbilicus, if needed.
HR-70 bpm SPO₂-67%	☐ Checks heart rate after 45-60 seconds of chest compressions ☐ Discontinues compressions ☐ Continues ventilations ☐ Adjusts oxygen based on oximetry and newborn's age	
RR-apneic HR-120 bpm SPO₂-74%	☐ After 30 seconds of PPV with endotracheal tube, checks respiratory effort, HR, and SPO₂ ☐ Adjusts oxygen based on oximetry and newborn's age	
RR-occasional gasp HR-140 bpm SPO₂-97%	☐ May continue PPV for 30 additional seconds. Adjust oxygen based on oximetry and newborn's age. Or ☐ Make a team decision to • Update family. • Secure endotracheal tube. • Move to post-resuscitation care.	
ALTERNATIVE AIRWAY: Placement of a laryngeal mask airway **"You have been unable to ventilate or intubate the baby. You decide to insert a laryngeal mask airway."**		
Sample Vital Signs	Performance Steps	Details
HR-50 bpm SPO₂ - - -	☐ Directs chest compressions to begin while preparing rescue airway	Newborn requires continued efforts at ventilation and chest compressions. Oxygen concentration should be at 100% during chest compressions.
	☐ Obtains size-1 laryngeal mask airway and 5-mL syringe	May consider placing orogastric tube to relieve gastric distention prior to placing laryngeal mask airway.
	☐ Using the 5-mL syringe, quickly inflates the cuff with no more than 4 mL of air to check for leaks or tears	Learner should be moving quickly to insert the rescue airway.
	☐ Withdraws air; however, leaves just enough air in cuff to remove the wrinkles	We have little experience using the laryngeal mask airway. This technique may keep the airway from folding over on itself during insertion.

Sample Vital Signs	Performance Steps	Details
	☐ Requests pause in chest compressions while placing airway	
	☐ Places baby's head in sniffing position ☐ Holding laryngeal mask airway like a pen, gently opens baby's mouth and inserts airway smoothly and quickly along the hard palate until resistance is met, just past the base of the tongue	Unlike placement of an adult laryngeal mask airway, the airway is inserted directly into the baby's hypopharynx in its intended position. It is not "flipped" into position at the back of the throat.
	☐ Holds airway in place with other hand and removes index finger without dislodging airway	
	☐ Ensures that airway stays in place by holding it against the hard palate; however, holds it gently enough so airway may rise and seat as cuff is inflated ☐ Inflates cuff with 5-mL syringe to total of no more than 4 mL of air	Airway may not rise and seat in the manikin. It also may be possible to insert the airway too far into the manikin, resulting in ineffective ventilation.
	☐ Connects airway to end-tidal CO_2 detector and PPV device ☐ Holds airway against baby's hard palate to protect from dislodgement	The provider holds the airway in place just as the endotracheal tube is held in place—with one finger against the baby's hard palate. The other hand holds the PPV device.
+ breath sounds + chest movement	☐ Begins PPV at 40-60 breaths/minute ☐ Confirms correct placement • Bilateral breath sounds • Chest movement • Color change on CO_2 detector	
HR-70 bpm SpO_2-67%	☐ Discontinues chest compressions ☐ Continues ventilations for 30 seconds	
HR-120 bpm Occasional respirations SpO_2-74%	☐ Slows PPV rate and stimulates baby to breathe ☐ Monitors pulse oximetry and decreases 100% oxygen to meet saturation target for baby's age	

Sample Vital Signs	Performance Steps	Details
HR-140 bpm Spontaneous respirations SpO_2-97%	☐ Suctions baby's mouth and throat with suction catheter ☐ Withdraws air from airway and removes laryngeal mask airway	Laryngeal mask airway could remain in place if desired. The baby can breathe spontaneously with the airway in place. The airway may be taped in place using the emergency endotracheal tube taping technique.
	☐ Monitors baby's respiratory efforts, heart rate, oximetry, and muscle tone ☐ Monitors pulse oximetry and adjusts oxygen if needed	
	☐ Indicates need for post-resuscitation care ☐ Updates family	

Instructor asks the learner Reflective Questions to enable self-assessment, such as

1 What went well during this resuscitation?

2 What was your main objective?

3 Who assumed the leadership role in this scenario? What skills did you use to ensure that your assistant understood what you needed? Give me an example of what you did or said that used that behavioral skill.

4 As the assistant, what suggestions might you make, if any, to help the team leader communicate clearly with team members?

5 Would you do anything differently when faced with this scenario again?

Neonatal Resuscitation Program Key Behavioral Skills

Know your environment.	Allocate attention wisely.
Anticipate and plan.	Use all available information.
Assume the leadership role.	Use all available resources.
Communicate effectively.	Call for help when needed.
Delegate workload optimally.	Maintain professional behavior.

Lesson 6: Medication Administration via Endotracheal Tube and Emergency Umbilical Venous Catheter

Performance Checklist

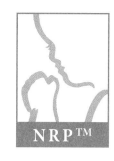

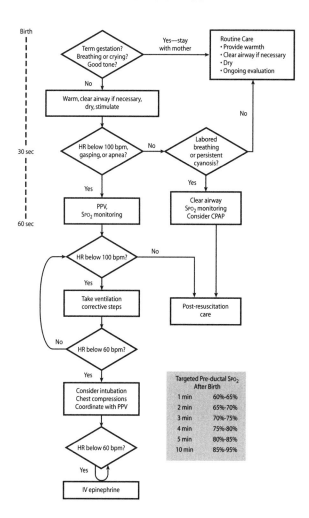

Targeted Pre-ductal SpO₂ After Birth	
1 min	60%-65%
2 min	65%-70%
3 min	70%-75%
4 min	75%-80%
5 min	80%-85%
10 min	85%-95%

The Performance Checklist Is a Learning Tool

The learner uses the checklist as a reference during independent practice or as a guide for discussion and practice with a Neonatal Resuscitation Program™ (NRP™) instructor. When the learner and instructor agree that the learner can perform the skills correctly and smoothly without coaching and within the context of a scenario, the learner may move on to the next lesson's Performance Checklist.

Knowledge Check

- What are the indications for epinephrine?

- What are the 2 routes? What are the 2 doses? Which route is preferred?

- What are indications for volume administration? What is used and what is the dose?

- How far is the emergency umbilical venous catheter (UVC) inserted into the vein?

Learning Objectives

1. Identify the newborn who requires epinephrine and/or volume during resuscitation.

2. Demonstrate correct technique for drawing up epinephrine.

3. Demonstrate correct technique for preparing/inserting an emergency UVC.

4. Demonstrate correct technique for administering epinephrine via endotracheal tube and UVC.

5. Demonstrate behavioral skills to ensure clear communication and teamwork during this critical component of newborn resuscitation.

"You are called to attend the emergency cesarean birth of a baby whose mother has sustained injuries in an automobile crash. Paramedics report intermittent detection of a "low fetal heart rate." How would you prepare for the resuscitation of this baby? As you work, say your thoughts and actions aloud so your assistant and I will know what you are thinking and doing."

This is a complex resuscitation. The learner and instructor decide how best to meet the learner's objectives. All learners taking Lesson 6 should know the correct concentration and dosage of epinephrine for both intratracheal and intravenous epinephrine. The learner and instructor may decide which additional skills are learning objectives: drawing up epinephrine, administering the medication, preparing and assisting with UVC insertion, and placing the UVC. Scope of practice may limit who may insert an umbilical catheter and order medication in the actual birth setting. The learner who is practicing medication administration and/or the leader of this resuscitation is not expected to perform all tasks, but may delegate tasks as required.

Participant Name:

Sample Vital Signs	Performance Steps	Details
	☐ Obtains relevant perinatal history	Gestational age? Fluid clear? How many babies? Other risk factors?
	☐ Performs equipment check ☐ Assembles resuscitation team (preferably 2-3 other people) and discusses plan and roles ☐ Based on risk factors, team may prepare items needs for complex resuscitation	**Warm, Clear airway, Auscultate, Oxygenate, Ventilate, Intubate, Medicate, Thermoregulate.** If there is time, team may prepare for intubation, umbilical venous catheter (UVC) placement, and medication/volume.
	"The baby has just been born."	
Term, Limp Apneic, Pale	Completes initial assessment when baby is born ☐ Asks 3 questions: Term? Tone? Crying or breathing?	
	☐ Receives baby at radiant warmer	
	☐ Performs initial steps	Warm, position airway, dry, remove wet linen, stimulate.
Respiratory Rate (RR)-apneic Heart Rate (HR)- 30 beats per minute (bpm)	☐ Evaluates respirations and heart rate	Auscultate pulse or palpates umbilicus.
	☐ Initiates positive-pressure ventilation (PPV) at 40-60 breaths per minute ☐ Calls for additional help if necessary ☐ Requests pulse oximetry	Begins with ___% oxygen per hospital protocol at about 20 cm H_2O pressure.
RR-apneic HR-40 bpm SPO_2 - - - - No breath sounds or chest movement	☐ Requests assessment of heart rate, pulse oximetry ☐ If not rising, requests assessment of bilateral breath sounds and chest movement	Pulse oximetry not functioning at low HR. Assistant must auscultate or palpate heart rate.

Sample Vital Signs	Performance Steps	Details
	☐ Takes ventilation corrective steps	**MR SOPA**
+ chest movement + breath sounds HR-30 bpm SpO$_2$ - - - -	☐ Requests evaluation of chest movement and breath sounds ☐ Evaluates heart rate and pulse oximetry	Ventilation corrective steps may result in chest movement and bilateral breath sounds at any point in the sequence.
	☐ Administers PPV by mask for 30 seconds	
HR-40 bpm SpO$_2$ - - - - + chest movement + breath sounds	☐ Evaluates heart rate and pulse oximetry	HR remains <60 bpm despite 30 seconds of effective ventilation.
	☐ Requests chest compressions ☐ Increases oxygen to 100% ☐ Indicates need for intubation ☐ Directs assistant to continue monitoring HR and SpO$_2$ (when SpO$_2$ functioning)	Chest compressions begin as intubator prepares equipment.
	☐ Requests pause in chest compressions (CC) while intubation occurs ☐ Takes corrective actions if signs of correct placement are not evident	If correct placement of endotracheal (ET) tube not evident: Repeat confirmation steps; Check tip-to-lip measurement; Reinsert laryngoscope and visualize placement; Remove ET tube and ventilate with mask; Repeat intubation or consider laryngeal mask airway.
	☐ CC resume after tube placement is confirmed ☐ CC and ventilations continue for at least 45-60 seconds	Compressor may move to head of bed after intubation to increase access to umbilicus for UVC placement.
HR-40 bpm SpO$_2$-63%	☐ Evaluates HR and pulse oximetry	Assistant monitors HR and SpO$_2$ (if possible) throughout procedure.
	☐ Requests epinephrine via ET tube while UVC is being placed ☐ Estimates baby's weight ☐ Orders dose of medication and route ☐ Asks medication person to repeat medication order (if necessary) ☐ Confirms that order was correctly received	Example: Leader states, "The baby weighs about 3 kg. Let's give 3 mL of 1:10,000 epinephrine down the endotracheal tube." Medication person repeats, "3 mL of 1:10,000 epinephrine down the ET tube." Leader: "That's right."

	☐ Draws up 1:10,000 epinephrine:
	  • Checks medication label
	  • Opens box
	  • Flips off yellow caps
	  • Twists 2 pieces together
	  • Removes needle guard cap
	  • Attaches 3-way stopcock or Luer lock syringe connector
	  • Attaches proper-size syringe to connector
	  • Draws up correct volume
	  • Labels syringe correctly
		Use a 5- or 6-mL syringe for intratracheal dose.

Sample Vital Signs	Performance Steps	Details
	☐ Administers intratracheal epinephrine • Verbalizes medication, dose, and intended route • Receives medication order confirmation • Removes PPV device from ET tube • Quickly gives drug directly into the tube • Re-attaches PPV device to ET tube • Announces that medication is in and may document dose, route, time, and response on code sheet	Example: "I have 3 mL of 1:10,000 epinephrine for the ET tube." If CO_2 detector gets wet, it is no longer reliable. May repeat epinephrine every 3-5 minutes.
	☐ Prepares emergency UVC • Obtains syringe with normal saline • Attaches 3-way stopcock to UVC • Flushes UVC and stopcock with saline • Closes stopcock to catheter	(if not already done with equipment check)
	☐ Inserts emergency UVC • Preps the base and lower 2 cm of the cord with antiseptic solution • Ties umbilical tape loosely on skin around base of cord • Cuts cord straight across not more than 2 cm above abdomen • Inserts catheter into vein 2-4 cm • Opens stopcock between baby and syringe and gently aspirates syringe to detect blood return • Advances catheter until blood return is detected • Clears any air from catheter and stopcock	Assistant may need to hold umbilicus up off abdomen with forceps or other instrument to allow cleaning, tying, and cutting of the umbilical cord. Ensure that team is aware when scalpel enters the field. Use sterile technique to the best of your ability under emergency circumstances.
HR-40 bpm SpO_2-63% + breath sounds + chest movement	☐ Evaluates HR and pulse oximetry ☐ May also re-evaluate effectiveness of ventilation	Re-evaluate heart rate and effectiveness of ventilation before each dose of epinephrine every 3 to 5 minutes.
	☐ Requests epinephrine via UVC ☐ Estimates baby's weight ☐ States medication, desired dose, and route ☐ Asks medication person to repeat medication order (if necessary) ☐ Confirms that order was correctly received	Example: Leader states, "The baby is about 3 kg. Let's give 0.9 mL of 1:10,000 epinephrine through the UVC." Medication person repeats, "0.9 mL of 1:10,000 epinephrine through the UVC." Leader: "That's right."
	☐ Administers epinephrine via UVC • Attaches proper-sized syringe (1-mL syringe) to connector • Draws up correct volume of medication • Labels syringe correctly	

Sample Vital Signs	Performance Steps	Details
	☐ Administers epinephrine via UVC • Verbalizes medication, dose, and intended route • Receives confirmation • Ensures that catheter is being held in place; attaches syringe to stopcock and gives rapidly without air bubbles • Flushes with .5 to 1 mL of normal saline Announces, "epinephrine is in" and may document dose, route, time, and response on code sheet	
	☐ Monitors HR and pulse oximetry (if functioning) ☐ Continues PPV and CC for at least 45-60 seconds after giving epinephrine	
HR-70 bpm SpO_2-67% RR-first gasps Pale, poor perfusion	☐ Evaluates HR and pulse oximetry in relation to baby's age ☐ Discontinues CC	
	☐ Requests volume expander • Reiterates estimated weight • Orders 10 mL/kg of normal saline per UVC over 5-10 minutes • Receives medication order confirmation • Confirms that order was correctly received	Example: Leader states, "The baby is about 3 kg. Let's give 30 mL of normal saline through the UVC over 5-10 minutes." Medication person repeats, "30 mL of normal saline through the UVC over 5-10 minutes." Leader: "That's right."
	☐ Administers normal saline per UVC • Draws up correct volume normal saline or uses prefilled syringes. Numbers more than one syringe (#1, #2) • Verbalizes medication, dose, and route • Receives confirmation • Ensures that catheter is being held in place; attaches syringe #1 to stopcock; gives entire dose in constant slow infusion over 5-10 minutes with no bubbles • Announces that medication is in, and may document dose, route, time, and response on code sheet	
Respirations-occasional gasp HR-120 bpm SpO_2-74%	☐ After 30 seconds of PPV with ET tube, checks respiratory effort, HR, and SpO_2 ☐ Adjusts oxygen based on oximetry and newborn's age	

Sample Vital Signs	Performance Steps	Details
RR-occasional gasp HR-140 bpm SPO_2-97%	☐ May continue PPV for 30 additional seconds to help ensure stability prior to transport to nursery ☐ Adjust oxygen based on oximetry and newborn's age ☐ Make a team decision to • Update family • Secure ET tube • Secure or remove UVC • Move to post-resuscitation care	

Instructor asks the learner Reflective Questions to enable self-assessment, such as the following:

1 What went well during this resuscitation?

2 Who assumed the leadership role in this scenario? What skills did you use to ensure that your assistants understood what you needed? Give me an example of what you did or said that used that behavioral skill.

3 As the assistant(s), what suggestions might you make (to the leader) to improve communication during a stressful resuscitation?

4 Would you do anything differently when faced with this scenario again?

Neonatal Resuscitation Program Key Behavioral Skills

Know your environment.
Anticipate and plan.
Assume the leadership role.
Communicate effectively.
Delegate workload optimally.

Allocate attention wisely.
Use all available information.
Use all available resources.
Call for help when needed.
Maintain professional behavior.

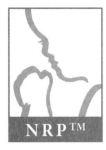

NRP™

Integrated Skills Station Performance Checklist (Basic)

The Integrated Skills Station is a required course component used for learner evaluation.

The instructor may use several scenarios to allow the learner to demonstrate all steps of the Neonatal Resuscitation Program™ (NRP™) Flow Diagram (Lessons 1 through 4) in correct order, using proper technique, without coaching from the instructor. If the learner makes significant errors in timing, sequence, or technique, the learner returns to the appropriate Performance Skills Station for additional help and practice.

If the instructor wants more detail and sample vital signs, Performance Checklist 4 may be used.

Participant Name: _____

Critical Performance Steps	Details
☐ Obtains relevant perinatal history	Gestational age, fluid, expected number of babies, additional risk factors?
☐ Performs Equipment Check	Warm, Clear airway, Auscultate, Oxygenate, Ventilate, Intubate, Medicate, Thermoregulate.
☐ Discusses plan and assigns team member roles	Use NRP Key Behavioral Skills throughout resuscitation to improve teamwork and communication.
☐ Completes initial assessment	Term, tone, crying, or breathing?
☐ *(option) Meconium management*	*If NOT vigorous, indicate need for endotracheal intubation and suction.*
☐ Performs initial steps	Warm, clear airway if necessary, dry, remove wet linen, stimulate.
☐ Evaluates respirations and heart rate (HR)	Auscultate apical pulse or palpate umbilicus. **Heart rate less than 60 beats per minute (bpm), apneic or gasping.**
☐ Initiates positive-pressure ventilation (PPV) with 21% oxygen	Apply mask correctly, rate 40-60/minute.
☐ Calls for additional help, if necessary	A minimum of 2 resuscitators necessary if PPV required.
☐ Requests pulse oximetry	Place probe on right hand before plugging into monitor.
☐ Assesses for rising heart rate and oxygen saturation within first 5-10 breaths.	**HR remains below 60 bpm.** Heart rate not rising. Pulse oximetry might not be functioning.
☐ Assesses chest movement and bilateral breath sounds.	Initially respond that **bilateral breath sounds are absent and chest is NOT moving with PPV.**
☐ Takes ventilation corrective steps (MR SOPA)	Instructor decides how many corrective steps are necessary. **M**ask adjustment and **R**eposition head. **S**uction mouth and nose and **O**pen mouth. Increase **P**ressure (do not exceed 40 cm H₂O). *Indicate need to* Use **A**lternative airway (endotracheal [ET] tube or laryngeal mask airway).
☐ Requests assessment of bilateral breath sounds and chest movement ☐ Performs 30 seconds of effective PPV	**Bilateral breath sounds and chest movement are present.**
☐ Evaluates HR, breathing, and oxygen saturation	**Heart rate remains below 60 bpm.** **Apneic.** **Pulse oximetry might not be functioning.**

Critical Performance Steps	Details
☐ Increases oxygen to 100% in preparation for chest compressions	**Increase oxygen concentration to 100% when chest compressions begin.**
☐ Initiates chest compressions coordinated with PPV	2 thumbs (preferred) on lower third of sternum, 3 compressions: 1 ventilation. Compress one-third of the anterior-posterior diameter of the chest.
☐ Calls for additional help	**Indicates need for help with intubation, line placement, and medication.**
☐ After at least 45-60 seconds of chest compressions, evaluates HR, breathing, and oxygen saturation	**Heart rate above 60 bpm. Occasional spontaneous breath. Pulse oximetry functioning.**
☐ Discontinues compressions, continues ventilation for 30 seconds	**Discontinue compressions if heart rate above 60 bpm. Reassess every 30 seconds.**
☐ Evaluates HR, breathing, and oxygen saturation. Continues/discontinues PPV appropriately. May provide free-flow oxygen and adjust oxygen concentration per oximetry.	**Adjust oxygen concentration based on oximetry and newborn's age. Continue PPV until HR above 100 bpm with adequate breathing.**
☐ Directs post-resuscitation care	Ongoing evaluation and monitoring. Communicate effectively with parent(s).

Reflective Questions:

1. What did you think you would need to do when this baby was placed on the radiant warmer?
2. What went well during this resuscitation? What would you do differently next time?
3. What NRP Key Behavioral Skills were used? Give examples.

Neonatal Resuscitation Program Key Behavioral Skills

Know your environment.   Delegate workload optimally.   Use all available resources.
Anticipate and plan.   Allocate attention wisely.   Call for help when needed.
Assume the leadership role.   Use all available information.   Maintain professional behavior.
Communicate effectively.

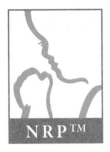

Integrated Skills Station Performance Checklist (Advanced)

The Integrated Skills Station is a required course component used for learner evaluation.

The instructor may use several scenarios to allow the learner to demonstrate all steps of the Neonatal Resuscitation Program™ (NRP™) Flow Diagram (Lessons 1 through 4 and additional lessons relevant to course objectives) in correct order, using proper technique, without coaching from the instructor. If the learner makes significant errors in timing, sequence, or technique, the learner returns to the appropriate Performance Skills Station for additional help and practice.

If the instructor wants more detail and sample vital signs, Performance Checklist 6 may be used.

Participant Name: _____

Critical Performance Steps	Details
☐ Obtains relevant perinatal history	Gestational age, fluid, expected number of babies, additional risk factors?
☐ Performs Equipment Check	Warm, Clear airway, Auscultate, Oxygenate, Ventilate, Intubate, Medicate, Thermoregulate.
☐ Discusses plan and assigns team member roles	Use NRP Key Behavioral Skills throughout resuscitation to improve teamwork and communication.
☐ Completes initial assessment	Term, tone, crying or breathing?
☐ *(option) Meconium management*	*If NOT vigorous, assist with/performs tracheal suction.*
☐ Performs initial steps	Warm, clear airway if necessary, dry, remove wet linen, stimulate.
☐ Evaluates respirations and heart rate (HR)	Auscultate apical pulse or palpate umbilicus. **Heart rate less than 60 beats per minute (bpm), apneic or gasping.**
☐ Initiates positive-pressure ventilation (PPV) with 21% oxygen	Apply mask correctly, rate 40-60/minute.
☐ Calls for additional help, if needed	A minimum of 2 resuscitators necessary if PPV required.
☐ Requests pulse oximetry	Place probe on right hand before plugging into monitor.
☐ Assesses for rising heart rate and oxygen saturation within first 5-10 breaths.	**HR remains below 60 bpm.** Heart rate not rising. Pulse oximetry might not be functioning.
☐ Assesses chest movement and bilateral breath sounds.	Initially respond that **bilateral breath sounds are absent and chest is NOT moving with PPV.**
☐ Takes ventilation corrective steps (MR SOPA)	Instructor decides how many corrective steps are necessary. **M**ask adjustment and **R**eposition head. **S**uction mouth and nose and **O**pen mouth. Increase **P**ressure (do not exceed 40 cm H₂O). Use **A**lternative airway (endotracheal [ET] tube or laryngeal mask airway).
☐ Requests assessment of bilateral breath sounds and chest movement ☐ Performs 30 seconds of effective PPV	**Bilateral breath sounds and chest movement are present.**
☐ Evaluates HR, breathing, and oxygen saturation	**Heart rate remains below 60 bpm.** **Apneic.** **Pulse oximetry might not be functioning.**

Critical Performance Steps	Details
☐ Intubates or directs intubation and assesses ET tube placement	Intubation is recommended prior to beginning chest compressions.
☐ Increases oxygen to 100% in preparation for chest compressions (CC)	**Increase oxygen concentration to 100% when chest compressions begin.**
☐ Initiates chest compressions coordinated with PPV	2 thumbs (preferred) on lower third of sternum, 3 compressions:1 ventilation. Compress one-third of the anterior-posterior diameter of the chest.
☐ Calls for additional help	Complex scenario may require more help.
☐ After at least 45-60 seconds of chest compressions, evaluates HR, breathing, and oxygen saturation	**HR remains below 60 bpm. Apneic. Pulse oximetry might not be functioning.**
☐ May consider intratracheal epinephrine while umbilical venous catheter (UVC) is being placed.	Epinephrine 1:10,000 (0.1 mg/kg). *Intratracheal dose:* 0.5 to 1 mL/kg. No response expected from intratracheal epinephrine for at least 1 minute and perhaps longer.
☐ Places or directs placement of UVC	CC may be performed from head of infant after intubation. Insert UVC 2-4 cm. Hold or tape catheter to avoid dislodgement.
☐ After at least 45-60 seconds of chest compressions, evaluates HR, breathing, and oxygen saturation	**Heart rate remains below 60 bpm. Apneic. Pulse oximeter might not be functioning.**
☐ Administers or directs administration of IV epinephrine	Epinephrine 1:10,000 (0.1 mg/kg). *IV dose:* 0.1 to 0.3 mL/kg. Flush UVC with 0.5-1 mL normal saline.
☐ After at least 45-60 seconds of chest compressions, evaluates HR, breathing, and oxygen saturation.	**Heart rate above 60 bpm. Occasional gasp. Pulse oximetry functioning.**
☐ Discontinues compressions, continues ventilation at 40-60 breaths/minute	Discontinue compressions if HR above 60 bpm. Reassess every 30 seconds.
☐ (Option) Based on scenario, identifies need for volume replacement (states solution, dose, route, rate)	*Risk factors:* Placenta previa, abruption, blood loss from umbilical cord. *Solutions:* Normal saline, Ringer's lactate or O Rh-negative packed cells. *Dose:* 10 mL/kg over 5-10 minutes. *Route:* Umbilical vein. *Rate:* Over 5-10 minutes.
☐ Continues to monitor HR, breathing, and oxygen saturation every 30 seconds during resuscitation	Adjust oxygen based on oximetry and newborn's age. Continue PPV until HR above 100 bpm with adequate respiratory effort (newborn may remain intubated).
☐ Directs post-resuscitation care	Ongoing evaluation and monitoring. Communicate effectively with parent(s).

Reflective Questions:
1. What did you think you would need to do when this baby was placed on the radiant warmer?
2. What went well during this resuscitation? What would you do differently next time?
3. What NRP Key Behavioral Skills were used? Give examples.

Neonatal Resuscitation Program Key Behavioral Skills

Know your environment. / Delegate workload optimally. / Use all available resources.
Anticipate and plan. / Allocate attention wisely. / Call for help when needed.
Assume the leadership role. / Use all available information. / Maintain professional behavior.
Communicate effectively.

List of Neonatal Resuscitation Program Resuscitation Skills Videos

Neonatal Resuscitation Program Resuscitation Skills Videos

These videos of selected resuscitation skills can be found on the *NRP Instructor DVD: An Interactive Tool for Facilitation of Simulation-based Learning,* and with enhanced graphics and animations on the DVD that accompanies the *Textbook of Neonatal Resuscitation, 6th Edition.* These DVDs may be viewed on a computer screen or through an LCD projector.

1. Equipment Check
2. Using a Meconium Aspirator
3. CPAP Administration
4. Using Pulse Oximetry
5. Using the T-piece Resuscitator
6. Positive-Pressure Ventilation With a Flow-Inflating Bag
7. MR SOPA: Ventilation Corrective Steps
8. Orogastric Tube Placement
9. Endotracheal Intubation
10. Using an End-Tidal CO_2 Detector
11. Endotracheal Tube: Emergency Tape Technique
12. Laryngeal Mask Airway Placement
13. Chest Compressions: Head of Infant Positioning
14. Preparing the Emergency UVC for Insertion
15. Placing an Emergency UVC
16. Securing and safeguarding the Emergency UVC
17. Drawing Up and Administering Epinephrine
18. Needle Thoracentesis
19. The ELBW Baby: Aspects of Delivery Room Management

Key Points in Lessons 1 Through 9 of the *Textbook of Neonatal Resuscitation, 6th Edition*

Lesson 1 Key Points

1. Most newly born babies are vigorous. Only about 10% require some kind of assistance and only 1% need major resuscitative measures (intubation, chest compressions, and/or medications) to survive.

2. The most important and effective action in neonatal resuscitation is to ventilate the baby's lungs.

3. Lack of ventilation of the newborn's lungs results in sustained constriction of the pulmonary arterioles, preventing systemic arterial blood from becoming oxygenated. Prolonged lack of

adequate perfusion and oxygenation to the baby's organs can lead to brain damage, damage to other organs, or death.

4. When a fetus/newborn first becomes compromised, an initial period of attempted rapid breathing is followed by primary apnea and decreasing heart rate that will improve with tactile stimulation. If compromise continues, secondary apnea ensues, accompanied by a continued fall in heart rate and blood pressure. Secondary apnea cannot be reversed with stimulation; assisted ventilation must be provided.

5. Initiation of effective positive-pressure ventilation during secondary apnea usually results in a rapid improvement in heart rate.

6. Many, but not all, babies who will require neonatal resuscitation can be anticipated by identifying the presence of antepartum and intrapartum risk factors associated with the need for neonatal resuscitation.

7. All newborns require initial assessment to determine whether resuscitation is required.

8. Every birth should be attended by at least 1 person whose only responsibility is the baby and who is capable of initiating resuscitation. Either that person or someone else who is immediately available should have the necessary additional skills required to perform a complete resuscitation. When resuscitation is anticipated, additional personnel should be present in the delivery room before the delivery occurs.

9. Resuscitation should proceed rapidly.
   - You have approximately 30 seconds to achieve a response from one step before deciding whether you need to go on to the next.
   - Evaluation and decision making are based primarily on respirations, heart rate, and oxygenation.

10. Behavioral skills such as teamwork, leadership, and effective communication are critical to successful resuscitation of the newborn.

11. The steps of neonatal resuscitation are as follows:
    A. Initial steps.
       - Provide warmth.
       - Position head and clear airway as necessary.*
       - Dry and stimulate the baby to breathe.
       - Evaluate respirations, heart rate, and oxygenation.
    B. Provide positive-pressure ventilation with a resuscitation positive-pressure device and apply pulse oximeter.*
    C. Provide chest compressions as you continue assisted ventilation and insert emergency umbilical venous catheter.*
    D. Administer epinephrine as you continue assisted ventilation and chest compressions.*

    *Consider intubation of the trachea at these points.

Lesson 2 Key Points

1. If meconium is present and the newborn *is not vigorous,* suction the baby's trachea before proceeding with any other steps. If the newborn *is vigorous,* suction the mouth and nose only, and proceed with taking the baby to the mother for your further assessment.

2. "Vigorous" is defined as a newborn who has strong respiratory efforts, good muscle tone, and a heart rate greater than 100 beats per minute.

3. Open the airway by positioning the newborn in a "sniffing" position.

4. Appropriate forms of tactile stimulation are
   • Slapping or flicking the soles of the feet
   • Gently rubbing the back

5. Continued use of tactile stimulation in an apneic newborn wastes valuable time. For persistent apnea, begin positive-pressure ventilation promptly.

6. A fetus has an oxygen saturation of approximately 60%, and it may take up to 10 minutes for a healthy newborn to increase saturation to the normal range of over 90%.

7. Acceptable methods for administering free-flow oxygen are
   • Oxygen mask held firmly over the baby's face
   • Mask from a flow-inflating bag or T-piece resuscitator held closely over the baby's mouth and nose
   • Oxygen tubing cupped closely over the baby's mouth and nose

8. Free-flow oxygen cannot be given reliably by a mask attached to a self-inflating bag.

9. Decisions and actions during newborn resuscitation are based on the newborn's
   • Respirations   • Heart rate   • Color (oxygenation)

10. Determine a newborn's heart rate by counting how many beats are in 6 seconds, then multiply by 10. For example, if you count 8 beats in 6 seconds, announce the baby's heart rate as 80 beats per minute.

11. Oxygen should be treated as a drug—either too little or too much can be injurious.

12. Use pulse oximetry:
    • When resuscitation is anticipated
    • When positive-pressure ventilation is required for more than a few breaths
    • When central cyanosis is persistent
    • When supplemental oxygen is administered
    • To confirm your perception of cyanosis

Lesson 3 Key Points

1. Ventilation of the lungs is the single most important and most effective step in cardiopulmonary resuscitation of the compromised newborn.

2. Indications for positive-pressure ventilation are
   - Apnea/gasping
   - Heart rate below 100 beats per minute even if breathing
   - Persistent central cyanosis and low SpO_2 despite free-flow supplemental oxygen increased to 100%

3. Resuscitation of term newborns may begin with 21% oxygen (room air); resuscitation of preterm newborns may begin with a somewhat higher oxygen concentration. Pulse oximetry is used to help adjust the amount of supplemental oxygen to avoid giving too much or too little oxygen.

4. Self-inflating bags
   - Fill spontaneously after they are squeezed, pulling oxygen or air into the bag
   - Remain inflated at all times
   - Must have a tight mask-to-face seal to inflate the lungs
   - Can deliver positive-pressure ventilation (PPV) without a compressed gas source; user must be certain the bag is connected to an oxygen source for the purpose of neonatal resuscitation
   - Require attachment of an oxygen reservoir to deliver high oxygen concentration
   - Cannot be used to administer free-flow oxygen reliably through the mask and cannot be used to deliver continuous positive airway pressure (CPAP)
   - Should have an integral pressure gauge, or, if there is a site for attaching a pressure gauge (manometer), it should be attached

5. Flow-inflating bags
   - Fill only when gas from a compressed source flows into them
   - Depend on a compressed gas source
   - Must have a tight mask-to-face seal to inflate
   - Use a flow-control valve to regulate pressure/inflation
   - Should have a pressure gauge (manometer)
   - Look like a deflated balloon when not in use
   - Can be used to administer free-flow oxygen and CPAP

6. The flow-inflating bag will not work if
   - The mask is not properly sealed over the newborn's nose and mouth.
   - There is a hole in the bag.
   - The flow-control valve is open too far.
   - The pressure gauge is missing or the port is not occluded.

7. T-piece resuscitators
   • Depend on a compressed gas source.
   • Must have a tight mask-to-face seal to inflate the lungs.
   • Require selection of a maximum pressure, peak inspiratory pressure, and positive-end expiratory pressure (PEEP).
   • May require adjustment of peak inspiratory pressure during resuscitation to achieve physiologic improvement, audible breath sounds, and perceptible chest movements.
   • Provide positive pressure when operator alternately occludes and opens the aperture in the PEEP cap.
   • Can be used to deliver free-flow oxygen and CPAP.

8. An oxygen reservoir must be attached to deliver high concentrations of oxygen using a self-inflating bag. Without the reservoir, the bag delivers a maximum of only about 40% oxygen, which may be insufficient for neonatal resuscitation.

9. The PPV device should be assembled and connected to a blender so that any concentration of oxygen from 21% (room air), up to 100% oxygen, can be provided.

10. If an oxygen blender and pulse oximeter are not immediately available, start PPV with 21% oxygen (room air) while you obtain an air-oxygen source and an oximeter.

11. Using pulse oximetry, supplemental oxygen concentration should be adjusted to achieve the target values for pre-ductal saturations summarized in the table on the Neonatal Resuscitation Program™ (NRP™) flow diagram.

12. If you cannot detect audible bilateral breath sounds and see no perceptible chest expansion during assisted ventilation, check or correct the following:
    • **M:** Mask adjustment.
    • **R:** Reposition airway.
    • **S:** Suction mouth and nose.
    • **O:** Open mouth.
    • **P:** Pressure increase.
    • **A:** Airway alternative.

13. The most important indicator of successful PPV is rising heart rate.

14. Effective ventilation is defined by the presence of
    • Bilateral breath sounds
    • Chest movement (heart rate may rise without visible chest movement, especially in preterm newborns)

15. Signs that PPV has been effective, and indications that PPV may be discontinued, are
    • Heart rate rises to over 100 breaths per minute
    • Improvement in oxygen saturation
    • Onset of spontaneous respirations

Lesson 4 Key Points

1. Chest compressions are indicated when the heart rate remains below 60 beats per minute, despite 30 seconds of effective positive-pressure ventilation.

2. Once the heart rate is below 60 beats per minute, the oximeter may stop working. You should increase the oxygen to 100% until return of the oximeter reading to guide you in the appropriate adjustment of delivered oxygen.

3. Chest compressions
   - Compress the heart against the spine.
   - Increase intrathoracic pressure.
   - Circulate blood to the vital organs, including the brain.

4. There are 2 acceptable techniques for chest compressions—the thumb technique and the 2-finger technique—but the thumb technique is preferred.

5. Locate the correct area for compressions by running your fingers along the lower edge of the rib cage until you locate the xiphoid. Then place your thumbs or fingers on the sternum, above the xiphoid and on a line connecting the nipples.

6. To ensure proper rate of chest compressions and ventilation, the compressor repeats "One-and-Two-and-Three-and-Breathe-and...."

7. During chest compressions, the breathing rate is 30 breaths per minute and the compression rate is 90 compressions per minute. This equals 120 "events" per minute. One cycle of 3 compressions and 1 breath takes 2 seconds.

8. If you anticipate that the baby will need medication by the umbilical route, you can continue chest compressions by moving to the head of the bed to continue giving compressions using the thumb technique. Performing chest compressions from the head of the bed is most easily accomplished if the trachea has been intubated.

9. During chest compressions, ensure that
   - Chest movement is adequate during ventilation.
   - Supplemental oxygen is being used.
   - Compression depth is one-third of the diameter of the chest.
   - Pressure is released fully to permit chest recoil during relaxation phase of chest compression.
   - Thumbs or fingers remain in contact with the chest at all times.
   - Duration of the downward stroke of the compression is shorter than duration of the release.
   - Chest compressions and ventilation are well coordinated.

10. After 45 to 60 seconds of chest compressions and ventilation, check the heart rate. If the heart rate is
    - Greater than 60 beats per minute, discontinue compressions and continue ventilation at 40 to 60 breaths per minute.
    - Greater than 100 beats per minute, discontinue compressions and gradually discontinue ventilation if the newborn is breathing spontaneously.
    - Less than 60 beats per minute, intubate the newborn (if not already done), and give epinephrine, preferably intravenously. Intubation provides a more reliable method of continuing ventilation.

Lesson 5 Key Points

1. A person experienced in endotracheal intubation should be immediately available to assist at every delivery.

2. Indications for endotracheal intubation include the following:
   - To suction the trachea in the presence of meconium when the newborn is not vigorous
   - To improve efficacy of ventilation if mask ventilation is ineffective
   - To improve efficacy of ventilation if mask ventilation is required for more than a few minutes
   - To facilitate coordination of chest compressions and ventilation and to maximize the efficiency of each ventilation
   - To improve ventilation in special conditions, such as extreme prematurity, surfactant administration, or suspected diaphragmatic hernia (see Lessons 7 and 8)

3. The laryngoscope is always held in the operator's left hand.

4. The correct-sized laryngoscope blade for a term newborn is No. 1. The correct-sized blade for a preterm newborn is No. 0 or, in extremely preterm infants, No. 00.

5. Choice of the proper endotracheal tube size is based on weight.

Weight (g)	Gestational Age (wks)	Tube Size (mm) (inside diameter)
Below 1,000	Below 28	2.5
1,000-2,000	28-34	3.0
2,000-3,000	34-38	3.5
Above 3,000	Above 38	3.5-4.0

6. The intubation procedure ideally should be completed within 30 seconds.

7. The steps for intubating a newborn are as follows:
   - Stabilize the newborn's head in the "sniffing" position.

- Slide the laryngoscope over the right side of the tongue, pushing the tongue to the left side of the mouth, and advancing the blade until the tip lies just beyond the base of the tongue.
- Lift the blade slightly. Raise the entire blade, not just the tip.
- Look for landmarks. Vocal cords should appear as vertical stripes on each side of the glottis or as an inverted letter "V". Suction with a large bore catheter, if necessary, for visualization.
- Insert the tube into the right side of the mouth with the curve of the tube lying in the horizontal plane so that the tube curves from left to right.
- If the cords are closed, wait for them to open. Insert the tip of the endotracheal tube until the vocal cord guide is at the level of the cords.
- Hold the tube firmly against the baby's palate while removing the laryngoscope. Hold the tube in place while removing the stylet if one was used.

8. Correct placement of the endotracheal tube is indicated by
   - Improved vital signs (heart rate, color/oximetry, activity)
   - Presence of exhaled CO_2 as determined by a CO_2 detector
   - Breath sounds over both lung fields but decreased or absent over the stomach
   - No gastric distention with ventilation
   - Vapor in the tube during exhalation
   - Chest movement with each breath
   - Tip-to-lip measurement: add 6 to newborn's estimated weight in kilograms
   - Direct visualization of the tube passing between the vocal cords
   - Chest x-ray confirmation if the tube is to remain in place past initial resuscitation

9. Placement of a laryngeal mask airway may be useful in the following situations:
   - When facial or upper airway malformations render ventilation by mask ineffective
   - When positive-pressure ventilation with a face mask fails to achieve effective ventilation and intubation is not possible

10. The limitations of a laryngeal mask airway are
    - Currently available devices are too large for small preterm babies (or babies less than approximately 32 weeks' gestational age).
    - The device cannot be used to suction meconium from the airway.
    - An air leak at the mask-larynx interface may result in delivery of insufficient pressure to the lungs.
    - Its use during chest compressions or to deliver medications to the lungs may not be as effective as with an endotracheal tube.
    - There is insufficient evidence to recommend the laryngeal mask airway for prolonged assisted ventilation in newborns.

Lesson 6 Key Points

1. Epinephrine is a cardiac stimulant that also increases blood pressure. Preferably, it should be given by umbilical venous catheter. Its administration is indicated when the heart rate remains below 60 beats per minute despite 30 seconds of effective assisted ventilation, followed by another 45 to 60 seconds of coordinated chest compressions and ventilations.

2. Recommended epinephrine
   - Concentration: 1:10,000 (0.1 mg/mL)
   - Route: Intravenously. Endotracheal administration may be considered while intravenous access is being established.
   - Dose: 0.1 to 0.3 mL/kg of a 1:10,000 concentration solution (consider higher dose, 0.5 to 1 mL/kg, for endotracheal route only)
   - Rate: *Rapidly*—as quickly as possible

3. Epinephrine should be given by umbilical vein. Administration via the endotracheal route is often faster and more accessible than placing an umbilical catheter, but is associated with unreliable absorption and is very likely not to be effective.

4. Indications for volume expansion during resuscitation include
   - Baby is not responding to resuscitation.

   AND
   - Baby appears in shock (pale color, weak pulses, persistently low heart rate, no improvement in circulatory status despite resuscitation efforts).

   OR
   - There is a history of a condition associated with fetal blood loss (eg, extensive vaginal bleeding, placenta previa, twin-to-twin transfusion, etc).

5. Recommended volume expander
   - Solution: Normal saline, Ringer's lactate, or O Rh-negative blood
   - Dose: 10 mL/kg
   - Route: Umbilical vein
   - Preparation: Correct volume drawn into a large syringe
   - Rate: Over 5 to 10 minutes

Lesson 7 Key Points

1. The appropriate action for a baby who fails to respond to resuscitation will depend on the presentation—failure to ventilate, persistent oxygen desaturation or bradycardia, or failure to initiate spontaneous breathing.

2. Respiratory distress due to choanal atresia can be helped by placing an oral airway.

3. Airway obstruction from Robin syndrome can be helped by inserting a nasopharyngeal tube and placing the baby prone.

4. In an emergency, a pneumothorax can be detected by transillumination and treated by aspirating air with a syringe attached to a needle inserted into the chest.

5. If diaphragmatic hernia is suspected, avoid positive-pressure ventilation by mask. Immediately intubate the trachea in the delivery room and insert an orogastric tube to decompress the stomach and intestines.

6. Persistent oxygen desaturation and/or bradycardia are rarely caused by congenital heart disease in a newborn. More commonly, the persistent desaturation and bradycardia are caused by inadequate ventilation.

7. A baby who has required resuscitation must have close monitoring and management of oxygenation, blood pressure, fluid status, respiratory effort, blood glucose, nutritional issues, and temperature.

8. Be careful not to overheat the baby during or following resuscitation.

9. If a mother has recently received narcotics and her baby fails to breathe, first provide effective positive-pressure ventilation to maintain a heart rate above 100 bpm, then you might consider giving naloxone to the baby.

10. Restoring adequate ventilation is the priority when resuscitating babies at birth in the delivery room or later in the nursery or other location.

11. Management steps for babies requiring resuscitation outside the delivery room include the following:
    - Maintain temperature by placing the baby skin-to-skin with the mother and raising the environmental temperature.
    - Clear airway with a bulb syringe or a cloth on your finger.
    - Use mouth-to-mouth-and-nose breathing for providing positive-pressure ventilation.
    - Obtain vascular access by cannulating a peripheral vein or placing an intraosseous needle in the intraosseous space in the tibia.

12. Therapeutic hypothermia following perinatal asphyxia should be
    - Used only for babies ≥36 weeks' gestation who meet previously defined criteria for this therapy
    - Initiated before 6 hours after birth
    - Used only according to specific protocols coordinated by centers with specialized programs equipped to provide the therapy

Lesson 8 Key Points

1. Preterm babies are at additional risk for requiring resuscitation because of their
   - Rapid heat loss
   - Vulnerability to hyperoxic injury
   - Immature lungs and diminished respiratory drive
   - Immature brains that are prone to bleeding
   - Vulnerability to infection
   - Small blood volume, increasing the implications of blood loss

2. Additional resources needed to prepare for an anticipated preterm birth include
   - Additional trained personnel, including someone with intubation and emergency umbilical venous catheterization expertise
   - Additional strategies for maintaining temperature
   - Compressed air source
   - Oxygen blender
   - Pulse oximeter

3. Premature babies are more vulnerable to hyperoxia; use an oximeter and blender to gradually achieve oxyhemoglobin saturations in the 85% to 95% range during and immediately following resuscitation.

4. Babies born very preterm are more susceptible to heat loss.
   - Increase temperature of room.
   - Preheat radiant warmer.
   - Consider using a chemically activated warming pad.
   - Use polyethylene wrap for babies less than approximately 29 weeks' gestation.
   - Use warmed transport incubator to transfer baby to nursery.

5. When assisting ventilation in preterm babies,
   - Follow the same criteria for initiating positive-pressure ventilation as with term babies.
   - Consider using continuous positive airway pressure (CPAP) if the baby is breathing spontaneously with a heart rate above 100 bpm, but has labored respirations or a low oxygen saturation. Use positive end-expiratory pressure if the baby has been intubated.
   - If positive-pressure ventilation is required, use the lowest inflation pressure necessary to achieve an adequate response.
   - Consider giving prophylactic surfactant.

6. Decrease the risk of brain injury by
   - Handling the baby gently
   - Avoiding the Trendelenburg position
   - Avoiding high airway pressures, when possible
   - Adjusting ventilation gradually, based on physical examination, oximetry, and blood gases

- Avoiding rapid intravenous fluid boluses and hypertonic solutions

7. After resuscitation of a preterm baby,
   - Monitor and control blood glucose.
   - Monitor for apnea, bradycardia, or oxygen desaturations, and intervene promptly.
   - Monitor and control oxygenation and ventilation.
   - Consider delaying feeding or initiating feeds cautiously if perinatal compromise was significant.
   - Have a high level of suspicion for infection.

Lesson 9 Key Points

1. The ethical principles regarding the resuscitation of a newborn should be no different from those followed in resuscitating an older child or adult.

2. Ethical and current national legal principles do not mandate attempted resuscitation in all circumstances, and withdrawal of critical care interventions and institution of comfort care are considered acceptable if there is agreement by health care professionals and the parents that further resuscitation efforts would be futile, would merely prolong dying, or would not offer sufficient benefit to justify the burdens imposed.

3. Parents are considered to be the appropriate surrogate decision makers for their own babies. For parents to fulfill this role responsibly, they must be given relevant and accurate information about the risks and benefits of each treatment option.

4. Where gestation, birth weight, and/or congenital anomalies are associated with almost certain early death, or unacceptably high morbidity is likely among the rare survivors, resuscitation is not indicated, although exceptions may be reasonable to comply with parental wishes.

5. In conditions associated with uncertain prognosis, where there is borderline survival and a high rate of morbidity, and where the burden to the child is high, parental desires regarding initiation of resuscitation should be supported.

6. Unless conception occurred via in vitro fertilization, techniques used for obstetrics dating are accurate to 3 to 5 days if applied in the first trimester, and only to ± 1 to 2 weeks subsequently. Estimates of fetal weight are accurate only to ± 15% to 20%. When counseling parents about the births of babies born at the extremes of prematurity, advise them that decisions made about neonatal management before birth may need to be modified in the delivery room, depending on the condition of the baby at birth and the postnatal gestational age assessment.

7. Discontinuation of resuscitation efforts should be considered after 10 minutes of absent heart rate. The decision to continue resuscitation efforts beyond this point should take into consideration factors such as the presumed etiology of the arrest, the gestational age of the baby, the presence or absence of complications, the potential role of therapeutic hypothermia, and the parents' previously expressed feelings about acceptable risk of morbidity.

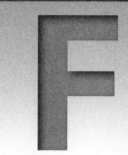

Scenario and Debriefing Tools

Neonatal Resuscitation Program Key Behavioral Skills

1. Know your environment.
2. Anticipate and plan.
3. Assume the leadership role.
4. Communicate effectively.
5. Delegate workload optimally.
6. Allocate attention wisely.
7. Use all available information.
8. Use all available resources.
9. Call for help when needed.
10. Maintain professional behavior.

From the Center for Advanced Pediatric and Perinatal Education (CAPE), Packard Children's Hospital at Stanford University (**http://www.cape.lpch.org**).

🖳**www**

Neonatal Resuscitation Program Key Behavioral Skills*	Examples of the Behavioral Skill in Action[†]
Know your environment.	Learners perform Equipment Check before newborn arrives. Learners know location of code cart or how to access it. Learners know to call for help and who is available.
Anticipate and plan.	All learners listen to circumstances of scenario. Resuscitation team "huddles" and assigns roles and responsibilities. Team discusses action plan in event of potential complications.
Assume the leadership role.	Learners "huddle" and assign leadership role(s). Leader clearly articulates goals. Leader effectively uses resources. Leader delegates tasks, as appropriate. Leader uses call-outs to communicate critical information. Leader asks for input from team members. Leader enables team members to challenge the plan when appropriate. Leader promotes teamwork and resolves conflict. Learners discuss plan in the event leadership role must shift due to the leader becoming engrossed in a task or procedure. Leader includes family in communication.
Communicate effectively.	Team members call each other by name. All team members actively share information. Team member orders medications by name, dose, and route. Team members verify information that is communicated. Team members ensure that changes in information are shared with all team members.
Delegate workload optimally.	Team members do not duplicate work or use more resources than necessary. • One person holds endotracheal tube and positive-pressure ventilation device. • One person holds emergency umbilical venous catheter and flush syringe. Team members agree to change task assignments depending on skill sets and what is required at the moment. Team members protect each other from work overload.
Allocate attention wisely.	Team members maintain situation awareness by scanning and assessing at all times. Team members monitor one another's actions in context of patient safety.
Use all available information.	Team members ask about prenatal, intrapartum history, including presence of meconium-stained amniotic fluid prior to birth. Team members ask about newborn history, if newborn is being resuscitated after first minutes of life.
Use all available resources.	Know human resources available. Know supplies and equipment availability.
Call for help when needed.	Team members call for help in timely manner. Team members know process for getting assistance of the right kind.
Maintain professional behavior.	Team members use respectful verbal and nonverbal behaviors. Team members actively seek and offer assistance. Team members support and promote teamwork. All team members are equally valued and respected.

*NRP Key Behavioral Skills are from the Center for Advanced Pediatric and Perinatal Education (CAPE), Lucile Packard Children's Hospital at Stanford University. Available at: http://cape.lpch.org/courses/logistics/skills.html. Accessed January 31, 2011.

†Selected information in column 2 derived from TeamSTEPPS™ Pocket Guide: Strategies & Tools to Enhance Performance and Patient Safety. Dept of Defense and Agency for Healthcare Research and Quality. *AHRQ.* Pub. No. 06-0020-2. Revised Nov 2008. Version 06.1.

Sample Ground Rules for Simulation and Debriefing	
The NRP instructor will	• Create a plausible scenario based on the participants' learning objectives. • Create a learning environment that resembles the birth setting as closely as possible, given the constraints of available resources. • Orient learners to supplies and equipment and how physiologic responses are demonstrated. • Promote learning in a safe and supportive environment where mistakes are considered an important part of the learning process. • Assume that learners are intelligent, doing their best, and striving to improve. • Maintain confidentiality. A learner's performance is never discussed outside the event, videotape is deleted after debriefing unless the instructor has each participant's written permission to use the film for a specified purpose, and aspects of a learner's performance are never used for an evaluation with a supervisor.
Neonatal Resuscitation Program learners will	• Participate fully in simulation and debriefing and maintain confidentiality as instructed. • Suspend disbelief and behave as they would during an actual resuscitation. • Think out loud and talk through interventions so that everyone knows what is happening. • Help each other in any way that is plausible to the scenario. Teamwork is expected. • Perform the actions. Pretending or "saying" the action without doing it is not acceptable. • Maintain professional behavior. Giggling and joking are not acceptable during resuscitation. • Treat others with respect. Support everyone's learning, even when it occurs by making mistakes. • Agree to play a role other than one's real-life • professional role, if necessary, remembering that the NRP does not certify or authorize learners to perform interventions outside their designated scope of practice.

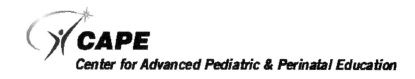

CONFIDENTIALITY AGREEMENT

During your participation in training in a simulated medical environment at the Center for Advanced Pediatric and Perinatal Education (CAPE) at Lucile Packard Children's Hospital at Stanford you will be both an active participant in realistic scenarios and an observer of others immersed in similar situations (either in real time or on videotape). The objective of this training program is to train individuals to better assess and improve their performance in difficult clinical situations. It is to be understood that the scenarios to which you and your colleagues will be exposed are designed to exacerbate the likelihood of lapses and errors in performance. Because of these issues you are asked to maintain strict confidentiality regarding both your performance and the performance of others, whether witnessed in real time or on videotape. Failure to maintain confidentiality may result in unwarranted and unfair defamation of character of the participants. This could cause irreparable harm to you and your colleagues and would seriously impair the effectiveness of this simulation-based training program.

While you are free to discuss in general terms the technical and behavioral skills acquired and maintained during training at CAPE, you are required to maintain strict confidentiality regarding the specific scenarios to which you are both directly and indirectly exposed. The development of challenging scenarios is extremely labor intensive and any foreknowledge by participants of what is to be presented to them will defeat the purpose of this type of training.

The bottom line: All that takes place in the simulator, stays in the simulator.

By signing below, you acknowledge having read and understood this statement and agree to maintain the strictest confidentiality about the performance of individuals and the details of scenarios to which you are exposed.

Signature: _____ Date: _____

Print name: _____

E-mail: _____

From the Center for Advanced Pediatric and Perinatal Education (CAPE), Packard Children's Hospital at Stanford University (**http://www.cape.lpch.org**).

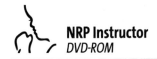 **NRP Instructor**
DVD-ROM

Appendix D
Sample Scenario Template

Title of Scenario: _____

Brief description for instructors: _____
_____

Learning objectives (cognitive, technical, and behavioral):

1. _____
_____

2. _____
_____

3. _____
_____

4. _____
_____

5. _____
_____

Pertinent history for learners:

Mother: _____ years old G_____ P_____ estimated gestational age: _____ weeks

Delivery: ☐ vaginal birth ☐ cesarean birth

Other (prenatal history, laboratory results, ultrasound results, pertinent maternal and social history, antepartum complications):

_____
_____

Scenario location:

☐ LDR ☐ OR ☐ ED ☐ ambulance ☐ parking lot ☐ other _____

Necessary equipment and supplies:

☐ Complete resuscitation setup

☐ Variance in setup (list additional supplies or equipment required): _____

Manikin preparation:

_____

Initial condition of neonate:

_____

Expected interventions during scenario:

_____

_____

_____

Skills demonstrated (cognitive, technical, behavioral):

Cognitive

1. _____

2. _____

3. _____

Technical

☐ Equipment check

☐ Initial steps

☐ Positive-pressure ventilation

    ☐ Self-inflating bag   ☐ Flow-inflating bag   ☐ T-piece resuscitator

    ☐ Management of oxygen concentration

    ☐ Rate and pressure

    ☐ MR SOPA

    ☐ Assessment of heart rate

    ☐ Assessment of breath sounds

    ☐ Use of pulse oximetry

    ☐ Administration of free-flow oxygen

    ☐ Use of orogastric tube as necessary

    ☐ Assessment of need for post-resuscitation care

☐ Chest compressions

☐ Endotracheal intubation (or assistance with intubation)

☐ Emergency umbilical venous catheter placement (or assistance with placement)

☐ Epinephrine administration (drawing up, routes, dosages)

☐ Laryngeal mask airway placement

Behavioral

☐ Know your environment.

☐ Anticipate and plan.

☐ Assume the leadership role.

☐ Communicate effectively.

☐ Delegate workload optimally.

☐ Allocate attention wisely.

☐ Use all available information.

☐ Use all available resources.

☐ Call for help when needed.

☐ Maintain professional behavior.

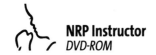

NRP Instructor
DVD-ROM

Appendix D
Sample Scenario Template

Title of Scenario: _Resuscitation with Bag and Mask_

Brief description for instructors: _This patient is born via vaginal delivery at 35 weeks' gestation & presents apneic; he begins to breathe spontaneously if bag-and-mask ventilation is properly administered._

Learning objectives (cognitive, technical, and behavioral):

1. _Identify the newborn who requires positive-pressure ventilation (PPV)._

2. _Demonstrate correct technique for PPV, including placement of mask on the newborn's face, rate and pressure, and corrective actions (MR SOPA) for ineffective PPV._

3. _Demonstrate correct placement and interpretation of pulse oximetry._

4. _Recognize improvement during PPV by noting improvement in increased heart rate, color and oxygen saturation, muscle tone, and spontaneous breathing._

5. _Demonstrate pertinent key behavioral skills to optimize team performance._

Pertinent history for learners:

Mother: _22_ years old   G_2_ P_1_   estimated gestational age: _35_ weeks

Delivery: ☒ vaginal birth   ☐ cesarean birth

Other (prenatal history, laboratory results, ultrasound results, pertinent maternal and social history, antepartum complications):

none

Scenario location:

☒ LDR   ☐ OR   ☐ ED   ☐ ambulance   ☐ parking lot   ☐ other _____

Necessary equipment and supplies:

☒ Complete resuscitation setup

☐ Variance in setup (list additional supplies or equipment required): _none_

Manikin preparation:

Blood, vernix

Initial condition of neonate:

Limp, apneic, cyanotic, Heart rate (HR) 50 beats per minute (bpm)

Expected interventions during scenario:

Equipment check, including presence and function of PPV device, initial steps, assessment of heart rate and breathing, call for assistance, initiation of PPV, pulse oximetry, assessment of effectiveness of PPV, corrective steps, 30 seconds of effective PPV, recognition of improving HR, tone, pulse oximetry, cessation of PPV, administration of free flow oxygen, assessment of need for post-resuscitation care.

Skills demonstrated (cognitive, technical, behavioral):

Cognitive

1. Recognize the infant who requires PPV.

2. Recall indications for effective ventilation (rising HR, rising oxygen saturation, bilateral breath sounds, chest movement).

3. Interpret pulse oximetry & adjust oxygen concentration according to the newborn's age & SpO2 target range.

Technical

- ☐ Equipment check
- ☐ Initial steps
- ☐ Positive-pressure ventilation
  - ☐ Self-inflating bag   ☐ Flow-inflating bag   ☐ T-piece resuscitator
  - ☐ Management of oxygen concentration
  - ☐ Rate and pressure
  - ☐ MR SOPA
  - ☐ Assessment of heart rate
  - ☐ Assessment of breath sounds
  - ☐ Use of pulse oximetry
  - ☐ Administration of free-flow oxygen
  - ☐ Use of orogastric tube as necessary
  - ☐ Assessment of need for post-resuscitation care
- ☐ Chest compressions
- ☐ Endotracheal intubation (or assistance with intubation)
- ☐ Emergency umbilical venous catheter placement (or assistance with placement)
- ☐ Epinephrine administration (drawing up, routes, dosages)
- ☐ Laryngeal mask airway placement

Behavioral

- ☐ Know your environment.
- ☐ Anticipate and plan.
- ☐ Assume the leadership role.
- ☐ Communicate effectively.
- ☐ Delegate workload optimally.
- ☐ Allocate attention wisely.
- ☐ Use all available information.
- ☐ Use all available resources.
- ☐ Call for help when needed.
- ☐ Maintain professional behavior.

Instructions for Using the Sample Scenario Template

Sample Scenario Template Section	Instructions and Notes for Use
Title of Scenario "Resuscitation With Bag and Mask"	The Title of Scenario is the name you give the scenario so that instructors can easily find this in a file by title. We call this one "Resuscitation With Bag and Mask."
Brief Description "This patient is born via vaginal delivery at 35 weeks' gestation and presents apneic; he begins to breathe spontaneously if bag-and-mask ventilation is properly administered."	Brief Description is one sentence that tells NRP instructors what occurs in the scenario.
Learning Objectives 1. Identify the newborn who requires positive-pressure ventilation (PPV). **(cognitive)** 2. Demonstrate correct technique for positive-pressure ventilation, including placement of the mask on the newborn's face, rate and pressure . . . **(cognitive and technical)** 3. Demonstrate correct placement and interpretation of pulse oximetry. **(cognitive and technical)** 4. Recognize improvement during PPV by noting improvement in increased heart rate, color and oxygen saturation . . . **(technical)** 5. Demonstrate pertinent key behavioral skills to optimize team performance. **(behavioral)**	These describe what you expect the learners to know/do during the scenario when they successfully integrate the cognitive, technical, and behavioral skills. Each scenario should encompass about 2-5 learning objectives in each of the three categories depending on the length and complexity of the scenario. This is a short and simple scenario with 5 learning objectives which encompass 3 cognitive objectives, 3 technical objectives, and 1 behavioral objective. The behavioral objective is written in general terms to capture any Key Behavioral Skill listed on the second page of the scenario template form. Other skills may indeed be demonstrated, but only the most important are listed so instructors and learners alike know on which ones to focus. You may wish to use selected Learning Objectives listed on each Performance Checklist.
Pertinent History for Learners Mother: *22* years old *G2 P1* Estimated gestational age: *35 weeks* Delivery: *x* vaginal birth Other: none	This section is more detailed than the Brief Description section above. Instructors need to know the details so they know how the newborn should respond (or not respond) to the learners' actions. The amount of information given to learners depends on the learning objectives. Sometimes a complete history is provided in the "Other" category, including maternal blood type, prenatal laboratory results, gestational age assessment methods, difficulties during pregnancy, ultrasound results, and pertinent maternal health and social issues. At other times, the learners are called to the delivery room, given limited information and limited time to prepare for the birth.
Scenario Location *X* LDR	Scenario location is usually the delivery room; however, the learning objectives may direct the birth setting to a different place such as the Operating Room, Emergency Department, ambulance, or parking lot.

Instructions for Using the Sample Scenario Template—*continued*

Sample Scenario Template Section	Instructions and Notes for Use
Necessary Equipment and Supplies *X* Complete resuscitation setup *X* Variance in setup: None	Scenarios that take place in the Delivery Room necessitate a complete resuscitation setup unless the learning objectives include improvisation or a work-around due to missing or malfunctioning equipment. "Variance in Setup" cues the instructor in the event that the usual setup is different, requiring either more or less equipment to match the learning objectives.
Manikin preparation *Blood, vernix*	Helps the instructor set the scene, especially if the newborn requires special effects besides blood, vernix, or meconium.
Page 2 of scenario template form	
Initial condition of the neonate *Limp, apneic, cyanotic, HR 50 beats per minute (bpm)*	Important to know so that learners begin the scenario with the correct physiologic feedback (eg, limp, apneic, cyanotic, HR 50 bpm in this case).
Expected interventions during the scenario **Equipment check, initial steps, assessment of heart rate and breathing, call for assistance, initiation of PPV, pulse oximetry, assessment of effectiveness of PPV, corrective steps, etc**	This is a list of what learners can be expected to do if they share the same mental model of the patient as the instructor, and if the learners perform resuscitation in competent manner. The Expected Interventions section is essentially an outline of what the instructor can expect to happen if all goes according to plan. The learners may not necessarily perform these listed interventions, but, instead, take a different path that requires the instructor to be alert for unexpected learning opportunities.
Skills Demonstrated: **Cognitive, Technical, and Behavioral** **Cognitive:** 1. Recognize the newborn who requires PPV. 2. Recall indications for effective ventilation . . . 3. Interpret pulse oximetry and adjust oxygen concentration . . . **Technical** (complete list) **Behavioral** (complete list)	These are printed on page 2 of the form so that instructors have room to make notes on this page in preparation for the debriefing. Three cognitive skills are listed. The Technical and Behavioral Skills are listed on each Scenario Template in this way so you can indicate when an objective has been met in any scenario. Use this information to guide your debriefing. Technical: The form includes the complete list of technical skills for PPV because this is a critical resuscitation skill; the form also lists headings for additional technical skills. Behavioral: The form includes the complete list of Key Behavioral Skills because any or all would be appropriate.

Scenario Building Tool

Choose the gestational age, weight, and mode of birth. Select a risk factor. Choose or create other descriptions of the newborn's condition at birth. The newborn's condition suggests the resuscitation interventions the team must perform.

Note: Meconium-stained newborns should be term or post-term.

Gestational Age	Estimated Weight	Mode of Delivery	Risk Factor	Condition of Newborn at Birth	Procedures Indicated	Lessons Evaluated
Term, post-term	>3,500 g	Vaginal birth	Shoulder dystocia	Apneic, heart rate 40 beats per minute (bpm)	Equipment Check, Initial steps, positive-pressure ventilation, pulse oximetry, chest compressions	Lessons 1 through 4
					Baby deteriorates: Add intubation, epinephrine	Lesson 5 Lesson 6
Term, post-term	>3,000 g	Emergency cesarean birth	Failed vacuum extraction	Apneic, heart rate 50 bpm	Equipment Check, initial steps, positive-pressure ventilation, pulse oximetry, chest compressions	Lessons 1 through 4
					Baby deteriorates: Add intubation, epinephrine, +/- volume	Lesson 5 Lesson 6
Term, post-term	>3,000 g	Vaginal or cesarean birth	Meconium-stained fluid	Irregular breathing, limp, heart rate 80 bpm then 40 bpm after tracheal suction	Equipment Check, initial steps, intubation, positive-pressure ventilation, pulse oximetry, chest compressions, re-intubation, epinephrine	Lessons 1 through 5 Lesson 6
Choose appropriate gestation	Choose appropriate weight for gestational age	Cesarean birth	Placenta previa	Apneic, heart rate 50 bpm, limp	Equipment Check, initial steps, positive-pressure ventilation, pulse oximetry, chest compressions	Lessons 1 through 4 Lesson 8 if preterm
					Baby deteriorates: Add intubation, epinephrine	Lesson 5 Lesson 6 Lesson 9 may be applicable

Gestational Age	Estimated Weight	Mode of Delivery	Risk Factor	Condition of Newborn at Birth	Procedures Indicated	Lessons Evaluated
Choose appropriate gestation	Choose appropriate weight for gestational age	Vaginal birth in mother's bed on antepartum unit	Amnionitis	Apneic, heart rate 80 bpm then falls to 50 bpm	Equipment Check, initial steps, positive-pressure ventilation, pulse oximetry, chest compressions	Lessons 1 through 4 Lesson 8 if preterm
					Baby deteriorates: Add intubation, epinephrine	Lesson 5 Lesson 6 Lesson 9 may be applicable
		2-day-old found in bassinet in mother's room	Unknown	Apneic, heart rate 40 bpm	Modified initial steps, positive-pressure ventilation, pulse oximetry, chest compressions	Lessons 1 through 4
					Baby deteriorates: Add intubation, epinephrine, +/- volume	Lesson 5 Lesson 6
		Cesarean birth	Cord entanglement	Apneic, heart rate 40 bpm, pale	Equipment Check, initial steps, positive-pressure ventilation, pulse oximetry, chest compressions	Lessons 1 through 4 Lesson 8 if preterm
					Baby deteriorates: Add intubation, epinephrine, +/- volume	Lesson 5 Lesson 6 Lesson 9 may be applicable
		Vaginal or cesarean birth	Congenital malformations	Breathing then apneic, heart rate 90 bpm then 50 bpm, persistent cyanosis	Equipment Check, initial steps, positive-pressure ventilation, pulse oximetry, chest compressions	Lessons 1 through 4 Lesson 8 if preterm
					Baby deteriorates: Add intubation, epinephrine	Lesson 5 Lesson 6 Lesson 9 may be applicable

Create Your Own Scenarios

Choose the gestational age, weight, and mode of birth. Select or create your own risk factor. Describe the condition of the newborn at birth to create a scenario in which selected procedures are necessary to resuscitate the newborn.

Note: Meconium-stained newborns should be term or post-term.

Appropriate weights for gestational age

28 weeks = 800 to 1,500 g   30 weeks = 1,000 to 1,750 g   32 weeks = 1,250 to 2,000 g

34 weeks = 1,500 to 2,700 g   36 weeks = 2,000 to 3,200 g   38 to 40 weeks = 2,500 to 3,700 g

Gestational Age	Estimated Weight	Mode of Delivery	Risk Factor	Potential Conditions of Newborn at Birth	Procedures Indicated	Lessons Evaluated

Procedure	Criteria
Intubate and suction trachea	Meconium in amniotic fluid or on the baby's skin/baby with depressed respirations or tone, or heart rate <100 beats per minute (bpm)
Free-flow oxygen	Heart rate >100 bpm after initial steps, breathing with perceived persistent cyanosis, low target oxygen saturation for age in minutes confirmed by pulse oximetry
Positive-pressure ventilation (PPV)	Apneic/gasping, heart rate <100 bpm even if breathing, or persistent cyanosis after free-flow oxygen and low target oxygen saturation for age in minutes confirmed by pulse oximetry
Chest compressions	Heart rate remains <60 bpm after 30 seconds of effective assisted ventilation
Intubation	Tracheal suctioning of meconium for non-vigorous newborn, bag-and-mask ventilation ineffective or prolonged, to facilitate coordination of chest compressions and ventilation, or as route for epinephrine pending establishment of emergency umbilical venous catheter (UVC)
Laryngeal mask airway placement	When ventilation is unsuccessful and intubation is not successful or not feasible
Placement of emergency UVC	When epinephrine or volume administration is indicated
Epinephrine administration	Intubated or UVC in place, heart rate <60 bpm after 30 seconds of effective assisted ventilation and another 45-60 seconds of coordinated chest compressions and effective PPV
Volume administration	Baby appears in shock and is not responding to resuscitation efforts or there is a history of a condition associated with fetal blood loss.

Simulation Preparation, Tips, and Sample Debriefing Questions

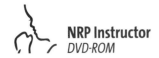

NRP Instructor
DVD-ROM

I. Prepare the Learners for Simulation Training

a. Orient to supplies and equipment and manikin's abilities as a simulation tool.

b. Learners must "get into it" and "think aloud."

c. Learners can't say they are doing something – they must actually do it.

d. The instructor sets up the scenario but does not coach, guide, or interrupt.

e. The instructor determines when the scenario is over. Most scenarios last 2-5 minutes.

II. Debriefing is NOT feedback from the instructor. Keep the discussion team-centered.

a. Self-discovery is key. Team members do most of the talking to EACH OTHER.

b. For complex debriefing, help team develop an agenda. What issues will be covered?

c. Link simulation to real-life practice.

d. Question: Statement ratio is 3:1. Ask WHAT, HOW, and WHY questions.

e. Use active listening – this is not an interrogation. Look and sound interested.

f. Use silence/pauses to encourage participation. Reword the question; do not give the answer.

g. Debrief constructively – hold your teaching points until team has finished. The debriefer enables the team to figure things out; then enhances understanding of the points they might have missed.

h. Maintain confidentiality. What happens here STAYS here.

i. A complex debriefing can last up to 30 minutes. You probably have 5-10 minutes. Choose the most important objectives to discuss. You may not be able to cover everything.

III. Sample debriefing questions

a. Tell me in a few sentences what happened to this baby.

b. What were your objectives? Which objectives were met? Not met?

c. What was your thought process when ...

d. What did the group do well? How did (those behaviors) help the team?

e. Who was the leader? How did you know?

f. What key behavioral skills did you use? When did you use (a behavioral skill)?

g. What could have gone better? What would you do differently next time?

h. How can you help when a team member's performance needs improvement?

i. What did you do to help the team? How did that help?

j. What did you learn?

k. Any additional comments?

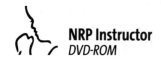

NRP Instructor
DVD-ROM

CAPE Debriefing Evaluation Tool©

Scenario description: _____

Before scenario:	• Reviews learning objectives and anticipated actions.
During scenario:	• Takes notes: performance of cognitive, technical, and behavioral skills.
After scenario:	• Briefs regarding performance issues/items on debriefing checklist.
Debriefing:	• Determines whether trainees share same mental model of patient.
	• Facilitates self-reflective learning.

Scenario start time: _____   Debriefing start time: _____

Scenario end time: _____   Debriefing end time: _____

Scenario length: _____   Debriefing length: _____

Time between end of scenario and start of debriefing: _____ min

Time when tape first rolls during debriefing: _____ min

Percentage of scenario covered during debriefing: _____ %

Percentage of learning objectives covered during debriefing: _____ %

Length of debriefing : Length of scenario ratio: _____

Number of times tape paused during debriefing: _____

Length of tape segments played: _____

Instructor Questions:	**Instructor Statements:**	**Trainee Responses:**
1. ☐☐☐☐☐☐☐☐☐☐	☐☐☐☐☐☐☐☐☐☐	☐☐☐☐☐☐☐☐☐☐
2. ☐☐☐☐☐☐☐☐☐☐	☐☐☐☐☐☐☐☐☐☐	☐☐☐☐☐☐☐☐☐☐
3. ☐☐☐☐☐☐☐☐☐☐	☐☐☐☐☐☐☐☐☐☐	☐☐☐☐☐☐☐☐☐☐
4. ☐☐☐☐☐☐☐☐☐☐	☐☐☐☐☐☐☐☐☐☐	☐☐☐☐☐☐☐☐☐☐
5. ☐☐☐☐☐☐☐☐☐☐	☐☐☐☐☐☐☐☐☐☐	☐☐☐☐☐☐☐☐☐☐
6. ☐☐☐☐☐☐☐☐☐☐	☐☐☐☐☐☐☐☐☐☐	☐☐☐☐☐☐☐☐☐☐
7. ☐☐☐☐☐☐☐☐☐☐	☐☐☐☐☐☐☐☐☐☐	☐☐☐☐☐☐☐☐☐☐
8. ☐☐☐☐☐☐☐☐☐☐	☐☐☐☐☐☐☐☐☐☐	☐☐☐☐☐☐☐☐☐☐
9. ☐☐☐☐☐☐☐☐☐☐	☐☐☐☐☐☐☐☐☐☐	☐☐☐☐☐☐☐☐☐☐
10. ☐☐☐☐☐☐☐☐☐☐	☐☐☐☐☐☐☐☐☐☐	☐☐☐☐☐☐☐☐☐☐
11. ☐☐☐☐☐☐☐☐☐☐	☐☐☐☐☐☐☐☐☐☐	☐☐☐☐☐☐☐☐☐☐
12. ☐☐☐☐☐☐☐☐☐☐	☐☐☐☐☐☐☐☐☐☐	☐☐☐☐☐☐☐☐☐☐
13. ☐☐☐☐☐☐☐☐☐☐	☐☐☐☐☐☐☐☐☐☐	☐☐☐☐☐☐☐☐☐☐
14. ☐☐☐☐☐☐☐☐☐☐	☐☐☐☐☐☐☐☐☐☐	☐☐☐☐☐☐☐☐☐☐
15. ☐☐☐☐☐☐☐☐☐☐	☐☐☐☐☐☐☐☐☐☐	☐☐☐☐☐☐☐☐☐☐

Instructor question : Instructor statement ratio: _____

Trainee responses : Instructor questions + statements ratio: _____

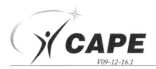

Instructions for Use of
CAPE Debriefing Evaluation Tool

Overview: This tool is designed to evaluate a debriefing following a simulation or drill. The tool can be used for self-evaluation when reviewing a taped debriefing session or by evaluators as the debriefing occurs.

Scenario Description: Indicate the name of the scenario as it is named on the Scenario script. Identifying the scenario gives the evaluator the option to review the written scenario during or after evaluation for specifics such as learning objectives.

Bulleted Items: These describe the role and activities of the instructor/debriefer.

Scenario/Debriefing Times and Length: The debriefing usually lasts about three times the length of the scenario. Shorter debriefing sessions should be evaluated to ensure that learning objectives were discussed. Long sessions should be evaluated to make sure time allotted for simulation was used effectively.

Time between end of scenario and start of debriefing: The recommended time period is 5-10 minutes. This short waiting period keeps learners engaged in the scenario and reduces anxiety of waiting for the tape to be viewed.

Time when tape first rolls during debriefing: A _brief_ discussion before rolling tape is optional, use video to discuss major learning objectives and incidental or unanticipated findings.

Percentage of scenario covered during debriefing: Majority of scenario should be reviewed but covering the learning objectives adequately is the main priority which is captured in the next area.

Percentage of learning objectives covered during debriefing: A copy of the scenario with learning objectives should be available to the evaluator during completion of this tool.

Length of debriefing: Length of scenario ratio: Calculation based on times listed in box at top of tool.

Number of times the tape is paused during debriefing: Each time the tape is paused place a tic mark. The tape should be paused to discuss learning objectives, other areas of interest for discussion or if the learners are talking among themselves while the tape is playing.

Length of tape segments played: The tape should be stopped at least every 90-120 seconds to keep learners engaged in the scenario.

Instructor Questions: The number of questions the instructor/debriefer asks is captured by checking a box for each question.

Instructor Statements: The number of statements the instructor/debriefer makes is captured by checking a box for each statement.

Trainee Responses: Each response from a trainee is counted by checking a box in this category. A response is considered an answer to a question or a question that is posed by a trainee. For example, if three trainees respond, three boxes are checked. If a trainee poses a new question during discussion, another box is checked.

Instructor question Instructor statement ratio: The instructor/debriefer guides the discussion, not dominate it. The ratio of questions to statements should be high with significantly more questions noted than statements.

Trainee responses Instructor questions + statements ratio: Add the debriefer's questions and statements together. That number is then compared to the number of trainee responses. Ideally, the trainees will be doing most of the talking with the instructor/debriefer guiding the discussion by asking questions designed to further discussion among the trainees.

Ready, Set, Go: Neonatal Resuscitation Program Instructor Prep Sheet for Simulation and Debriefing

READY

- ❏ Scenario is based on learning objectives, is plausible, and useful to these learners.
- ❏ Instructors have agreed on responsibilities (eg, vital signs, filming, taking notes).
- ❏ Instructors have prepared the setting with key visual, tactile, and auditory cues.
- ❏ Learners have been oriented to
  - a. Location of supplies and equipment
  - b. Each other (names and usual roles during a resuscitation in their birth setting)
  - c. How they will know the manikin's heart rate, breathing, tone, pulse oximetry, etc.
- ❏ Learners are given a chance to touch and handle the supplies and arrange them as desired.
- ❏ Learners are given a chance to do a short "practice" scenario with instructor's guidance.
- ❏ Learners understand that they
  - a. Think out loud.
  - b. Do the actions, not pretend them.
  - c. Act as a team and help each other.

SET

- ❏ Learners' roles are designated based on the needs of the scenario (as determined by the instructor) or their usual team composition. Learners wear name tags designating roles (eg, RN, MD, RT, NNP, etc).
- ❏ Begin filming the scenario.
- ❏ Instructor reads the scenario.
- ❏ Instructor (or "obstetric [OB] provider") provides additional information if learners ask questions.
- ❏ Learners may appoint a leader, determine the plan of care, and delegate tasks.
- ❏ Learners may check equipment, if not already done.

GO

- ❏ Obstetric provider arrives at radiant warmer with the newborn, or gives the newborn to a resuscitation team member. If manikin must be on the radiant warmer during learner preparation, cover the manikin with a towel until the scenario begins.
- ❏ Instructor gives vital signs information only if cued by the learner (when learner auscultates or palpates heart rate) or when learner asks about breathing, tone, etc, if necessary.
- ❏ Instructor stays out of the way and allows the learners to take the scenario down its own path.
- ❏ Instructor signals the end of the scenario without judgment (eg, "That ends your scenario. Let's debrief now."). Learners do not end the scenario.
- ❏ **Instructor does not lecture or give feedback. The instructor guides self-discovery and discussion among team members.**
  - a. Tell me in a few sentences about this baby. What did you think you would need to do?
  - b. What were your objectives? Which objectives were met? Not met?
  - c. What was your thought process when . . .
  - d. Who was the leader? How did you know?
  - e. What key behavioral skills did you use? Give examples. How did that help?
  - f. What could have gone better? What would you do differently next time?
  - g. What did you learn? Any additional comments?
- ❏ Instructor uses strategies to encourage more in-depth discussion, such as
  - a. "Tell us more about that."
  - b. "What would have happened if . . . ?"
  - c. "What caused the disagreement?"
  - d. "How would that sound? What could he or she have said to make it more clear for you?"
  - e. "Who else observed this behavior? What did you notice and what were you thinking about?"
  - f. "Why was that helpful?"
  - g. "How could your team have helped you at that point?"
  - h. How can you help when a team member's performance needs improvement?

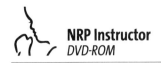

NRP Instructor Simulation and Debriefing Checklist

Scenario start time: _____ Scenario end time: _____ Length of scenario: _____ min

Debrief start time: _____ Debrief end time: _____ Length of debrief: _____ min

Component	Yes	Notes About Variance

Scenario Development

The scenario is based on learning objectives tailored to learners' needs. _____ _____

The scenario is plausible. _____ _____

Supplies and equipment are present that enable learners to resuscitate the newborn with correct technique. _____ _____

Learner Orientation

Learners introduce themselves and describe their roles, if necessary. _____ _____

Learners receive orientation to manikin and its functions. _____ _____

Learners receive orientation to location and function of supplies if necessary. _____ _____

Learners receive orientation to how they will get feedback pertaining to manikin's breathing, heart rate, muscle tone, pulse oximetry, color, or special circumstances. _____ _____

Instructor reviews learner responsibilities (suspend disbelief, think out loud, perform actions instead of pretending actions). _____ _____

Instructor allows the learners a few minutes to practice using the supplies and equipment before beginning. _____ _____

Instructor tells learners the cue for beginning the scenario and reminds learners that the instructor will end the scenario. _____ _____

During the Scenario

The instructor allows the learners to proceed through the scenario without coaching, interference, or assistance. _____ _____

The instructor takes notes about performance of cognitive, technical, and behavioral skills. _____ _____

The instructor ends the scenario without judgmental comments or feedback. _____ _____

Component	Yes	Notes About Variance

Debriefing

Instructor begins by ensuring a shared mental model of the patient (learners are asked to describe the clinical situation they faced).

Instructor assists the team to formulate a discussion agenda if necessary for a complex scenario.

Instructor promotes discussion about what went well, and what could be improved, and how.

Instructor allows silence after asking a question; if no response, instructor rephrases the question.

Instructor is sincere, approachable, uses active listening, uses open body language.

Instructor keeps the discussion positive and constructive.

Instructor keeps the learners focused on the learning objectives. Instructor encourages learners to list their objectives: cognitive, technical (hands-on) and behavioral.

Instructor involves quiet learners by asking them questions directly.

Instructor encourages learners to talk to each other, not to the instructor.

Instructor helps learners link scenario to real-life experience.

Instructor encourages learners to talk about what they were thinking as they made decisions and performed interventions.

Instructor asks learners to discuss how they were affected by each others' actions.

Instructor shows video segments for purpose of discussion.

Video paused when instructor asks questions and during comments and discussion.

Instructor ends scenario by briefly summarizing important issues and clarifying any plans for follow-up.

Instructor uses at least 3 questions: 1 statement.

Comments: _____

_____

_____

_____

The Art of Moulage: Guidelines, Recipes, and Easy Techniques

Guidelines for moulage

A little goes a long way. For example, do not drench the manikin in simulated blood unless you are providing a visual cue for extreme maternal blood loss.

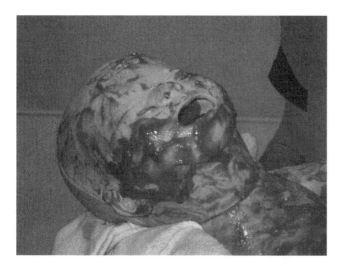

This heavy application of blood and meconium makes the scenario less plausible.

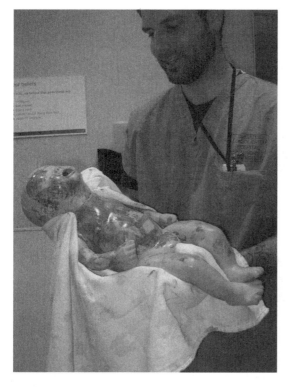

This moderate application of simulated blood and baby oil helps learners "suspend disbelief" and treat this manikin as an actual newborn.

Choose one of your manikins for moulage practice until you are confident with your techniques. It is easier to prepare and clean one manikin than several.

If you do not wish to put simulated fluids directly onto the manikin, put the fluids on the towel or blanket on the radiant warmer. You may wish to use a spray bottle of simulated blood to wet the blanket. Consider a light spray of simulated blood on the manikin in a few small, but visible, areas, such as the forehead or abdomen. This is an easy way to provide an important visual cue, and it cleans up quickly.

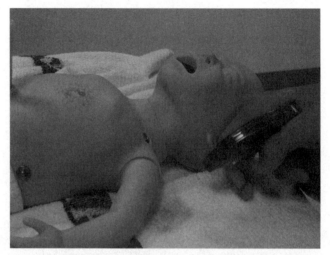

For quick and easy visual cue of blood on the newborn and wet linen, use a spray bottle of simulated blood to lightly wet the manikin and moisten the blanket.

Test colored fluids on the manikin's back or the bottom of a foot to determine if permanent staining results. To avoid staining your manikin, do not use food coloring in your recipes, and clean the manikin's surface thoroughly after each use.

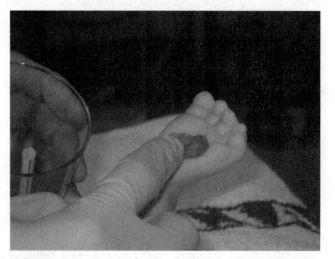

Make sure that your recipe for blood will not permanently stain the manikin by testing it first on an inconspicuous area, such as the sole of the foot.

Allow any wet areas of the manikin to dry thoroughly before storing. It may be necessary to remove the manikin's chest skin or lungs to allow drying. If the manikin is stored wet, it may develop moldy surfaces.

If you decide to put simulated body fluids down the airway of your traditional (nonelectronic) manikin, be prepared for the cleanup and reassembly involved.

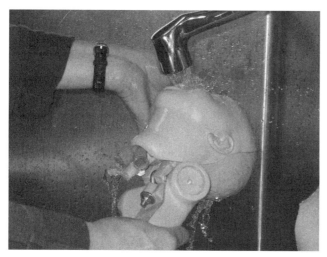

Substances such as baby food or split pea soup applied down the manikin's airway call for extensive disassembly and clean-up.

Check manufacturer recommendations carefully before putting liquids down the airway of an electronic simulator. This may cause serious damage.

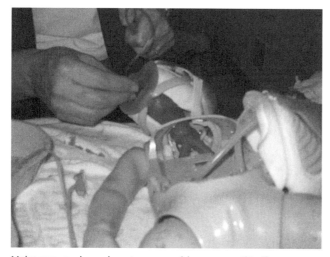

Make sure you know how to reassemble your manikin if you must disassemble it for cleaning.

Recipes for Blood, Vernix, Meconium

Experiment with your own ingredients and determine what works best for you. Simulated blood also may be purchased. The following recipes will give you a good start for creating your own simulated fluids.

Blood:

1. Red water-based paint

   Green water-based paint

   Blue dishwashing liquid

   Baby oil or mineral oil

2. Purchase simulated blood (liquid or powder)

Vernix:

1. Heavy unscented hand cream

   Mashed potato flakes (optional)

2. Baby diaper rash cream

Meconium:

1. Single-use baby food jars/cartons of pureed split peas or green beans

   Baby oil or mineral oil

2. Dry oatmeal

   Green and brown finger paint

   Baby oil or mineral oil

3. Split pea soup

   Baby oil or mineral oil

Acrocyanosis

Apply blue eye shadow to manikin's hands and feet.

Simulated acrocyanosis helps determine if learners know the difference between acrocyanosis and central cyanosis (photo courtesy of Cynthia Jensen, Intensive Care Nursery, University of California San Francisco).

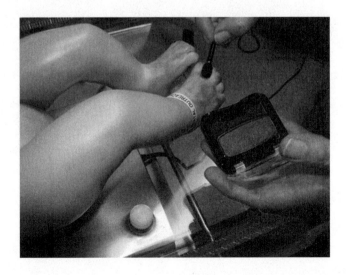

Abdominal Defect (also can be used in smaller size for spinal defect)

1. Tie off the fingers of a surgical glove.

2. Fill the glove with small dried beans, such as pinto beans.

3. Add a squirt of red finger paint and mineral oil or baby oil.

4. Tie off the glove to keep the beans inside.

5. Remove the umbilicus from the manikin and insert the omphalocele into the umbilicus hole. You may wish to place the umbilicus In the opening right next to the abdominal defect.

6. It may be necessary to use double stick, clear tape to secure the underside of the omphalocele to the manikin's abdomen.

7. When the manikin is prepped for the scenario, include the defect in the prep by wetting it with simulated blood and mineral or baby oil.

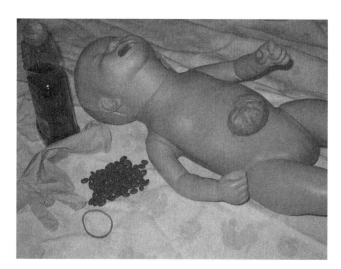

This omphalocele looks more realistic when simulated blood and baby oil are applied to the skin and abdominal defect. The umbilicus protrudes from the umbilical opening on the other side of the defect.

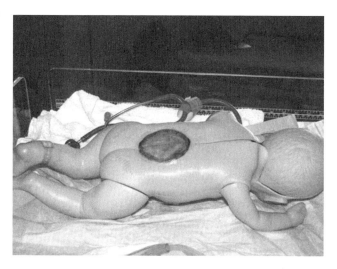

The myelomeningocele is made of children's soft modeling clay, shaped and painted and affixed with a large clear adhesive dressing. (Photo courtesy of Cynthia Jensen, Intensive Care Nursery, University of California San Francisco.)

Chest "Glow" With Transillumination

How to make one side of the chest "glow" for a pneumothorax (as demonstrated in the Resuscitation Skills video titled "Thoracentesis")

1. Carefully remove the manikin's chest skin. It may be necessary to unscrew the manikin's arms to prevent tearing the chest skin.

2. Insert a piece of paper over the lung area on that side (the side that will NOT be needled to aspirate air).

3. Replace the chest skin.

4. When the transilluminator is used in a darkened room, the papered side of the chest will be dark and the side with the pneumothorax will "glow."

Make a Pulse Oximeter Out of a Box

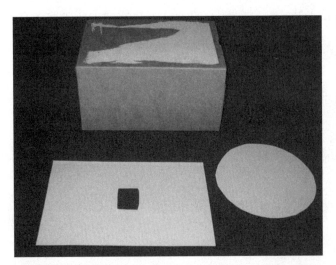

Start with a strong cardboard board that is about the same size as an actual oximeter. You may wish to cover the box in paper for a clean look. Cut a circular wheel from heavy paper the same height as the cardboard box. Cut a paper square the same size as the front of the box. You will cut a window in the paper cover for viewing the heart rate and SpO_2 after you place the wheel on the box.

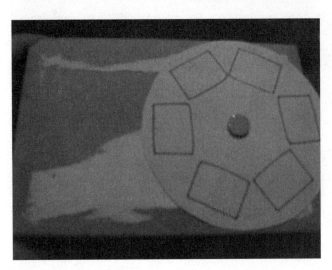

Position the wheel on the right side of the box with a thumbtack or brad. Allow the edge of the wheel to overhang the edge of the box on the right to enable the operator to easily grasp the wheel and turn it. Lay out 6 (or more) squares on the wheel. Write or type the SpO_2 and heart rate (HR) values in each square. **This pulse oximeter uses the following:**

— — — **no oximeter signal**

HR 50, SpO_2 63

HR 70, SpO_2 67

HR 120, SpO_2 74

HR 140, SpO_2 84

HR 160, SpO_2 96

The Performance Checklists in the *Textbook of Neonatal Resuscitation, 6ᵗʰ Edition,* use:

— — — no oximeter signal

HR 40, Sᴘo₂ 63

HR 70, Sᴘo₂ 67

HR 120, Sᴘo₂ 74

HR 140, Sᴘo₂ 97

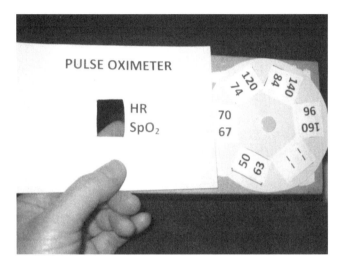

Glue the oximeter cover onto the top of the box. Do not glue the oximeter cover onto the wheel, or the wheel will not turn.

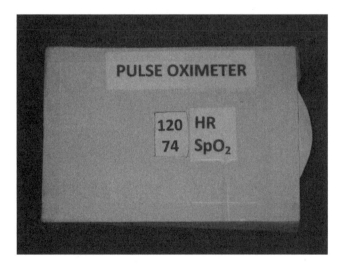

You may wish to cut a hole or create a connection site for the pulse oximeter probe on the bottom right edge of the box.

Make a Pulse Oximeter From a Desktop Card File

A small card file (see photos below) can make an easy-to-use visual cue that simulates pulse oximeter readings. For easy access by the instructor, the "levels" of heart rate and oxygen saturation are written on the tabbed cards. The heart rate and SpO_2 are written on the index cards.

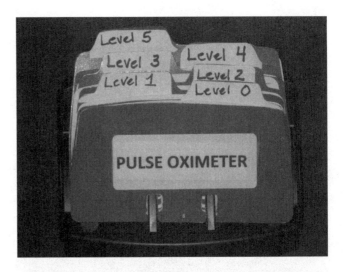

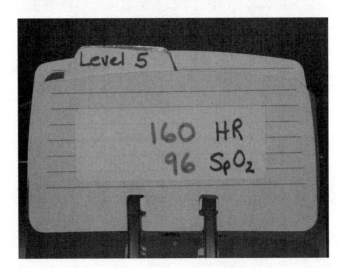

The Neonatal Mock Code

A simulated neonatal code is a highly recommended optional activity. Conducted in a realistic setting and in real time, a mock code provides resuscitation team members with the opportunity to improve skills, practice teamwork, and troubleshoot problems with systems or personnel. In settings where neonatal resuscitation is infrequent, the mock code is especially important for maintaining skills and increasing self-efficacy.

How often should I conduct a mock code?

This depends on the team's level of resuscitation proficiency. It may be necessary to conduct a mock code as often as twice per month to give all staff an opportunity to participate 2 or 3 times per year. A mock code offered less than twice per year makes it difficult to work on problem areas and track improvements.

What kind of supplies and location are required for a neonatal mock code?

This depends, in part, on how complex and realistic you wish the code to be. At a minimum, you need the setup you use for an Advanced Integrated Skills Station. Ideally, the mock code uses a realistic scenario in the intrapartum area or in an area where resuscitation may occur so that participants are able to "suspend disbelief" and feel as if they are truly involved in an actual resuscitation.

How long does a mock code last?

That depends on your learning objectives and your participants. If you are planning an in-service education program prior to the code, plan to spend from 30 to 60 minutes. If the mock code is spontaneous and involves people who are already in the vicinity and have patient assignments, you should plan to be finished (including evaluation and discussion) in 15 minutes or less.

What are the steps for conducting a neonatal mock code?

- Assess unit activity. (If it is a period of high activity, no one will be able to attend.)

- Choose the location.

- Give participants 30 to 60 minutes of advance notice (optional).

- Assemble the equipment that would normally be available at the resuscitation scene. Use items from your course supply bag or box, if possible, and leave actual equipment undisturbed.

- Use the NRP Scenario Template (pages 104-105) to create or select a scenario you have already created based on staff learning objectives.

- Begin the mock code by announcing a mock code overhead, paging participants, or assembling people via telephone or word of mouth.

- Videotape the exercise. Visual feedback is an important adjunct to education and provides an objective record of the actions and communication skills of the resuscitation team.

- Allow a team member, a staff member trained in debriefing techniques, or an NRP instructor to debrief the team after the resuscitation. The person conducting the debriefing may find it helpful to use the Debriefing Reference Form (page 336) or any of the other debriefing tools found in Appendix F.

How should people organize their roles prior to a mock code?

It is important that the members of the team know who is responsible for specific activities. The team leader needs to assign duties to resuscitation team members prior to the baby's birth, even if resuscitation is practiced frequently and roles of the various disciplines are established and understood. In any case, it is a good idea to establish a plan. For example,

- Physicians or neonatal nurse practitioners may assess the patient's condition and direct the resuscitation.

- Nurses may make the clinical assessments, such as auscultating breath sounds, counting the heart rate, and preparing and administering medications.

- Respiratory care practitioners, anesthesiologists, or nurse anesthetists may assist with airway management.

- When assigning tasks and discussing the plan, the person in charge might say the following:
  "When the baby comes to the warmer, I will clear and maintain the airway. We both can dry the baby, then I will lift him, and you will remove the wet towels. I will be responsible for oxygen and ventilation; you will be responsible for checking heart rate and breath sounds. Either tap the heart rate out where I can see it, or tell me the actual heart rate. You are responsible for attaching the pulse oximeter probe to the baby, then to the oximeter. If we proceed to chest compressions, we will need help. You call for help before starting compressions. Are we set?"

Who debriefs the team?

The neonatal mock code debriefer may be an NRP instructor, the resuscitation team leader, a member of the resuscitation team, or an observer who did not participate in the scenario, Ideally, we want to encourage teams to use both real-time, on-site, short debriefings after signficant events in the delivery room and/or nursery and more structured, comprehensive debriefings (with video, etc) as part of their ongoing NRP education. The mock code could be used to model either of these.

If the instructor always leads the debriefings, then team members may not develop the skills to become comfortable leading short debriefings after real-life significant events. On the other hand, if the team leader facilitates the debriefing, it may discourage participants from honestly discussing leadership issues. If an NRP instructor is not present for a mock code (eg, the mock code is organized by the team), the team leader does not have to be the one leading the debriefing. Any member of the team can be empowered to facilitate the debriefing.

My staff members are very afraid of neonatal resuscitation, even during a mock code. Some people are so frightened that they actually feel sick or are not able to think clearly. How can I help them?

Resuscitation is a stressful event. Discussing past experiences and acknowledging that everyone feels nervous prior to and during resuscitation can help alleviate anxiety prior to a mock code. It is helpful for participants to know that simulation-based training is not a "test," but a way to assess weaknesses and work on ways to improve performance. As staff become accustomed to simulation-based training and receive supportive nonjudgmental assistance for improving skills, anxiety should dissipate.

How should I evaluate the mock code performance?

- The team should be debriefed immediately.

- Debrief the team using the Neonatal Mock Code Debriefing Reference Form (page 336) or another debriefing tool that is helpful for guiding a team-centered discussion.

- Reinforce that the purpose of the mock code is to find areas that need clarification or problem solving. Remind participants that sometimes the best learning occurs through errors.

- Enable the team to make suggestions for improved performance.

Documentation seems like the final step of neonatal resuscitation. How can I help participants learn to chart accurately and objectively?

Documentation is important at every birth. The resuscitation record does not give the whole picture. The narrative note re-creates the resuscitation with details that you may not remember clearly if you are ever asked to review the events.

Actual narrative writing may take more time than you have to spend on your mock code; therefore, discuss the essential components of documentation while you write them on a white board or large piece of paper taped to the wall. The code record must correlate with the narrative charting. A sample code record and the corresponding narrative note are in Appendix H. Essential elements of the record include the following:

- Identification of the baby (eg, "male, term, SGA")

- Time of birth

- Type of birth (cesarean, vaginal, vacuum extraction, etc)

- Description of what was happening when you arrived, if you were not there at the time of birth

- Interventions in order of occurrence and the newborn's response to each

- Description of what support was offered to the family

Neonatal Mock Code Debriefing Reference Form

Date: _____ Location: _____ Start time: _____ Stop time: _____

Persons participating: _____

Person debriefing and role (NRP instructor, team member, staff debriefer):

_____

Title of Scenario: _____ **Newborn's estimated weight:** _____

Risk factor(s): _____

Skills	Done	Comments
Performed Equipment Check.		
Notified team members per protocol.		
Team leader was identified.		
• Team leader stated overall plan for resuscitation.		
• Team leader clarified responsibilities of each team member.		
• Team members asked questions, clarified the plan, if necessary.		
• Met time criteria for arrival at code scene.		
Performed initial steps.		
• Suctioned meconium with good technique, if necessary.		
Evaluated respirations and heart rate.		
If indicated: provided free-flow oxygen and/or continuous positive airway pressure (CPAP).		
• Used pulse oximetry and interpreted appropriately.		
If indicated: positive-pressure ventilation (PPV)		
• Checked effectiveness of PPV by assessing heart rate, bilateral breath sounds, chest movement (MR SOPA, if required).		
• Ventilated at correct rate and pressure.		
If indicated: chest compressions performed correctly at correct depth and rate.		
If indicated: endotracheal intubation		
• Used correct-sized tube for weight and gestation.		
• Performed procedure with correct technique.		
• Confirmed placement by auscultation and CO_2 detector		
• Secured tube at correct tip-to-lip marking.		
If indicated, use of additional device such as		
• Laryngeal mask airway.		
If indicated: medications and volume		
• Ordered correct medication, dose, and route.		
• Administered medication correctly.		
If indicated: problem solved newborn's poor response to resuscitative efforts.		
Documented times, events, and newborn's response.		
Team communication: Used Key Behavioral Skills.		
Communicated effectively with family.		
The debriefer:		
Asked questions to promote a team-centered discussion.		
Team assessed strengths and weaknesses of performance.		

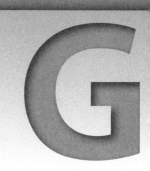

APPENDIX

Instructor Courses

Hospital-based Instructor Course

Regional Trainer Course

Hospital-based Instructor Course
Sample Curriculum

1. **Welcome and Introductions**
   Lead regional trainer asks hospital-based instructor candidates if there are any questions about the NRP Instructor Self-assessment content.

2. **Group Skills Review (all learners together)**
   Lead regional trainer talks through important points and demonstrates
   - Equipment Check
   - Initial Steps
   - Positive-Pressure Ventilation with a bag and mask, T-piece resuscitator if applicable to learners' needs, and use of pulse oximetry and MR SOPA
   - Chest Compressions

   The lead regional trainer may choose to show Resuscitation Skills videos from the NRP Instructor DVD or the DVD that accompanies the *Textbook of Neonatal Resuscitation, 6th Edition*, especially to help ensure standardized and accurate information about the least familiar procedures, such as use of pulse oximetry, laryngeal mask airway placement, and emergency umbilical venous catheter (UVC) placement.

3. **Practice Session in Teams:**
   Learners break into groups of at least 2 learners and no more than 4 learners. Each team is coached by a regional trainer or hospital-based instructor who is an experienced assistant instructor for the course.

   Each learner practices and demonstrates these skills at a complete skills station
   - Equipment Check
   - Initial Steps
   - Positive-Pressure Ventilation with a bag and mask, T-piece resuscitator (if applicable to learners' needs), and use of pulse oximetry and MR SOPA
   - Chest Compressions

4. **Group Skills Review (all learners together)**
   Lead regional trainer talks through important points and demonstrates laryngeal mask airway placement, intubation, UVC preparation and insertion, and medication administration. The regional trainer also may lead a discussion about how to incorporate additional aspects of neonatal resuscitation into the Provider Course (management of the preterm newborn, special resuscitation circumstances, and ethics).

5. **Practice Session in Teams**
   Performance Skills Stations are set up so that 3 to 4 learners may practice the skill at a time. Learners rotate to each station with their team and assistant instructor.
   - Laryngeal mask airway placement
   - Intubation
   - Umbilical venous catheter preparation and insertion
   - Medication administration

6. **Group Skills Review (all learners together)**
   - Review use of Experience Survey. Discuss NRP Provider Course agenda development to ensure that hospital-based instructor candidates understand the core elements of an NRP Provider Course and how to choose optional elements to meet the course participants' learning objectives.
   - Review purpose of and how to administer Performance Skills Checklists and Integrated Skills Station Checklist.
   - Review how to convey physiologic feedback (heart rate, breathing, muscle tone, oximetry). If using an electronic simulator, orient learners to the simulator capabilities. If using a traditional manikin, remind hospital-based instructor candidates that physiologic cues are not revealed using a traditional manikin unless the learner palpates the umbilicus or auscultates the apical pulse for heart rate, or listens to breath sounds, or asks about muscle tone and oxygen saturation.
   - Observe a demonstration of the Basic Integrated Skills Station Checklist, including Reflective Questions.

7. **Practice Session in Teams**
   Teams return to complete skills stations. With coaching and feedback from the assistant instructor, the team members practice administering the Performance Skills Stations Checklists to one another and end by administering the Integrated Skills Station to one another, using the Advanced Integrated Skills Station checklist and asking Reflective Questions.

Simulation and Debriefing

8. **Group Skills Review (all learners)**
   Lead regional trainer introduces how Simulation and Debriefing Training session works.
   - Review use of Scenario Template and discuss how to design a scenario.
   - Each team designs a scenario for the practice session.
   - Lead regional trainer or assistant hospital-based instructor demonstrates basic moulage techniques for blood, meconium, and vernix. This "Baby Prep" station includes supplies for making and applying the appropriate body fluids, and for cleaning up the manikin between scenarios.
   - Lead regional trainer or assistant hospital-based instructor points out the key cues at the Simulation area.
     A. Radiant warmer (or conference room table with *Simply NRP* kit control board or other visual cues to make the setting resemble the birth setting as closely as possible)
     B. Scrub tops or cover gowns and gloves for participants
     C. Metronome for heart rate when learner listens or palpates for heart rate in a traditional manikin
     D. Pulse oximetry (per *Simply NRP* kit control board, flash cards, dry-erase board, etc)

9. **Simulation and Debriefing Practice**
   - Lead regional trainer appoints
     A. Team 1: Learners who facilitate the scenario, prepare the newborn with bodily fluids, and debrief the learners.
     B. Team 2: Learners who are the resuscitation team.
     C. Team 3: Learners who operate the camera and film the team, then prepare the video for group viewing.
     D. Team 4: If there are additional hospital-based instructor candidates, they are assigned to watch the team facilitate the scenario and debrief the learners, using a tool that works for you (pages 319-324).

   Teams rotate roles until all hospital-based instructor candidates have had a chance to facilitate and debrief a scenario, be part of the resuscitation team, operate the video camera and set up to view the film, and, if possible, debrief the debriefers, using the tool you prefer on pages 319-324.

10. **Group Discussion (all learners)**
   At the conclusion of the Simulation and Debriefing practice, the lead regional trainer
   - Reviews high points of the day.
   - Polls learners about what they found most valuable about the course.
   - Recommends that novice hospital-based instructors co-teach at least one Provider Course with an experienced instructor or regional trainer to further develop their instructor skills, if possible.
   - Reminds learners that the regional trainer is available to answer questions and serve as a resource in the future. (See sample letter on page 161.)
   - Reminds hospital-based instructor candidates that their NRP Instructor Card will come to them in the mail from the AAP. At that time, the new instructor must go online and register as an instructor. This is important for being able to complete NRP Provider Course Rosters and receive information about NRP from the AAP Division of Life Support.

11. **Course Conclusion**
   Course participants
   - Turn in their completed course evaluations
   - Takes resource letter from regional trainer (optional, see page 161)

   Lead Regional Trainer

   - Completes online Course Roster for the Hospital-based Instructor Course as soon as possible after the course. See the form on page 172 for what information the regional trainer needs to know about each course participant to complete the online Course Roster form.

   - Summarizes course evaluation results and sends to appropriate people

SAMPLE LETTER "Eligibility Confirmation"

Hospital letterhead or logo

We have received your *intent* to complete registration requirements for the American Academy of Pediatrics Neonatal Resuscitation Program™ (NRP™) Hospital-based Instructor Course scheduled for **(date) and (time)**.

DO NOT DELAY completing your registration prerequisites. Your space in this course is not confirmed until you have submitted the items listed below.

Class size is limited. If the class fills to capacity with registrants who complete all registration materials before you finish submitting your required materials, you will not have a space in the course. You will be given the option of being placed on the waiting list in the event of a cancellation on this date, being moved to the next course date, or receiving a full refund of your registration fee. Refunds cannot be issued for purchased books or DVDs.

To complete your course registration, submit the following items immediately:

- Photocopy of both sides of your current NRP Provider Card (Lessons 1 through 9)

- Photocopy of verification of your professional licensure as an RN, MD or DO, RT, or PA

- Letter of support from your manager or supervisor (link to this form at _____ _____) or see the form on the following page

Fax or mail these 3 items to: (name, contact information)

After your registration is complete, you will receive a confirmation letter with driving/parking directions. The NRP Instructor Course requires the following prerequisites, which must be complete on the course date:

- Self-study the *Textbook of Neonatal Resuscitation, 6th Edition.*

- Take and pass the NRP online examination, Lessons 1 through 9, *during the 30 days before* the Instructor Course. You will be sent directions for how to access the online examination after your 3 course registration items have been received and registration is complete.

- View the *NRP Instructor DVD during the 30 days before* the Instructor Course.

- Self-study the *Instructor Manual for Neonatal Resuscitation.*

- Take the NRP Instructor Self-assessment (Appendix A of the *Instructor Manual for Neonatal Resuscitation*).

For additional course content information, contact _____ at _____. For registration information/assistance, contact _____ at _____.

SAMPLE Hospital-based Instructor Course

Letter of support from applicant's manager/supervisor/hospital administrator

This letter supports the intent of _____

(Print applicant's name)

to become a Neonatal Resuscitation Program™ (NRP™) hospital-based instructor for

_____

(Print name of institution, city)

The applicant meets eligibility requirements:

❑ Current NRP Provider Card, Lessons 1 through 9

❑ Current licensure as an RN, MD or DO, RT, or physician assistant

❑ Experience working with newborns in a hospital setting

❑ Current educational or clinical responsibility within a hospital setting

I am confident that this applicant

• Will implement our hospital Neonatal Resuscitation Program enthusiastically

• Will demonstrate good interpersonal skills and the self-confidence necessary to work with all levels of health care professionals

• Will meet the time commitment necessary to implement NRP in our institution

I am aware that course prerequisites include purchasing the *NRP Instructor DVD* for this individual and passing the online NRP examination during the 30 days before the Instructor Course.

My institution will provide administrative support for a hospital-based Neonatal Resuscitation Program, including components such as space, resources, and personnel.

_____   _____

Print name   Signature

_____   _____   _____

Title   Date   Phone Number or E-mail

Return this form to: _____ at _____ or fax to _____

SAMPLE LETTER "REGISTRATION CONFIRMATION IN INSTRUCTOR COURSE"

Hospital letterhead or logo

Thank you for completing your registration prerequisites for the NRP Hospital-based Instructor Course.

We are expecting you: **Date:**   **Time:**   **Location:**

See the attached information for driving directions and parking information.

Lunch on your own (brown bag encouraged due to short time for lunch; a microwave is available).

These course prerequisites must be complete by the course date:

- Self-study the *Textbook of Neonatal Resuscitation, 6th Edition.*

- Take and pass the Neonatal Resuscitation Program™ (NRP™) online examination, Lessons 1 through 9, *during the 30 days before* the Instructor Course.

- View the *NRP Instructor DVD during the 30 days before* the Instructor Course.

- Self-study the *Instructor Manual for Neonatal Resuscitation.*

- Take the NRP Instructor Self-assessment (Appendix A of the *Instructor Manual for Neonatal Resuscitation*).

To gain admittance to the course, you must bring your:

- Examination verification for the NRP online examination, Lessons 1 through 9

- Certificate of Completion for the *NRP Instructor DVD*

- Copy of the completed NRP Instructor Self-assessment Answer Sheet

This is a hands-on interactive course. You successfully pass the course after you

- Identify core components of a Provider Course and accompanying administrative duties.

- Demonstrate the ability to facilitate participants' learning at the Performance Skills Stations.

- Demonstrate the basic steps of creating a scenario and conducting a simulation and debriefing.

- Identify resources for NRP instructor assistance and continued learning.

Neonatal Resuscitation Program course attendance does not guarantee successful course completion and attainment of NRP instructor status. If a participant cannot demonstrate basic abilities to perform and evaluate critical skills of neonatal resuscitation with adult learners, the learner may be asked to repeat the Instructor Course at a later date.

If you have questions about this NRP course, contact: _____

Neonatal Resuscitation Program

Hospital-based Instructor Course
SAMPLE Individual Recording Sheet

Name: _____ Credentials: RN   MD   DO   RT   PA

Work Phone: _____ **Home Phone (optional:)** _____

Address (the American Academy of Pediatrics [AAP] will use this address to correspond with you and mail Neonatal Resuscitation Program™ [NRP™] Provider Course Completion Cards):

_____

E-mail address: _____

Institution: _____ **Department:** _____

> For Regional Trainer Use:
>
> _____ Evidence of current licensure as RN, MD, DO, RT, or PA (required)
>
> _____ Evidence of current NRP provider status, Lessons 1 through 9 (required)
>
> _____ Letter of Support from supervisor or administrator (required)
>
> _____ Examination verification for NRP online examination, Lessons 1 through 9 (required)
>
> _____ Certificate of Completion for *NRP Instructor DVD*
>
> _____ NRP Instructor Self-assessment (strongly recommended)

At the end of this course, you should be able to demonstrate

- Technical skills at all Performance Skills Stations and at the Integrated Skills Station
- Excellent communication skills and ability to facilitate the student's learning
- Developing skills at creating and conducting a scenario and facilitating a debriefing

❑ Set up Performance Skills Stations (Performance Skills Stations and Integrated Skills Station).

❑ Communicate indications for each skill and facilitate learning for participants.

❑ Equipment check   ❑ Initial steps   ❑ Positive-pressure ventilation including use of oximetry   ❑ Chest compressions

❑ Intubation   ❑ Laryngeal mask airway   ❑ Emergency umbilical venous catheter   ❑ Medication administration

❑ Ability to ask reflective questions and help learners improve performance

❑ Demonstrate administration of the Integrated Skills Station Checklist.

❑ Create a scenario for simulation-based training based on learning objectives.

❑ Set up and prepare for a scenario including construction of visual and auditory cues.

❑ Prepare learners for simulation-based training (ground rules, orientation, method of giving physiologic feedback from manikin) and conduct a scenario.

❑ Conduct a debriefing and demonstrate developing debriefing skills.

❑ Observe demonstration or discuss how to submit a Provider Course Roster to the AAP.

SAMPLE LETTER of Resources

For participants who successfully completed the Hospital-based Instructor Course

Hospital Logo or Letterhead

Thank you for attending our Neonatal Resuscitation Program™ (NRP™) Hospital-based Instructor Course.

As your regional trainer, I'm happy to assist you with NRP questions or topics anytime.

You can reach me at: _____

The American Academy of Pediatrics (AAP) will mail you an AAP/American Heart Association (AHA) Hospital-based Instructor Card that is valid for 2 years.

Maintain your instructor status by

- Teaching or assisting with at least 2 NRP courses during the 2 years for which your Instructor Card is valid.

- Taking and passing all 9 lessons of the NRP online examination every 2 years as part of instructor maintenance, beginning January 2013.

American Academy of Pediatrics Resources for Hospital-based Instructors

Be the first to receive broadcast information about new educational programs, administrative updates, new NRP course materials, program revision information, and much more.

NRP broadcast e-mail list: www.aap.org/nrp

Share your views with other NRP instructors.

NRP discussion groups: www.aap.org/nrp

Receive the *NRP Instructor Update* newsletter, which is your primary source of current NRP information.

NRP Instructor Update: **www.aap.org/nrp**

Let the AAP Life Support staff know if you change your hospital base or home address.

Begin at **www.aap.org/nrp,** click on "Courses and Instructors," then "Instructor Only." Click on "Update Info."

**Neonatal Resuscitation Program™ Hospital-based Instructor
Course Evaluation
Sample**

(hospital name)

Date: _____

Course Title: Neonatal Resuscitation Program (NRP™) Hospital-based Instructor Course

Course Objectives

1. Demonstrate understanding of neonatal resuscitation key concepts by successfully completing the NRP online examination.
2. Identify core components of a Provider Course and accompanying administrative duties.
3. Demonstrate the ability to facilitate participants' learning at the Performance Skills Stations.
4. Demonstrate the basic steps of creating a scenario and conducting a simulation and debriefing session.
5. Identify resources for NRP instructor assistance and continued learning.

1. Did the course meet the written objectives? ❑ Yes ❑ No
2. Did the course meet your personal objectives? ❑ Yes ❑ No

Please rate the following with 1=lowest/5=highest.   *Low*   *High*

3. Course expectations and requirements were clear.   1   2   3   4   5
4. The course prepared me to be an NRP instructor.   1   2   3   4   5
5. My regional trainer was knowledgeable, supportive, and facilitated my learning.   1   2   3   4   5
6. The hands-on practice exercises were useful.   1   2   3   4   5
7. The environment was conducive to learning.   1   2   3   4   5
8. The information was useful to your work setting.   1   2   3   4   5
9. What was the best part of this course?

10. What needs improvement?

SAMPLE LETTER "Registration Confirmation in Regional Trainer Course"

Hospital letterhead or logo

Thank you for registering for the Neonatal Resuscitation Program™ (NRP™) Regional Trainer Course. To complete your registration, send:

- Evidence of current licensure as an RN, MD (or DO), Respiratory Care Practitioner, or Physician Assistant

- Photocopy of both sides of your current NRP Hospital-based Instructor Card

We are expecting you: **Date:**   **Time:**   **Location:**

See the attached information for driving directions and parking information.

Lunch on your own (brown bag encouraged due to short time for lunch; a microwave is available).

These course prerequisites must be complete by the course date:

- Self-study the *Textbook of Neonatal Resuscitation, 6th Edition*

- Take and pass the NRP online examination, Lessons 1 through 9, *during the 30 days before* the Regional Trainer Course.

- View the *NRP Instructor DVD*. Review the DVD if you already viewed it and completed the education activity as a Hospital-based Instructor.

- Self-study the *Instructor Manual for Neonatal Resuscitation*.

- Take the NRP Instructor Self-assessment (Appendix A of the *Instructor Manual for Neonatal Resuscitation*).

To gain admittance to the course, you must bring your

- Examination verification for NRP Online Examination, Lessons 1 through 9

- Certificate of Completion for the *NRP Instructor DVD (you may bring your certificate from the first time you completed this requirement as a hospital-based instructor)*

- Copy of the completed NRP Instructor Self-assessment Answer Sheet

This is a hands-on interactive course. You successfully pass the course after you

- Can identify and discuss the role as conceptualized by the American Academy of Pediatrics.

- Demonstrate developing abilities to plan and implement all levels of NRP instruction.

- Demonstrate knowledge of NRP in the region and explain expectations of the role.

- Demonstrate excellent interpersonal skills and the ability to facilitate learning to diverse groups.

- Demonstrate excellent NRP cognitive, technical, and communication skills.

- Demonstrate developing abilities at simulation and debriefing skills.

If you have questions about this NRP course, contact: _____

Neonatal Resuscitation Program

Neonatal Resuscitation Program™ Regional Trainer Course

SAMPLE Individual Recording Sheet

Name: _____ Credentials: RN   MD   DO   RT   PA

Work Phone: _____ Home Phone (optional): _____

Address (American Academy of Pediatrics [AAP] will use this address to correspond with you and mail Neonatal Resuscitation Program [NRP™] Provider Course Completion Cards):

_____

E-mail address: _____

Institution: _____ Department: _____

> For Regional Trainer Use:
>
> _____ Evidence of current NRP hospital-based instructor status (required)
>
> _____ Examination verification for NRP online examination, Lessons 1 through 9 (required)
>
> _____ Certificate of Completion for the **NRP Instructor DVD** (may be from a previous viewing)
>
> _____ NRP Instructor Self-assessment Answer Sheet (strongly recommended)

_____ Learner can identify and discuss the role as conceptualized by the AAP.

_____ Learner demonstrates abilities (or developing abilities) to plan and implement all levels of NRP instruction, if this is a region-specific expectation of the role.

_____ Learner demonstrates knowledge of NRP in the region and can explain the expectations of the role.

_____ Learner demonstrates excellent interpersonal skills, ability to facilitate learning to a diverse group of learners with different learning styles and abilities, and is ready to represent the region's NRP as an expert resource and respected leader.

The regional trainer should be able to demonstrate

_____ Technical skills at all Performance Stations and at the Integrated Skills Station

_____ Excellent communication skills and ability to facilitate the trainee's learning

_____ Developing skills at creating and conducting a scenario and facilitating a debriefing

**Neonatal Resuscitation Program™ Regional Trainer
Course Evaluation
Sample**

(hospital name)

Date: _____

Course Title: Neonatal Resuscitation Program (NRP™) Regional Trainer Course

Course Objectives

1. Identify and discuss the role as conceptualized by the American Academy of Pediatrics.
2. Demonstrate developing abilities to plan and implement all levels of NRP instruction.
3. Demonstrate knowledge of NRP in the region and explain expectations of the role.
4. Demonstrate excellent interpersonal skills and the ability to facilitate learning to diverse groups.
5. Demonstrate excellent NRP cognitive, technical, and communication skills.
6. Demonstrate developing abilities at simulation and debriefing skills.

1. Did the course meet the written objectives?	❏ Yes	❏ No
2. Did the course meet your personal objectives?	❏ Yes	❏ No

Please rate the following with 1=lowest/5=highest.

	Low				High
3. Course expectations and requirements were clear.	1	2	3	4	5
4. The course prepared me to be an NRP regional trainer.	1	2	3	4	5
5. My regional trainer was knowledgeable, supportive, and facilitated my learning.	1	2	3	4	5
6. The teaching methods were informative and useful.	1	2	3	4	5
7. The environment was conducive to learning.	1	2	3	4	5
8. The information was useful to your work setting.	1	2	3	4	5

9. What was the best part of this course?

10. What needs improvement?

Managing Challenging Classroom Situations

The monopolizer
This individual makes a comment before anyone else has a chance. He or she may tell long stories about past experiences.

- Thank this person for participating.
- Try some humor by asking if anyone besides this person would like to participate in the class discussion.
- Hold up your hand to interrupt the story, highlight one part of it, and answer the apparent question. If the story has no question, tell the person you appreciate the comments but must move on. Tell the person you would love to hear the rest of the story at the break.
- Ask participants to write down 2 ideas or comments, then call on the people who have not participated as much to share their ideas.
- Listen to the monopolizer's stories one-on-one at the break.

Your friends and colleagues
This group wishes to take advantage of you as their instructor.

- Let them know there are certain standards that must be met.
- Be friendly and polite, but do not bend the rules for a friend. Once it happens, you will have difficulty regaining control.
- Let them know this is their class—you facilitate their learning.

The negative participant
This person has closed body language and makes comments such as "Oh, sure. I'm supposed to do that in real life."

- Listen, ask questions, and evaluate the source of the problem.
- Try not to disagree. Find something you do agree with, and get this person on your side.
- Separate negative people and group them with positive class participants.

The questioner
This person has a "what if" question for many scenarios or asks difficult questions outside the scope of your course curriculum.

- Do not get defensive. Thank the participant for asking the question.
- Restate the question to be sure you understand the intent.
- Try, "I'd like to try to answer your question. Is there some background I should know about what prompted this question?"
- Do not try to bluff an answer if you do not know. Poll the course participants—maybe someone else can help. If not, consider telling the person you will research the answer or find some further resources. Get the person's name, and provide information or resources at a later date.

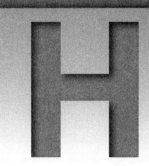
Neonatal Code Forms and Documentation

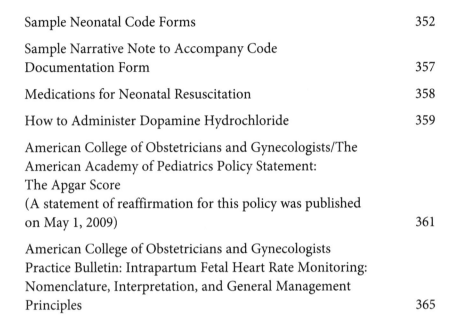

Neonatal Code Documentation Form: Sample 1

Neonatal Resuscitation Record

Side 1 of 2

Neonatal Code Documentation Form Sample 1

Baby's Last Name: _____   Sex: ☐ Male ☐ Female   Birth Date: _____   Time: _____

Estimated Gestational Age: _____   Estimated Weight: _____ kg

Apgars:
_____ 1 minute
_____ 5 minutes
_____ 10 minutes
_____ 15 minutes

☐ Meconium Present   Tracheal Suction: ☐ Yes ☐ No

Reason for Attending Birth: _____

OR

Patient history and events for baby requiring post-birth resuscitation: (note baby's age at resuscitation) _____

_____

_____

Comments: _____

_____

_____

_____

_____

_____

_____

_____

MD or RN Signature: _____

Who Attended: Physician (maternal) _____   RT _____

                 Physician (newborn) _____   Other _____

Outcome: ☐ Routine Care ☐ Nursery Observation ☐ Nursery Admittance   Time Transferred   to _____

ADDRESSOGRAPH

**NEONATAL
RESUSCITATION RECORD**
Side 1 of 2

Side 2 of 2

Complete this side when intubation/chest compressions are required.

DATE	Vital Signs					O₂ THERAPY				CPR	MEDICATIONS / DOSE					OTHER			REMARKS
Time	Resp. Rate	Heart Rate	Color	Preductal SpO₂	Tone	Free-flow O₂	Positive-pressure ventilation	Intubation	Endotracheal tube cm marking at lip	Chest Compressions	1:10,000 Epinephrine	Normal Saline	4.2% Sodium Bicarbonate			ABGs Drawn	Laryngeal Mask Airway		Note: Include such items as significant events, laboratory, ABG results, who intubated, and medication route.

Signatures: _____   Signatures: _____   Signatures: _____

_____   _____   _____

ADDRESSOGRAPH	**NEONATAL RESUSCITATION RECORD**
	Side 2 of 2
	KEY ✓ in accordance with policy/procedure manual
	COLOR: TONE:
	P – pink D - dusky + – active with stimulation
	W – pale C - cyanotic – – limp, floppy
	R – ruddy M - mottled J – jittery
	Sz – seizures

Neonatal Code Documentation Form: Sample 2

(Consider using Extended Apgar Score Reporting Form on page 35 of the Textbook of Neonatal Resuscitation, 6th Edition, *and on page 363 of this Instructor Manual.)*

Newborn Code Record

Side 1 of 2

Neonatal Code Documentation Form Sample 2

Date _____

Location _____

Time _____

Staff Present _____

Resuscitation required
☐ Tracheal suction for meconium
☐ Free-flow oxygen
☐ Positive-pressure ventilation
☐ Intubation tube size: _____
☐ Chest compressions
☐ Medications
☐ Volume infusion
☐ Laryngeal Mask Airway

HISTORY OF EVENTS PRIOR TO ARREST:

_____
_____
_____

APGAR SCORE			1	5	10	15	20
Color	Completely pink	2					
	Acrocyanotic	1					
	Blue/pale	0					
Heart Rate	>100	2					
	<100	1					
	Absent	0					
Reflex Irritability	Cry/active withdrawal	2					
	Grimace	1					
	No response	0					
Muscle Tone	Active motion	2					
	Some flexion	1					
	Limp	0					
Respiration	Good, crying	2					
	Weak cry; hypoventilation	1					
	Absent	0					
TOTAL							

PATIENT CARD IMPRINT

CODE TEAM

Charge MD or NNP _____

RN _____

RN _____

Other _____

Recorder _____

TIME	VITAL SIGNS/INTERVENTIONS										MEDS			OTHER									PATIENT'S RESPONSE	OUTCOME
	BREATHING (APNEIC, GASP, SPONT.)	POSITIVE-PRESSURE VENTILATION	VENTILATED RATE	HEART RATE	COLOR (PINK, WHITE, MOTTLED, BLUE)	TONE (+ –)/REFLEXES (+ –)	CHEST COMPRESSIONS	INTUBATION	EXTUBATION	FREE-FLOW OXYGEN	EPINEPHRINE DOSE/ ROUTE	NORMAL SALINE DOSE/ ROUTE	SODIUM BICARB DOSE/ ROUTE	HR/RR PER MONITOR	PREDUCTAL SpO₂	TEMPERATURE	SERVO CONTROL SETTING	GLUCOSE SCREEN	MAP	LARYNGEAL MASK AIRWAY			• Lab Results • Procedures (CXR, Line placement) • Activity/movement (seizures, etc.) • Urine output EST'D WEIGHT _____ Kg	Code terminated by
																								Code terminated at
																								Transferred to
																								Time
																								Time expired (if applicable)

SAMPLE

NEWBORN CODE

RECORD

SIDE 1 OF 2

Side 2 of 2

TIME	BREATHING (APNEIC, GASP, SPONT.)	POSITIVE-PRESSURE VENTILATION	VENTILATED RATE	HEART RATE	COLOR (PINK, WHITE, MOTTLED, BLUE)	TONE (+-)/REFLEXES (+-)	CHEST COMPRESSIONS	INTUBATION	EXTUBATION	FREE-FLOW OXYGEN	EPINEPHRINE DOSE/ ROUTE	NORMAL SALINE DOSE/ ROUTE	SODIUM BICARB DOSE/ ROUTE	HR/RR PER MONITOR	PREDUCTAL SpO₂	TEMPERATURE	SERVO CONTROL SETTING	GLUCOSE SCREEN	MAP	LARYNGEAL MASK AIRWAY				

VITAL SIGNS/INTERVENTIONS — MEDS — OTHER

- Lab Results
- Procedures (CXR, Line placement)
- Activity/movement (seizures, etc.)
- Urine output

EST'D WEIGHT _____ Kg

Neonatal Code Documentation Form: Sample 3

(Consider using Extended Apgar Score Reporting Form on page 35 of the Textbook of Neonatal Resuscitation, 6th Edition, *and on page 363 of this Instructor Manual.)*

NEONATAL RESUSCITATION RECORD

Date: _____

Patient Name: _____

Est. Wt.: _____ grams   Sex: _____

Time of Birth _____ AM/PM

Time of Transfer to Radiant Heater: _____ AM/PM _____

Resuscitation Procedures Initiated At:

Resuscitation Procedures Completed At:

Perinatal History:

Amniotic Fluid: Clear/Meconium Stained

APGAR SCORE

			1	5	10	15	20
Color	Completely pink	2					
	Acrocyanotic	1					
	Blue/pale	0					
Heart Rate	>100	2					
	<100	1					
	Absent	0					
Reflex Irritability	Cry/active withdrawal	2					
	Grimace	1					
	No response	0					
Muscle Tone	Active motion	2					
	Some flexion	1					
	Limp	0					
Respiration	Good, crying	2					
	Weak cry; hypoventilation	1					
	Absent	0					
TOTAL							

PROCEDURE

PROCEDURE	START	END	BY WHOM			
UVC or UAC				UA / UV Size:	3½ 5 8	
Intubation				ETT Size:	2.5 3.0 3.5 4.0	
Intubation With Ventilation				Total Minutes:		
Intubation/Suctioning Only				Total Minutes:		
Chest Compressions				Total Minutes:		
Positive-Pressure Ventilation				Total Minutes:		
Free-Flow Oxygen				Total Minutes: @ _____ L/min.		
Suction						
O/G Tube in: Yes No						
Laryngeal Mask Airway				Size: _____		

DRUGS

DRUGS	TIME/AMT	TIME/AMT	ROUTE	FLUSH SOLUTIONS
Epinephrine 1:10,000 0.1 to 0.3 mL/kg per IV 0.5 to 1 mL/kg per ET tube				_____ Normal Saline
Volume Expander: Normal saline 10 mL/kg Ringer's lactate				_____ Other
Sodium Bicarbonate 0.5 mEq/mL 2 mEq/kg (4.2% solution)				**BASE IV Solution** _____ 10% G/W
Blood Products				_____ 5% G/W
Others				

CLINICAL OBSERVATIONS

CLINICAL OBSERVATIONS	TIME/NOTED	Condition at completion of Code
First Gasp		(Circle one.)
Spontaneous Respirations		
First Grimace		Good Fair Guarded
HR >100 bpm		Expired

COMMENTS: _____

_____

_____

_____

Resuscitation Personnel Signatures:

MD _____

RN _____

Recording RN _____

RT _____

Admission to Nursery:

Temp: _____ HR _____ RR _____

Glucose _____ BP _____

Hct: _____ O₂ Sat. _____

Transferred to:

_____ Newborn Nursery

_____ Transitional Level Care Nursery

_____ NICU

Adapted from an original by Barbara Gerwatosky

Sample Narrative Note to Accompany Code Documentation Form

Documentation is a crucial skill for members of the resuscitation team. Your documentation should objectively re-create the resuscitation. A documentation sheet is filled out during the resuscitation by the "recorder." It is important for the recorder to know enough about neonatal resuscitation so that he or she knows what is most important to write down. Your narrative note accompanies the documentation sheet to ensure a complete record of the resuscitation. The narrative note includes at least

- Identification of the baby (sex, gestation)

- Time of birth

- Mode of birth

- Risk factor(s)

- What was happening when you arrived, if you were not there at the time of birth

- Interventions in order of occurrence and the baby's response to each

- What happened to support the family

4/20/11 0600

Term male newborn delivered per cesarean section at 0520 for breech presentation and meconium-stained amniotic fluid. Baby limp with no respiratory effort. Immediately placed on preheated radiant warmer. Dr Cook visualized cords, intubated, and suctioned meconium from trachea x1. (See Dr Cook's dictation.) Baby then dried with warm linen and repositioned on dry towel. Baby remained apneic. Bag-and-mask ventilation begun with room air at rate of 60/minute for approximately 30 seconds. Breath sounds and chest movement noted. Pulse oximeter placed on right wrist; no signal. Heart rate assessed at approximately 40 bpm. Chest compressions begun and PPV continued. F_{IO_2} increased to 100%. After 60 seconds, heart rate assessed at approximately 50 bpm. Baby intubated with 3.5 ET tube. CO_2 detector turned yellow. Breath sounds audible bilaterally. Chest compressions continued. After an additional 45 seconds of chest compressions and PPV per ET tube and bag, heart rate had increased to approximately 80 bpm. Pulse oximeter achieved signal (see flow sheet). Chest compressions discontinued, PPV continued. At 5 minutes of age, baby's heart rate 140 bpm. F_{IO_2} decreased to 40% to achieve target saturation (see flow sheet). Improving color and wet bilateral breath sounds; however, baby remained limp. No spontaneous respirations. Tube secured. Baby transported to nursery on radiant warmer with PPV in progress. Arrived in nursery at 0540. Social worker with father of baby and will give updates to parents from nursery. See accompanying resuscitation documentation sheet.

Sylvia Bettingford, RN

Medications for Neonatal Resuscitation

Medication	Concentration to Administer	Route	Dosage/Prep	Rate/Precautions
Epinephrine Caution: 2 ROUTES 2 DOSAGES	1:10,000	Umbilical vein	0.1 to 0.3 mL/kg IV. Draw up in 1-mL syringe.	Give rapidly. Follow with a 0.5- to 1-mL flush of normal saline to ensure the drug reaches the blood.
	1:10,000	Intratracheal route acceptable while IV access is being established	0.5 to 1 mL/kg via endotracheal tube. Draw up in a 5-mL or 6-mL syringe.	Give rapidly. Give directly into endotracheal tube. Follow with positive-pressure ventilation.
Volume expanders	Normal saline (recommended) Acceptable: Ringer's lactate O Rh-negative packed red blood cells	Umbilical vein	10 mL/kg. Draw estimated volume needed into large syringe(s).	Give over 5 to 10 minutes. Give by syringe or infusion pump.
Post-resuscitation Medications				
Sodium bicarbonate	0.5 mEq/mL (4.2% solution)	Large vein with good blood return; usually the umbilical vein	2 mEq/kg/dose. Prepare 20-mL prefilled syringe or two 10-mL prefilled syringes.	Give slowly, no faster than 1 mEq/kg/min. Give only if newborn lungs are being adequately ventilated. Never give via ET tube.
Naloxone hydrochloride	1.0 mg/mL	IV route preferred IM route acceptable, but delayed onset of action	0.1 mg/kg. Prepare 1 mL of 1.0-mg/mL solution in a 1-mL syringe.	Give rapidly. Do not give to newborn of mother suspected of being addicted to narcotics or on methadone maintenance. This may result in the newborn having seizures.

How to Administer Dopamine Hydrochloride

Dopamine

One of the effects of asphyxia is to decrease cardiac contractility with a consequent decrease in cardiac output. If a newborn undergoes a prolonged resuscitation, including administration of epinephrine and a volume expander, and continues to have poor peripheral perfusion, thready pulses, and evidence of shock, a continuous infusion of a catecholamine may help raise the blood pressure. Dopamine hydrochloride is a catecholamine widely used with newborns for this purpose.

The main effect of dopamine is to increase systemic vascular resistance, thereby raising the newborn's blood pressure.

When dopamine is required, the newborn is very sick indeed. It is suggested that a neonatologist or referral nursery be consulted at this point, if not before, about the continuing care of the newborn.

Additional Considerations

The administration of dopamine has some additional considerations. It must be given as a continuous infusion, with the flow rate carefully controlled with an infusion pump. Since dopamine affects cardiac output and blood pressure, the newborn receiving dopamine requires continuous monitoring and frequent assessment of heart rate and blood pressure.

Indications

After a prolonged resuscitation, consider the administration of dopamine **if the newborn has poor peripheral perfusion and thready pulses and continues to show evidence of shock.**

Preparation and Administration

The preparation and administration of dopamine is very different from that of other medications. Dopamine is administered only as a continuous infusion. An intravenous solution containing dopamine must be prepared.

The concentration of the solution prepared will vary based on the

- Dosage desired
- Newborn's weight
- Volume of fluid considered desirable or safe to administer

Dosage

Since dopamine is given as a continuous infusion, **the dosage *is always* expressed as the *amount of dopamine* to be infused per kilogram per minute** (eg, 5 µg/kg per minute, not 5 µg/kg or 5 µg).

Infusing Solution

Infusing the solution at the desired mL/hour provides the newborn with the desired dose per minute. Remember that an infusion pump must always be used to ensure a controlled infusion rate.

Be sure to clear all the dead space in the intravenous tubing. Because the infusion rates, in terms of mL/min, are relatively slow, it may take some time before the newborn actually begins receiving dopamine if the dead space is not cleared first.

Effects

- Increases peripheral vascular resistance
- Strengthens cardiac contractions and thus increases cardiac output to some degree
- Increases heart rate, thus increasing cardiac output to some degree
- Raises blood pressure

Expected Signs

- Blood pressure should rise.
- Heart rate should stabilize; tachycardia often present.

Infusion rates are usually increased in increments of 3 to 5 µg/kg/min if the blood pressure and perfusion do not improve. Consultation with a neonatologist is advised.

Follow-up

First 15 minutes

- Check the heart rate every 30 to 60 seconds.
- Check blood pressure every 2 minutes.

After 15 minutes

- Check heart rate and blood pressure at least every 3 to 5 minutes until the blood pressure is stabilized.

The administration of a dopamine drip may need to be continued for several hours. As you attempt to decrease the infusion, be sure that heart rate and blood pressure stay within a normal range.

Caution

If newborn has an insufficient response to 20 µg/kg/min of dopamine, it is highly unlikely that raising the dose further will make a difference.

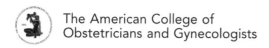 The American College of
Obstetricians and Gynecologists

 American Academy
of Pediatrics

DEDICATED TO THE HEALTH OF ALL CHILDREN™

POLICY STATEMENT

The Apgar Score

American Academy of Pediatrics
Committee on Fetus and Newborn
American College of Obstetricians and Gynecologists
Committee on Obstetric Practice

Organizational Principles to Guide and
Define the Child Health Care System and/or
Improve the Health of All Children

ABSTRACT

The Apgar score provides a convenient shorthand for reporting the status of the
newborn infant and the response to resuscitation. The Apgar score has been used
inappropriately to predict specific neurologic outcome in the term infant. There are
no consistent data on the significance of the Apgar score in preterm infants. The
Apgar score has limitations, and it is inappropriate to use it alone to establish the
diagnosis of asphyxia. An Apgar score assigned during resuscitation is not equivalent to a score assigned to a spontaneously breathing infant. An expanded Apgar
score reporting form will account for concurrent resuscitative interventions and
provide information to improve systems of perinatal and neonatal care.

INTRODUCTION

In 1952, Dr Virginia Apgar devised a scoring system that was a rapid method of
assessing the clinical status of the newborn infant at 1 minute of age and the need
for prompt intervention to establish breathing.[1] A second report evaluating a larger
number of patients was published in 1958.[2] This scoring system provided a
standardized assessment for infants after delivery. The Apgar score comprises 5
components: heart rate, respiratory effort, muscle tone, reflex irritability, and
color, each of which is given a score of 0, 1, or 2. The score is now reported at 1
and 5 minutes after birth. The Apgar score continues to provide a convenient
shorthand for reporting the status of the newborn infant and the response to
resuscitation. The Apgar score has been used inappropriately in term infants to
predict specific neurologic outcome. Because there are no consistent data on the
significance of the Apgar score in preterm infants, in this population the score
should not be used for any purpose other than ongoing assessment in the delivery
room. The purpose of this statement is to place the Apgar score in its proper
perspective.

The neonatal resuscitation program (NRP) guidelines[3] state that "Apgar scores
should not be used to dictate appropriate resuscitative actions, nor should interventions for depressed infants be delayed until the 1-minute assessment." However, an Apgar score that remains 0 beyond 10 minutes of age may be useful in
determining whether additional resuscitative efforts are indicated.[4] The current
NRP guidelines[3] state that "if there is no heart rate after 10 minutes of complete
and adequate resuscitation efforts, and there is no evidence of other causes of
newborn compromise, discontinuation of resuscitation efforts may be appropriate.
Current data indicate that, after 10 minutes of asystole, newborns are very unlikely to survive, or the rare survivor is likely to survive with severe disability."

www.pediatrics.org/cgi/doi/10.1542/
peds.2006-0325

doi:10.1542/peds.2006-0325

All policy statements from the American
Academy of Pediatrics automatically
expire 5 years after publication unless
reaffirmed, revised, or retired at or
before that time.

Key Words
Apgar score, asphyxia, neurologic
outcome, resuscitation, cerebral palsy

Abbreviation
NRP—neonatal resuscitation program

PEDIATRICS (ISSN Numbers: Print, 0031-4005;
Online, 1098-4275). Copyright © 2006 by the
American Academy of Pediatrics and the
American College of Obstetricians and
Gynecologists

Previously, an Apgar score of 3 or less at 5 minutes was considered an essential requirement for the diagnosis of perinatal asphyxia. *Neonatal Encephalopathy and Cerebral Palsy: Defining the Pathogenesis and Pathophysiology*,[5] produced in 2003 by the American College of Obstetricians and Gynecologists in collaboration with the American Academy of Pediatrics, lists an Apgar score of 0 to 3 beyond 5 minutes as one suggestive criterion for an intrapartum asphyxial insult. However, a persistently low Apgar score alone is not a specific indicator for intrapartum compromise. Further, although the score is used widely in outcome studies, its inappropriate use has led to an erroneous definition of asphyxia. Intrapartum asphyxia implies fetal hypercarbia and hypoxemia, which, if prolonged, will result in metabolic acidemia. Because the intrapartum disruption of uterine or fetal blood flow is rarely, if ever, absolute, asphyxia is an imprecise, general term. Descriptions such as hypercarbia, hypoxia, and metabolic, respiratory, or lactic acidemia are more precise for immediate assessment of the newborn infant and retrospective assessment of intrapartum management.

LIMITATIONS OF THE APGAR SCORE

It is important to recognize the limitations of the Apgar score. The Apgar score is an expression of the infant's physiologic condition, has a limited time frame, and includes subjective components. In addition, the biochemical disturbance must be significant before the score is affected. Elements of the score such as tone, color, and reflex irritability partially depend on the physiologic maturity of the infant. The healthy preterm infant with no evidence of asphyxia may receive a low score only because of immaturity.[6] A number of factors may influence an Apgar score, including but not limited to drugs, trauma, congenital anomalies, infections, hypoxia, hypovolemia, and preterm birth.[7] The incidence of low Apgar scores is inversely related to birth weight, and a low score is limited in predicting morbidity or mortality.[8] Accordingly, it is inappropriate to use an Apgar score alone to establish the diagnosis of asphyxia.

APGAR SCORE AND RESUSCITATION

The 5-minute Apgar score, and particularly a change in the score between 1 and 5 minutes, is a useful index of the response to resuscitation. If the Apgar score is less than 7 at 5 minutes, the NRP guidelines state that the assessment should be repeated every 5 minutes up to 20 minutes.[3] However, an Apgar score assigned during a resuscitation is not equivalent to a score assigned to a spontaneously breathing infant.[9] There is no accepted standard for reporting an Apgar score in infants undergoing resuscitation after birth, because many of the elements contributing to the score are altered by resuscitation. The concept of an "assisted" score that accounts for

resuscitative interventions has been suggested, but the predictive reliability has not been studied. To describe such infants correctly and provide accurate documentation and data collection, an expanded Apgar score report form is proposed (Fig 1).

PREDICTION OF OUTCOME

A low 1-minute Apgar score alone does not correlate with the infant's future outcome. A retrospective analysis concluded that the 5-minute Apgar score remained a valid predictor of neonatal mortality, but using it to predict long-term outcome was inappropriate.[10] On the other hand, another study[11] stated that low Apgar scores at 5 minutes are associated with death or cerebral palsy, and this association increased if both 1- and 5-minute scores were low.

An Apgar score at 5 minutes in term infants correlates poorly with future neurologic outcomes. For example, a score of 0 to 3 at 5 minutes was associated with a slightly increased risk of cerebral palsy compared with higher scores.[12] Conversely, 75% of children with cerebral palsy had normal scores at 5 minutes.[12] In addition, a low 5-minute score in combination with other markers of asphyxia may identify infants at risk of developing seizures (odds ratio: 39; 95% confidence interval: 3.9–392.5).[13] The risk of poor neurologic outcomes increases when the Apgar score is 3 or less at 10, 15, and 20 minutes.[7]

A 5-minute Apgar score of 7 to 10 is considered normal. Scores of 4, 5, and 6 are intermediate and are not markers of increased risk of neurologic dysfunction. Such scores may be the result of physiologic immaturity, maternal medications, the presence of congenital malformations, and other factors. Because of these other conditions, the Apgar score alone cannot be considered evidence or a consequence of asphyxia. Other factors including nonreassuring fetal heart rate monitoring patterns and abnormalities in umbilical arterial blood gases, clinical cerebral function, neuroimaging studies, neonatal electroencephalography, placental pathology, hematologic studies, and multisystem organ dysfunction need to be considered when defining an intrapartum hypoxic-ischemic event as a cause of cerebral palsy.[5]

OTHER APPLICATIONS

Monitoring of low Apgar scores from a delivery service can be useful. Individual case reviews can identify needs for focused educational programs and improvement in systems of perinatal care. Analyzing trends allows assessment of the impact of quality improvement interventions.

CONCLUSION

The Apgar score describes the condition of the newborn infant immediately after birth[14] and, when properly ap-

APGAR SCORE

Gestational Age _____ weeks

SIGN	0	1	2		1 minute	5 minute	10 minute	15 minute	20 minute
COLOR	Blue or Pale	Acrocyanotic	Completely Pink						
HEART RATE	Absent	<100 minute	>100 minute						
REFLEX IRRITABILITY	No Response	Grimace	Cry or Active Withdrawal						
MUSCLE TONE	Limp	Some Flexion	Active Motion						
RESPIRATION	Absent	Weak Cry; Hypoventilation	Good, crying						
			TOTAL						

Comments:

Resuscitation					
Minutes	1	5	10	15	20
Oxygen					
PPV/NCPAP					
ETT					
Chest Compressions					
Epinephrine					

FIGURE 1

Expanded Apgar score form. Record the score in the appropriate place at specific time intervals. The additional resuscitative measures (if appropriate) are recorded at the same time that the score is reported using a check mark in the appropriate box. Use the comment box to list other factors including maternal medications and/or the response to resuscitation between the recorded times of scoring. PPV/NCPAP indicates positive-pressure ventilation/nasal continuous positive airway pressure; ETT, endotracheal tube.

plied, is a tool for standardized assessment. It also provides a mechanism to record fetal-to-neonatal transition. An Apgar score of 0 to 3 at 5 minutes may correlate with neonatal mortality but alone does not predict later neurologic dysfunction. The Apgar score is affected by gestational age, maternal medications, resuscitation, and cardiorespiratory and neurologic conditions. Low 1- and 5-minute Apgar scores alone are not conclusive markers of an acute intrapartum hypoxic event. Resuscitative interventions modify the components of the Apgar score. There is a need for perinatal health care professionals to be consistent in assigning an Apgar score during a resuscitation. The American Academy of Pediatrics and the American College of Obstetricians and Gynecologists propose use of an expanded Apgar score reporting form that accounts for concurrent resuscitative interventions.

AAP COMMITTEE ON FETUS AND NEWBORN, 2005–2006
Ann R. Stark, MD, Chairperson
David H. Adamkin, MD
Daniel G. Batton, MD
Edward F. Bell, MD
Vinod K. Bhutani, MD
Susan E. Denson, MD
William A. Engle, MD
*Gilbert I. Martin, MD
Lillian R. Blackmon, MD, Past Chairperson

LIAISONS
Keith J. Barrington, MD
    Canadian Paediatric Society
Gary D.V. Hankins, MD
    American College of Obstetricians and Gynecologists
Tonse N.K. Raju, MD, DCH
    National Institutes of Health
Kay M. Tomashek, MD, MPH
    Centers for Disease Control and Prevention
Carol Wallman, MSN, RNC, NNP
    National Association of Neonatal Nurses and
    Association of Women's Health, Obstetric and
    Neonatal Nurses
Laura E. Riley, MD, Past Liaison
    American College of Obstetricians and Gynecologists

STAFF
Jim Couto, MA

ACOG COMMITTEE ON OBSTETRIC PRACTICE
*Gary D.V. Hankins, MD, Chairperson
Sarah J. Kilpatrick, MD, Vice-Chairperson
Angela L. Bell, MD
Jeanne M. Coulehan, CNM
Susan Hellerstein, MD
Jack Ludmir, MD
Carol A. Major, MD
Sean McFadden, MD
Susan M. Ramin, MD
Russell R. Snyder, Col, MC, USAF

LIAISONS

Hani K. Atrash, MD, MPH
Centers for Disease Control and Prevention

William Callaghan, MD
Centers for Disease Control and Prevention

Joshua A. Copel, MD
Association for Medical Ultrasound

Gary A. Dildy III, MD
Society for Maternal-Fetal Medicine

William Herbert, MD
Committee on Practice Bulletins-Obstetrics Liaison

Samuel C. Hughes, MD
American Society of Anesthesiologists

Bruce Patsner, MD, JD
Food and Drug Administration

Colin Pollard
Food and Drug Administration

Phill Price, MD
Food and Drug Administration

Catherine Y. Spong, MD
National Institute of Child Health and Human Development

Ann Stark, MD
American Academy of Pediatrics

John S. Wachtel, MD
Committee on Quality Improvement and Patient Safety

STAFF

Stanley Zinberg, MD, MS
Beth Steele
Debra Hawks, MPH

*Lead authors

REFERENCES

1. Apgar V. A proposal for a new method of evaluation of the newborn infant. *Curr Res Anesth Analg.* 1953;32:260–267
2. Apgar V, Holiday DA, James LS, Weisbrot IM, Berrien C. Evaluation of the newborn infant: second report. *JAMA.* 1958;168:1985–1988
3. American Academy of Pediatrics and American Heart Association. *Textbook of Neonatal Resuscitation.* Elk Grove Village, IL: American Academy of Pediatrics and American Heart Association; 2005
4. Jain L, Ferre C, Vidyasagar D, Nath S, Sheftel D. Cardiopulmonary resuscitation of apparently stillborn infants: survival and long-term outcome. *J Pediatr.* 1991;118:778–782
5. American College of Obstetrics and Gynecology, Task Force on Neonatal Encephalopathy and Cerebral Palsy; American Academy of Pediatrics. *Neonatal Encephalopathy and Cerebral Palsy: Defining the Pathogenesis and Pathophysiology.* Washington, DC: American College of Obstetricians and Gynecologists; 2003
6. Catlin EA, Carpenter MW, Brann BS IV, et al. The Apgar score revisited: influence of gestational age. *J Pediatr.* 1986;109:865–868
7. Freeman JM, Nelson KB. Intrapartum asphyxia and cerebral palsy. *Pediatrics.* 1988;82:240–249
8. Hegyi T, Carone T, Anwar M, et al. The Apgar score and its components in the preterm infant. *Pediatrics.* 1998;101:77–81
9. Lopriore E, van Burk F, Walther F, Arnout J. Correct use of the Apgar score for resuscitated and intubated newborn babies: questionnaire study. *BMJ.* 2004;329:143–144
10. Casey BM, McIntire DD, Leveno KJ. The continuing value of the Apgar score for the assessment of the newborn infants. *N Engl J Med.* 2001;344:467–471
11. Moster D, Lie RT, Irgens LM, Bjerkedal T, Markestad T. The association of Apgar score with subsequent death and cerebral palsy: a population-based study in term infants. *J Pediatr.* 2001;138:798–803
12. Nelson KB, Ellenberg JH. Apgar scores as predictors of chronic neurologic disability. *Pediatrics.* 1981;68:36–44
13. Perlman JM, Risser R. Can asphyxiated infants at risk for neonatal seizures be rapidly identified by current high-risk markers? *Pediatrics.* 1996;97:456–462
14. Papile LA. The Apgar score in the 21st century. *N Engl J Med.* 2001;344:519–520

ACOG PRACTICE BULLETIN

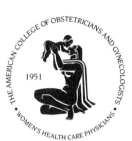

CLINICAL MANAGEMENT GUIDELINES FOR OBSTETRICIAN–GYNECOLOGISTS

NUMBER 106, JULY 2009

Replaces Practice Bulletin Number 70, December 2005

Intrapartum Fetal Heart Rate Monitoring: Nomenclature, Interpretation, and General Management Principles

This Practice Bulletin was developed by the ACOG Committee on Practice Bulletins with the assistance of George A. Macones, MD. The information is designed to aid practitioners in making decisions about appropriate obstetric and gynecologic care. These guidelines should not be construed as dictating an exclusive course of treatment or procedure. Variations in practice may be warranted based on the needs of the individual patient, resources, and limitations unique to the institution or type of practice.

In the most recent year for which data are available, approximately 3.4 million fetuses (85% of approximately 4 million live births) in the United States were assessed with electronic fetal monitoring (EFM), making it the most common obstetric procedure (1). Despite its widespread use, there is controversy about the efficacy of EFM, interobserver and intraobserver variability, nomenclature, systems for interpretation, and management algorithms. Moreover, there is evidence that the use of EFM increases the rate of cesarean deliveries and operative vaginal deliveries. The purpose of this document is to review nomenclature for fetal heart rate assessment, review the data on the efficacy of EFM, delineate the strengths and shortcomings of EFM, and describe a system for EFM classification.

Background

A complex interplay of antepartum complications, suboptimal uterine perfusion, placental dysfunction, and intrapartum events can result in adverse neonatal outcome. Known obstetric conditions, such as hypertensive disease, fetal growth restriction, and preterm birth, predispose fetuses to poor outcomes, but they account for a small proportion of asphyxial injury. In a study of term pregnancies with fetal asphyxia, 63% had no known risk factors (2).

The fetal brain modulates the fetal heart rate through an interplay of sympathetic and parasympathetic forces. Thus, fetal heart rate (FHR) monitoring can be used to determine if a fetus is well oxygenated. It was used among 45% of laboring women in 1980, 62% in 1988, 74% in 1992, and 85% in 2002 (1).

THE AMERICAN COLLEGE OF OBSTETRICIANS AND GYNECOLOGISTS
WOMEN'S HEALTH CARE PHYSICIANS

Despite the frequency of its use, limitations of EFM include poor interobserver and intraobserver reliability, uncertain efficacy, and a high false-positive rate.

Fetal heart rate monitoring may be performed externally or internally. Most external monitors use a Doppler device with computerized logic to interpret and count the Doppler signals. Internal FHR monitoring is accomplished with a fetal electrode, which is a spiral wire placed directly on the fetal scalp or other presenting part.

Guidelines for Nomenclature and Interpretation of Electronic Fetal Heart Rate Monitoring

In 2008, the *Eunice Kennedy Shriver* National Institute of Child Health and Human Development partnered with the American College of Obstetricians and Gynecologists and the Society for Maternal–Fetal Medicine to sponsor a workshop focused on electronic FHR monitoring (3). This 2008 workshop gathered a diverse group of investigators with expertise and interest in the field to accomplish three goals: 1) to review and update the definitions for FHR pattern categorization from the prior workshop; 2) to assess existing classification systems for interpreting specific FHR patterns and make recommendations about a system for use in the United States; and 3) to make recommendations for research priorities for EFM. A complete clinical understanding of EFM necessitates discussion of uterine contractions, baseline FHR rate and variability, presence of accelerations, periodic or episodic decelerations, and the changes in these characteristics over time. A number of assumptions and factors common to FHR interpretation in the United States are central to the proposed system of nomenclature and interpretation (3). Two such assumptions are of particular importance. First, the definitions are primarily developed for visual interpretation of FHR patterns, but should be adaptable to computerized systems of interpretation. Second, the definitions should be applied to intrapartum patterns, but also are applicable to antepartum observations.

Uterine contractions are quantified as the number of contractions present in a 10-minute window, averaged over a 30-minute period. Contraction frequency alone is a partial assessment of uterine activity. Other factors such as duration, intensity, and relaxation time between contractions are equally important in clinical practice.

Listed as follows is terminology used to describe uterine activity:

Normal: five contractions or less in 10 minutes, averaged over a 30-minute window

Tachysystole: more than five contractions in 10 minutes, averaged over a 30-minute window

Characteristics of uterine contractions

- The terms hyperstimulation and hypercontractility are not defined and should be abandoned.
- Tachysystole should always be qualified as to the presence or absence of associated FHR decelerations.
- The term tachysystole applies to both spontaneous and stimulated labor. The clinical response to tachysystole may differ depending on whether contractions are spontaneous or stimulated.

Table 1 provides EFM definitions and descriptions based on the 2008 National Institute of Child Health and Human Development Working Group findings. Decelerations are defined as recurrent if they occur with at least one half of the contractions.

Classification of Fetal Heart Rate Tracings

A variety of systems for EFM interpretation have been used in the United States and worldwide (4–6). Based on careful review of the available options, a three-tiered system for the categorization of FHR patterns is recommended (see box). It is important to recognize that FHR tracing patterns provide information only on the current acid–base status of the fetus. Categorization of the FHR tracing evaluates the fetus at that point in time; tracing patterns can and will change. An FHR tracing may move back and forth between the categories depending on the clinical situation and management strategies used.

Category I FHR tracings are normal. Category I FHR tracings are strongly predictive of normal fetal acid–base status at the time of observation. Category I FHR tracings may be monitored in a routine manner, and no specific action is required.

Category II FHR tracings are indeterminate. Category II FHR tracings are not predictive of abnormal fetal acid–base status, yet presently there is not adequate evidence to classify these as Category I or Category III. Category II FHR tracings require evaluation and continued surveillance and reevaluation, taking into account the entire associated clinical circumstances. In some circumstances, either ancillary tests to ensure fetal well-being or intrauterine resuscitative measures may be used with Category II tracings.

Category III FHR tracings are abnormal. Category III tracings are associated with abnormal fetal acid–base status at the time of observation. Category III FHR tracings require prompt evaluation. Depending on the clinical situation, efforts to expeditiously resolve the

Table 1. Electronic Fetal Monitoring Definitions

Pattern	Definition

Baseline	• The mean FHR rounded to increments of 5 beats per minute during a 10-minute segment, excluding:
	  —Periodic or episodic changes
	  —Periods of marked FHR variability
	  —Segments of baseline that differ by more than 25 beats per minute
	• The baseline must be for a minimum of 2 minutes in any 10-minute segment, or the baseline for that time period is indeterminate. In this case, one may refer to the prior 10-minute window for determination of baseline.
	• Normal FHR baseline: 110–160 beats per minute
	• Tachycardia: FHR baseline is greater than 160 beats per minute
	• Bradycardia: FHR baseline is less than 110 beats per minute

Baseline variability	• Fluctuations in the baseline FHR that are irregular in amplitude and frequency
	• Variability is visually quantitated as the amplitude of peak-to-trough in beats per minute.
	  —Absent—amplitude range undetectable
	  —Minimal—amplitude range detectable but 5 beats per minute or fewer
	  —Moderate (normal)—amplitude range 6–25 beats per minute
	  —Marked—amplitude range greater than 25 beats per minute

Acceleration	• A visually apparent abrupt increase (onset to peak in less than 30 seconds) in the FHR • At 32 weeks of gestation and beyond, an acceleration has a peak of 15 beats per minute or more above baseline, with a duration of 15 seconds or more but less than 2 minutes from onset to return. • Before 32 weeks of gestation, an acceleration has a peak of 10 beats per minute or more above baseline, with a duration of 10 seconds or more but less than 2 minutes from onset to return. • Prolonged acceleration lasts 2 minutes or more but less than 10 minutes in duration. • If an acceleration lasts 10 minutes or longer, it is a baseline change.
Early deceleration	• Visually apparent usually symmetrical gradual decrease and return of the FHR associated with a uterine contraction • A gradual FHR decrease is defined as from the onset to the FHR nadir of 30 seconds or more. • The decrease in FHR is calculated from the onset to the nadir of the deceleration. • The nadir of the deceleration occurs at the same time as the peak of the contraction. • In most cases the onset, nadir, and recovery of the deceleration are coincident with the beginning, peak, and ending of the contraction, respectively.
Late deceleration	• Visually apparent usually symmetrical gradual decrease and return of the FHR associated with a uterine contraction • A gradual FHR decrease is defined as from the onset to the FHR nadir of 30 seconds or more. • The decrease in FHR is calculated from the onset to the nadir of the deceleration. • The deceleration is delayed in timing, with the nadir of the deceleration occurring after the peak of the contraction. • In most cases, the onset, nadir, and recovery of the deceleration occur after the beginning, peak, and ending of the contraction, respectively.
Variable deceleration	• Visually apparent abrupt decrease in FHR • An abrupt FHR decrease is defined as from the onset of the deceleration to the beginning of the FHR nadir of less than 30 seconds. • The decrease in FHR is calculated from the onset to the nadir of the deceleration. • The decrease in FHR is 15 beats per minute or greater, lasting 15 seconds or greater, and less than 2 minutes in duration. • When variable decelerations are associated with uterine contractions, their onset, depth, and duration commonly vary with successive uterine contractions.
Prolonged deceleration	• Visually apparent decrease in the FHR below the baseline • Decrease in FHR from the baseline that is 15 beats per minute or more, lasting 2 minutes or more but less than 10 minutes in duration. • If a deceleration lasts 10 minutes or longer, it is a baseline change.
Sinusoidal pattern	• Visually apparent, smooth, sine wave-like undulating pattern in FHR baseline with a cycle frequency of 3–5 per minute which persists for 20 minutes or more.

Abbreviation: FHR, fetal heart rate.

Macones GA, Hankins GD, Spong CY, Hauth J, Moore T. The 2008 National Institute of Child Health and Human Development workshop report on electronic fetal monitoring: update on definitions, interpretation, and research guidelines. Obstet Gynecol 2008;112:661–6.

Three-Tiered Fetal Heart Rate Interpretation System

Category I
- Category I FHR tracings include all of the following:
- Baseline rate: 110–160 beats per minute
- Baseline FHR variability: moderate
- Late or variable decelerations: absent
- Early decelerations: present or absent
- Accelerations: present or absent

Category II
Category II FHR tracings includes all FHR tracings not categorized as Category I or Category III. Category II tracings may represent an appreciable fraction of those encountered in clinical care. Examples of Category II FHR tracings include any of the following:

Baseline rate
- Bradycardia not accompanied by absent baseline variability
- Tachycardia

Baseline FHR variability
- Minimal baseline variability
- Absent baseline variability with no recurrent decelerations
- Marked baseline variability

Accelerations
- Absence of induced accelerations after fetal stimulation

Periodic or episodic decelerations
- Recurrent variable decelerations accompanied by minimal or moderate baseline variability
- Prolonged deceleration more than 2 minutes but less than 10 minutes
- Recurrent late decelerations with moderate baseline variability
- Variable decelerations with other characteristics such as slow return to baseline, overshoots, or "shoulders"

Category III
Category III FHR tracings include either
- Absent baseline FHR variability and any of the following:
  - Recurrent late decelerations
  - Recurrent variable decelerations
  - Bradycardia
- Sinusoidal pattern

Abbreviation: FHR, fetal heart rate

Macones GA, Hankins GD, Spong CY, Hauth J, Moore T. The 2008 National Institute of Child Health and Human Development workshop report on electronic fetal monitoring: update on definitions, interpretation, and research guidelines. Obstet Gynecol 2008;112:661–6.

abnormal FHR pattern may include but are not limited to provision of maternal oxygen, change in maternal position, discontinuation of labor stimulation, treatment of maternal hypotension, and treatment of tachysystole with FHR changes. If a Category III tracing does not resolve with these measures, delivery should be undertaken.

Guidelines for Review of Electronic Fetal Heart Rate Monitoring

When EFM is used during labor, the nurses or physicians should review it frequently. In a patient without complications, the FHR tracing should be reviewed approximately every 30 minutes in the first stage of labor and every 15 minutes during the second stage. The corresponding frequency for patients with complications (eg, fetal growth restriction, preeclampsia) is approximately every 15 minutes in the first stage of labor and every 5 minutes during the second stage. Health care providers should periodically document that they have reviewed the tracing. The FHR tracing, as part of the medical record, should be labeled and available for review if the need arises. Computer storage of the FHR tracing that does not permit overwriting or revisions is reasonable, as is microfilm recording.

Clinical Considerations and Recommendations

▶ *How efficacious is intrapartum electronic fetal heart rate monitoring?*

The efficacy of EFM during labor is judged by its ability to decrease complications, such as neonatal seizures, cerebral palsy, or intrapartum fetal death, while minimizing the need for unnecessary obstetric interventions, such as operative vaginal delivery or cesarean delivery. There are no randomized clinical trials to compare the benefits of EFM with any form of monitoring during labor (7). Thus, the benefits of EFM are gauged from reports comparing it with intermittent auscultation.

A meta-analysis synthesizing the results of the randomized clinical trials comparing the modalities had the following conclusions (8):

- The use of EFM compared with intermittent auscultation increased the overall cesarean delivery rate (relative risk [RR], 1.66; 95% confidence interval [CI], 1.30–2.13) and the cesarean delivery rate for abnormal FHR or acidosis or both (RR, 2.37; 95% CI, 1.88–3.00).

- The use of EFM increased the risk of both vacuum and forceps operative vaginal delivery (RR, 1.16; 95% CI, 1.01–1.32).

- The use of EFM did not reduce perinatal mortality (RR, 0.85; 95% CI, 0.59–1.23).

- The use of EFM reduced the risk of neonatal seizures (RR, 0.50; 95% CI, 0.31–0.80).

- The use of EFM did not reduce the risk of cerebral palsy (RR, 1.74; 95% CI, 0.97–3.11).

There is an unrealistic expectation that a nonreassuring FHR tracing is predictive of cerebral palsy. The positive predictive value of a nonreassuring pattern to predict cerebral palsy among singleton newborns with birth weights of 2,500 g or more is 0.14%, meaning that out of 1,000 fetuses with a nonreassuring FHR pattern, only one or two will develop cerebral palsy (9). The false-positive rate of EFM for predicting cerebral palsy is extremely high, at greater than 99%.

Available data, although limited in quantity, suggest that the use of EFM does not result in a reduction in cerebral palsy (8). This is consistent with data that suggest that the occurrence of cerebral palsy has been stable over time, despite the widespread introduction of EFM (10). The principal explanation for why the prevalence of cerebral palsy has not diminished despite the use of EFM is that 70% of cases occur before the onset of labor; only 4% of cases of encephalopathy can be attributed solely to intrapartum events (11, 12).

Given that the available data do not show a clear benefit for the use of EFM over intermittent auscultation, either option is acceptable in a patient without complications. Logistically, it may not be feasible to adhere to guidelines for how frequently the heart rate should be auscultated. One prospective study noted that the protocol for intermittent auscultation was successfully completed in only 3% of the cases (13). The most common reasons for unsuccessful intermittent auscultation included the frequency of recording and the requirements for recording.

Intermittent auscultation may not be appropriate for all pregnancies. Most of the clinical trials that compare EFM with intermittent auscultation have excluded participants at high risk of adverse outcomes, and the relative safety of intermittent auscultation in such cases is uncertain. The labor of women with high-risk conditions (eg, suspected fetal growth restriction, preeclampsia, and type 1 diabetes) should be monitored with continuous FHR monitoring.

There are no comparative data indicating the optimal frequency at which intermittent auscultation should be performed in the absence of risk factors. One method is to evaluate and record the FHR at least every 15 minutes in the active phase of the first stage of labor and at least every 5 minutes in the second stage (14).

▶ *What is the interobserver and intraobserver variability of intrapartum electronic fetal heart rate monitoring assessment?*

There is high interobserver and intraobserver variability in the interpretation of FHR tracings. For example, when four obstetricians examined 50 cardiotocograms, they agreed in only 22% of the cases (15). Two months later, during the second review of the same 50 tracings, the clinicians interpreted 21% of the tracings differently than they did during the first evaluation. In another study, five obstetricians independently interpreted 150 cardiotocograms (16). The obstetricians interpreted the tracings similarly in 29% of the cases, suggesting poor interobserver reliability.

The interpretation of cardiotocograms is more consistent when the tracing is normal (17). With retrospective reviews, the foreknowledge of neonatal outcome may alter the reviewer's impressions of the tracing. Given the same intrapartum tracing, a reviewer is more likely to find evidence of fetal hypoxia and criticize the obstetrician's management if the outcome was poor versus good (18). Therefore, reinterpretation of the FHR tracing, especially if neonatal outcome is known, may not be reliable.

▶ *When should the very preterm fetus be monitored?*

The decision to monitor the very preterm fetus requires a discussion between the obstetrician, pediatrician, and patient concerning the likelihood of survival or severe morbidity of the preterm child (based on gestational age, estimated fetal weight, and other factors) and issues related to mode of delivery. If a patient undergoes a cesarean delivery for indications related to a preterm fetus, continuous monitoring should be used rather than intermittent auscultation. The earliest gestational age that this will occur may vary.

Nonreassuring FHR patterns may occur with up to 60% of women with preterm labor, with the most common abnormality being deceleration and bradycardia, followed by tachycardia and minimal or absent baseline variability (19). Variable decelerations are more common among preterm (55–70%) deliveries than term (20–30%) deliveries (20). If FHR abnormalities are persistent, intrauterine resuscitation, ancillary tests to ensure fetal well-being, and possibly delivery should be undertaken (21).

▶ What medications can affect the fetal heart rate?

Fetal heart rate patterns can be influenced by the medications administered in the intrapartum period. Most often, these changes are transient, although they sometimes lead to obstetric interventions.

Epidural analgesia with local anesthetic agents (ie, lidocaine, bupivacaine) can lead to sympathetic blockade, maternal hypotension, transient uteroplacental insufficiency, and alterations in the FHR. Parenteral narcotics also may affect the FHR. A randomized trial comparing epidural anesthesia with 0.25% of bupivacaine and intravenous meperidine reported that the variability was decreased, and FHR accelerations were significantly less common with parenteral analgesia compared with regional analgesia (22). The rates of decelerations and cesarean delivery for "nonreassuring" FHR tracings were similar for the two groups. A systematic review of five randomized trials and seven observational studies also noted that the rate of cesarean delivery for nonreassuring FHR was similar between those who did and those who did not receive epidural analgesia during labor (23).

Concern has been raised about combined spinal–epidural anesthesia during labor. An intent-to-treat analysis of 1,223 laboring women randomized to combined spinal–epidural anesthesia (10 mcg of intrathecal sufentanil, followed by epidural bupivacaine and fentanyl at the next request for analgesia) or intravenous meperidine (50 mg on demand, maximum 200 mg in 4 hours) noted a significantly higher rate of bradycardia and emergent cesarean delivery for abnormal FHR in the group randomized to combined spinal–epidural anesthesia (24). Neonatal outcome, however, was not significantly different between the two groups. There are some methodological concerns with this study. Another randomized controlled trial compared the occurrence of FHR tracing abnormalities in laboring women who received combined spinal–epidural anesthesia (n=41) to epidural anesthesia (n=46). In this study, FHR abnormalities were more common in women receiving combined spinal–epidural anesthesia (25). Additional trials are necessary to determine the potential safety and efficacy of the combined spinal–epidural technique.

Other medications that influence FHR tracing have been studied (see Table 2). Of note, multiple regression analysis indicated that decreased variability attributed to the use of magnesium sulfate was related to early gestational age but not the serum magnesium level (26). Studies report different findings with regard to the effect of magnesium on FHR patterns. Some show no independent effect; others show small changes in baseline or variability. In general, however, caution should be used in ascribing unfavorable findings on EFM to the use of magnesium alone.

Transient sinusoidal FHR patterns occurred in 75% of patients who received butorphanol during labor, but this was not associated with adverse outcomes (27). Fetuses exposed to cocaine did not exhibit any characteristic changes in the heart rate pattern, although they did have frequent contractions even when labor was unstimulated (28). As determined by computer analysis of cardiotocograms, a randomized trial reported that compared with meperidine, nalbuphine used for intrapartum analgesia decreased the likelihood of two 15-second accelerations over 20 minutes (29). In antepartum patients, administration of morphine decreased not only the fetal breathing movement but also the number of accelerations (30).

The effect of corticosteroids, which are used to enhance pulmonary maturity of fetuses during preterm labor, on FHR has been studied (Table 2). Among twins (31) and singletons (32, 33), the use of betamethasone transiently decreased the FHR variability, which returned to pretreatment status by the fourth to seventh day. There also may be a decrease in the rate of accelerations with the use of betamethasone. These changes, however, were not associated with increased obstetric interventions or with adverse outcomes (31). The biologic mechanism of this is unknown. Computerized analysis of the cardiotocograms indicates that use of dexamethasone is not associated with a decrease in the FHR variability (33).

▶ What findings on EFM are consistent with normal fetal acid–base status?

The presence of FHR accelerations generally ensures that the fetus is not acidemic. The data relating FHR variability to clinical outcomes, however, are sparse. Results of an observational study suggest that moderate FHR variability is strongly associated with an arterial umbilical cord pH higher than 7.15 (34). One study reported that in the presence of late or variable decelerations, the umbilical arterial pH was higher than 7.00 in 97% of the cases if the FHR tracing had normal variability (35). In another retrospective study, most cases of adverse neonatal outcome demonstrated normal FHR variability (36). This study is limited because it did not consider other characteristics of the FHR tracing, such as the presence of accelerations or decelerations. However, in most cases, normal FHR variability provides reassurance about fetal status and the absence of metabolic acidemia.

Table 2. Effects of Commonly Used Medications on Fetal Heart Rate Patterns

Medications	Comments	References
Narcotics	At equivalent doses, all narcotics (with or without added antiemetics) have similar effects: a decrease in variability and a decrease in the frequency of accelerations 75 mg meperidine = 10 mg morphine = 0.1 mg fentanyl = 10 mg nalbuphine	1–7
Butorphanol	Transient sinusoidal FHR pattern, slight increased mean heart rate compared with meperidine	8, 9
Cocaine	Decreased long-term variability	10, 11
Corticosteroids	Decrease in FHR variability with beta-methasone but not dexamethasone, abolishment of diurnal fetal rhythms, increased effect at greater than 29 weeks of gestation	12–15
Magnesium sulfate	A significant decrease in short-term variability, clinically insignificant decrease in FHR, inhibits the increase in accelerations with advancing gestational age	16, 17
Terbutaline	Increase in baseline FHR and incidence of fetal tachycardia	18, 19
Zidovudine	No difference in the FHR baseline, variability, number of accelerations, or decelerations	20

Abbreviation: FHR, fetal heart rate.

References

1. Hill JB, Alexander JM, Sharma SK, McIntire DD, Leveno KJ. A comparison of the effects of epidural and meperidine analgesia during labor on fetal heart rate. Obstet Gynecol 2003;102:333–7.

2. Panayotopoulos N, Salamalekis E, Kassanos D, Vitoratos N, Loghis C, Batalias L. Intrapartum vibratory acoustic stimulation after maternal meperidine administration. Clin Exp Obstet Gynecol 1998;25:139–40.

3. Zimmer EZ, Divon MY, Vadasz A. Influence of meperidine on fetal movements and heart rate beat-to-beat variability in the active phase of labor. Am J Perinatol 1988;5:197–200.

4. Kopecky EA, Ryan ML, Barrett JF, Seaward PG, Ryan G, Koren G, et al. Fetal response to maternally administered morphine. Am J Obstet Gynecol 2000;183:424–30.

5. Rayburn W, Rathke A, Leuschen MP, Chleborad J, Weidner W. Fentanyl citrate analgesia during labor. Am J Obstet Gynecol 1989;161:202–6.

6. Nicolle E, Devillier P, Delanoy B, Durand C, Bessard G. Therapeutic monitoring of nalbuphine: transplacental transfer and estimated pharmacokinetics in the neonate. Eur J Clin Pharmacol 1996;49:485–9.

7. Poehlmann S, Pinette M, Stubblefield P. Effect of labor analgesia with nalbuphine hydrochloride on fetal response to vibroacoustic stimulation. J Reprod Med 1995;40:707–10.

8. Hatjis CG, Meis PJ. Sinusoidal fetal heart rate pattern associated with butorphanol administration. Obstet Gynecol 1986;67:377–80.

9. Quilligan EJ, Keegan KA, Donahue MJ. Double-blind comparison of intravenously injected butorphanol and meperidine in parturients. Int J Gynaecol Obstet 1980;18:363–7.

10. Chazotte C, Forman L, Gandhi J. Heart rate patterns in fetuses exposed to cocaine. Obstet Gynecol 1991;78:323–5.

11. Tabor BL, Soffici AR, Smith-Wallace T, Yonekura ML. The effect of maternal cocaine use on the fetus: changes in antepartum fetal heart rate tracings. Am J Obstet Gynecol 1991;165:1278–81.

12. Senat MV, Minoui S, Multon O, Fernandez H, Frydman R, Ville Y. Effect of dexamethasone and betamethasone on fetal heart rate variability in preterm labour: a randomised study. Br J Obstet Gynaecol 1998;105:749–55.

13. Rotmensch S, Liberati M, Vishne TH, Celentano C, Ben-Rafael Z, Bellati U. The effect of betamethasone and dexamethasone on fetal heart rate patterns and biophysical activities. A prospective randomized trial. Acta Obstet Gynecol Scand 1999;78:493–500.

14. Koenen SV, Mulder EJ, Wijnberger LD, Visser GH. Transient loss of the diurnal rhythms of fetal movements, heart rate, and its variation after maternal betamethasone administration. Pediatr Res 2005;57:662–6.

15. Mulder EJ, Koenen SV, Blom I, Visser GH. The effects of antenatal betamethasone administration on fetal heart rate and behaviour depend on gestational age. Early Hum Dev 2004;76:65–77.

16. Hallak M, Martinez-Poyer J, Kruger ML, Hassan S, Blackwell SC, Sorokin Y. The effect of magnesium sulfate on fetal heart rate parameters: a randomized, placebo-controlled trial. Am J Obstet Gynecol 1999;181:1122–7.

17. Wright JW, Ridgway LE, Wright BD, Covington DL, Bobitt JR. Effect of MgSO4 on heart rate monitoring in the preterm fetus. J Reprod Med 1996;41:605–8.

18. Mawaldi L, Duminy P, Tamim H. Terbutaline versus nifedipine for prolongation of pregnancy in patients with preterm labor. Int J Gynaecol Obstet 2008;100:65–8.

19. Roth AC, Milsom I, Forssman L, Ekman LG, Hedner T. Effects of intravenous terbutaline on maternal circulation and fetal heart activity. Acta Obstet Gynecol Scand 1990;69:223–8.

20. Blackwell SC, Sahai A, Hassan SS, Treadwell MC, Tomlinson MW, Jones TB, et al. Effects of intrapartum zidovudine therapy on fetal heart rate parameters in women with human immunodeficiency virus infection. Fetal Diagn Ther 2001;16:413–6.

▶ *Are there ancillary tests that can aid in the management of Category II or Category III fetal heart rate tracings?*

There are some ancillary tests available that help to ensure fetal well-being in the face of a Category II or Category III FHR tracing, thereby reducing the high false-positive rate of EFM.

In the case of an EFM tracing with minimal or absent variability and without spontaneous acceleration, an effort should be made to elicit one. A meta-analysis of 11 studies of intrapartum fetal stimulation noted that four techniques are available to stimulate the fetus: 1) fetal scalp sampling, 2) Allis clamp scalp stimulation, 3) vibroacoustic stimulation, and 4) digital scalp stimulation (37). Because vibroacoustic stimulation and digital scalp stimulation are less invasive than the other two methods, they are the preferred methods. When there is an acceleration following stimulation, acidemia is unlikely and labor can continue.

When a Category III FHR tracing is persistent, a scalp blood sample for the determination of pH or lactate may be considered. However, the use of scalp pH assessment has decreased (38), and this test may not even be available at some tertiary hospitals (39). There are likely many reasons for this decrease, including physician experience, difficulty in obtaining and processing an adequate sample in a short amount of time, and the need for routine maintenance and calibration of laboratory equipment that may be used infrequently. More importantly, scalp stimulation, which is less invasive, provides similar information about the likelihood of fetal acidemia as does scalp pH.

In one study, the sensitivity and positive predictive value of a low scalp pH (defined in the study as less than 7.21 because it is the 75th percentile) to predict umbilical arterial pH less than 7.00 was 36% and 9%, respectively (40). More importantly, the sensitivity and positive predictive value of a low scalp pH to identify a newborn with hypoxic–ischemic encephalopathy was 50% and 3%, respectively. However, the greater utility of scalp pH is in its high negative predictive value (97–99%). There are some data to suggest that fetal scalp lactate levels have higher sensitivity and specificity than scalp pH (40). However, a recent large randomized clinical trial that compared the use of scalp pH assessment to scalp lactate level assessment in cases of intrapartum fetal distress did not demonstrate a difference in the rate of acidemia at birth, Apgar scores, or neonatal intensive care unit admissions (41). Although scalp stimulation has largely replaced scalp pH and scalp lactate assessment in the United States, if available, these tests may provide additional information in the setting of a Category III tracing.

Pulse oximetry has not been demonstrated to be a clinically useful test in evaluating fetal status (42–44).

▶ *Are there methods of intrauterine resuscitation that can be used for Category II or Category III tracings?*

A Category II or Category III FHR tracing requires evaluation of the possible causes. Initial evaluation and treatment may include the following:

- Discontinuation of any labor stimulating agent
- Cervical examination to determine umbilical cord prolapse, rapid cervical dilation, or descent of the fetal head
- Changing maternal position to left or right lateral recumbent position, reducing compression of the vena cava and improving uteroplacental blood flow
- Monitoring maternal blood pressure level for evidence of hypotension, especially in those with regional anesthesia (if present, treatment with volume expansion or with ephedrine or both, or phenylephrine may be warranted)
- Assessment of patient for uterine tachysystole by evaluating uterine contraction frequency and duration

Supplemental maternal oxygen commonly is used in cases of an indeterminate or abnormal pattern. There are no data on the efficacy or safety of this therapy. Often, the FHR patterns persist and do not respond to change in position or oxygenation. In such cases, the use of tocolytic agents has been suggested to stop uterine contractions and perhaps avoid umbilical cord compression. A meta-analysis reported the pooled results of three randomized clinical trials that compared tocolytic therapy (terbutaline, hexoprenaline, or magnesium sulfate) with untreated controls in the management of a suspected nonreassuring FHR tracing (45). Compared with no treatment, tocolytic therapy more commonly improved the FHR tracing. However, there were no differences in rates of perinatal mortality, low 5-minute Apgar score, or admission to the neonatal intensive care unit between the groups (possibly because of the small sample size). Thus, although tocolytic therapy appears to reduce the number of FHR abnormalities, there is insufficient evidence to recommend it.

Tachysystole with associated FHR changes can be successfully treated with β_2-adrenergic drugs (hexoprenaline or terbutaline). A retrospective study suggested that 98% of such cases respond to treatment with a β-agonist (46).

When the FHR tracing includes recurrent variable decelerations, amnioinfusion to relieve umbilical cord compression may be considered (47). A meta-analysis of 12 randomized trials that allocated patients to no treatment or transcervical amnioinfusion noted that placement of fluid in the uterine cavity significantly reduced the rate of decelerations (RR, 0.54; 95% CI, 0.43–0.68) and cesarean delivery for suspected fetal distress (RR, 0.35; 95% CI, 0.24–0.52) (48). Because of the lower rate of cesarean delivery, amnioinfusion also decreased the likelihood that either the patient or the newborn will stay in the hospital more than 3 days (48). Amnioinfusion can be done by bolus or continuous infusion technique. A randomized trial compared the two techniques of amnioinfusion and concluded that both have a similar ability to relieve recurrent variable decelerations (49).

Another common cause of a Category II or Category III FHR pattern is maternal hypotension secondary to regional anesthesia. If maternal hypotension is identified and suspected to be secondary to regional anesthesia, treatment with volume expansion or intravenous ephedrine or both is warranted.

Summary of Recommendations and Conclusions

The following recommendations and conclusions are based on good and consistent scientific evidence (Level A):

▶ The false-positive rate of EFM for predicting cerebral palsy is high, at greater than 99%.

▶ The use of EFM is associated with an increased rate of both vacuum and forceps operative vaginal delivery, and cesarean delivery for abnormal FHR patterns or acidosis or both.

▶ When the FHR tracing includes recurrent variable decelerations, amnioinfusion to relieve umbilical cord compression should be considered.

▶ Pulse oximetry has not been demonstrated to be a clinically useful test in evaluating fetal status.

The following conclusions are based on limited or inconsistent scientific evidence (Level B):

▶ There is high interobserver and intraobserver variability in interpretation of FHR tracing.

▶ Reinterpretation of the FHR tracing, especially if the neonatal outcome is known, may not be reliable.

▶ The use of EFM does not result in a reduction of cerebral palsy.

The following recommendations are based on expert opinion (Level C):

▶ A three-tiered system for the categorization of FHR patterns is recommended.

▶ The labor of women with high-risk conditions should be monitored with continuous FHR monitoring.

▶ The terms hyperstimulation and hypercontractility should be abandoned.

References

1. Martin JA, Hamilton BE, Sutton PD, Ventura SJ, Menacker F, Munson ML. Births: final data for 2002. Natl Vital Stat Rep 2003;52:1–113. (Level II-3)

2. Low JA, Pickersgill H, Killen H, Derrick EJ. The prediction and prevention of intrapartum fetal asphyxia in term pregnancies. Am J Obstet Gynecol 2001;184:724–30. (Level II-2)

3. Macones GA, Hankins GD, Spong CY, Hauth J, Moore T. The 2008 National Institute of Child Health and Human Development workshop report on electronic fetal monitoring: update on definitions, interpretation, and research guidelines. Obstet Gynecol 2008;112:661–6. (Level III)

4. Royal College of Obstetricians and Gynaecologists. The use of electronic fetal monitoring: the use and interpretation of cardiotocography in intrapartum fetal surveillance. Evidence-based Clinical Guideline No. 8. London (UK): RCOG; 2001. http://www.rcog.org.uk/files/rcog-corp/uploaded-files/NEBEFMGuidelineFinal2may2001.pdf (Level III)

5. Liston R, Sawchuck D, Young D. Fetal health surveillance: antepartum and intrapartum consensus guideline. Society of Obstetrics and Gynaecologists of Canada; British Columbia Perinatal Health Program [published erratum appears in J Obstet Gynaecol Can 2007;29:909]. J Obstet Gynaecol Can 2007;29(suppl 4):S3–56. (Level III)

6. Parer JT, Ikeda T. A framework for standardized management of intrapartum fetal heart rate patterns. Am J Obstet Gynecol 2007;197:26.e1–26.e6. (Level III)

7. Freeman RK. Problems with intrapartum fetal heart rate monitoring interpretation and patient management. Obstet Gynecol 2002;100:813–26. (Level III)

8. Alfirevic Z, Devane D, Gyte GML. Continuous cardiotocography (CTG) as a form of electronic fetal monitoring (EFM) for fetal assessment during labour. Cochrane Database of Systematic Reviews 2006, Issue 3. Art. No.: CD006066. DOI: 10.1002/14651858.CD006066. (Meta-analysis)

9. Nelson KB, Dambrosia JM, Ting TY, Grether JK. Uncertain value of electronic fetal monitoring in predicting cerebral palsy. N Engl J Med 1996;334:613–8. (Level II-2)

10. Clark SL, Hankins GD. Temporal and demographic trends in cerebral palsy—fact and fiction. Am J Obstet Gynecol 2003;188:628–33. (Level III)

11. Hankins GD, Speer M. Defining the pathogenesis and pathophysiology of neonatal encephalopathy and cerebral palsy. Obstet Gynecol 2003;102:628–36. (Level III)

12. Badawi N, Kurinczuk JJ, Keogh JM, Alessandri LM, O'Sullivan F, Burton PR, et al. Antepartum risk factors for newborn encephalopathy: the Western Australian case-control study. BMJ 1998;317:1549–53. (Level II-2)

13. Morrison JC, Chez BF, Davis ID, Martin RW, Roberts WE, Martin JN Jr, et al. Intrapartum fetal heart rate assessment: monitoring by auscultation or electronic means. Am J Obstet Gynecol 1993;168:63–6. (Level III)

14. Vintzileos AM, Nochimson DJ, Antsaklis A, Varvarigos I, Guzman ER, Knuppel RA. Comparison of intrapartum electronic fetal heart rate monitoring versus intermittent auscultation in detecting fetal acidemia at birth. Am J Obstet Gynecol 1995;173:1021–4. (Level II-1)

15. Nielsen PV, Stigsby B, Nickelsen C, Nim J. Intra- and inter-observer variability in the assessment of intrapartum cardiotocograms. Acta Obstet Gynecol Scand 1987;66: 421–4. (Level III)

16. Beaulieu MD, Fabia J, Leduc B, Brisson J, Bastide A, Blouin D, et al. The reproducibility of intrapartum cardiotocogram assessments. Can Med Assoc J 1982;127: 214–6. (Level III)

17. Blix E, Sviggum O, Koss KS, Oian P. Inter-observer variation in assessment of 845 labour admission tests: comparison between midwives and obstetricians in the clinical setting and two experts. BJOG 2003;110:1–5. (Level III)

18. Zain HA, Wright JW, Parrish GE, Diehl SJ. Interpreting the fetal heart rate tracing. Effect of knowledge of neonatal outcome. J Reprod Med 1998;43:367–70. (Level III)

19. Ayoubi JM, Audibert F, Vial M, Pons JC, Taylor S, Frydman R. Fetal heart rate and survival of the very premature newborn. Am J Obstet Gynecol 2002;187:1026–30. (Level II-2)

20. Westgren M, Holmquist P, Svenningsen NW, Ingemarsson I. Intrapartum fetal monitoring in preterm deliveries: prospective study. Obstet Gynecol 1982;60:99–106. (Level II-2)

21. Westgren M, Hormquist P, Ingemarsson I, Svenningsen N. Intrapartum fetal acidosis in preterm infants: fetal monitoring and long-term morbidity. Obstet Gynecol 1984;63: 355–9. (Level II-2)

22. Hill JB, Alexander JM, Sharma SK, McIntire DD, Leveno KJ. A comparison of the effects of epidural and meperidine analgesia during labor on fetal heart rate. Obstet Gynecol 2003;102:333–7. (Level I)

23. Lieberman E, O'Donoghue C. Unintended effects of epidural analgesia during labor: a systematic review. Am J Obstet Gynecol 2002;186(suppl 1):S31–68. (Level III)

24. Gambling DR, Sharma SK, Ramin SM, Lucas MJ, Leveno KJ, Wiley J, et al. A randomized study of combined spinal-epidural analgesia versus intravenous meperidine during labor: impact on cesarean delivery rate. Anesthesiology 1998;89:1336–44. (Level I)

25. Abrao KC, Francisco RP, Miyadahira S, Cicarelli DD, Zugaib M. Elevation of uterine basal tone and fetal heart rate abnormalities after labor analgesia: a randomized controlled trial. Obstet Gynecol 2009;113:41–7. (Level I)

26. Wright JW, Ridgway LE, Wright BD, Covington DL, Bobitt JR. Effect of MgSO4 on heart rate monitoring in the preterm fetus. J Reprod Med 1996;41:605–8. (Level II-2)

27. Hatjis CG, Meis PJ. Sinusoidal fetal heart rate pattern associated with butorphanol administration. Obstet Gynecol 1986;67:377–80. (Level II-2)

28. Chazotte C, Forman L, Gandhi J. Heart rate patterns in fetuses exposed to cocaine. Obstet Gynecol 1991;78: 323–5. (Level II-3)

29. Giannina G, Guzman ER, Lai YL, Lake MF, Cernadas M, Vintzileos AM. Comparison of the effects of meperidine and nalbuphine on intrapartum fetal heart rate tracings. Obstet Gynecol 1995;86:441–5. (Level I)

30. Kopecky EA, Ryan ML, Barrett JF, Seaward PG, Ryan G, Koren G, et al. Fetal response to maternally administered morphine. Am J Obstet Gynecol 2000;183:424–30. (Level II-2)

31. Ville Y, Vincent Y, Tordjman N, Hue MV, Fernandez H, Frydman R. Effect of betamethasone on the fetal heart rate pattern assessed by computerized cardiotocography in normal twin pregnancies. Fetal Diagn Ther 1995;10: 301–6. (Level II-3)

32. Subtil D, Tiberghien P, Devos P, Therby D, Leclerc G, Vaast P, et al. Immediate and delayed effects of antenatal corticosteroids on fetal heart rate: a randomized trial that compares betamethasone acetate and phosphate, betamethasone phosphate, and dexamethasone. Am J Obstet Gynecol 2003;188:524–31. (Level I)

33. Senat MV, Minoui S, Multon O, Fernandez H, Frydman R, Ville Y. Effect of dexamethasone and betamethasone on fetal heart rate variability in preterm labour: a randomised study. Br J Obstet Gynaecol 1998;105:749–55. (Level I)

34. Parer JT, King T, Flanders S, Fox M, Kilpatrick SJ. Fetal acidemia and electronic fetal heart rate patterns: is there evidence of an association? J Matern Fetal Neonatal Med 2006;19:289–94. (Level III)

35. Williams KP, Galerneau F. Intrapartum fetal heart rate patterns in the prediction of neonatal acidemia. Am J Obstet Gynecol 2003;188:820–3. (Level II-3)

36. Samueloff A, Langer O, Berkus M, Field N, Xenakis E, Ridgway L. Is fetal heart rate variability a good predictor of fetal outcome? Acta Obstet Gynecol Scand 1994;73: 39–44. (Level II-2)

37. Skupski DW, Rosenberg CR, Eglinton GS. Intrapartum fetal stimulation tests: a meta-analysis. Obstet Gynecol 2002;99:129–34. (Meta-analysis)

38. Goodwin TM, Milner-Masterson L, Paul RH. Elimination of fetal scalp blood sampling on a large clinical service. Obstet Gynecol 1994;83:971–4. (Level II-3)

39. Hendrix NW, Chauhan SP, Scardo JA, Ellings JM, Devoe LD. Managing nonreassuring fetal heart rate patterns before cesarean delivery. Compliance with ACOG recommendations. J Reprod Med 2000;45:995–9. (Level III)

40. Kruger K, Hallberg B, Blennow M, Kublickas M, Westgren M. Predictive value of fetal scalp blood lactate concentration and pH as markers of neurologic disability. Am J Obstet Gynecol 1999;181:1072–8. (Level II-3)

41. Wiberg-Itzel E, Lipponer C, Norman M, Herbst A, Prebensen D, Hansson A, et al. Determination of pH or lactate in fetal scalp blood in management of intrapartum fetal distress: randomised controlled multicentre trial. BMJ 2008;336:1284–7. (Level I)

42. Garite TJ, Dildy GA, McNamara H, Nageotte MP, Boehm FH, Dellinger EH, et al. A multicenter controlled trial of fetal pulse oximetry in the intrapartum management of nonreassuring fetal heart rate patterns. Am J Obstet Gynecol 2000;183:1049–58. (Level I)

43. Bloom SL, Spong CY, Thom E, Varner MW, Rouse DJ, Weininger S, et al. Fetal pulse oximetry and cesarean delivery. National Institute of Child Health and Human Development Maternal-Fetal Medicine Units Network. N Engl J Med 2006;355:2195–202. (Level I)

44. East CE, Chan FY, Colditz PB, Begg L. Fetal pulse oximetry for fetal assessment in labour. Cochrane Database of Systematic Reviews 2007, Issue 2. Art. No.: CD004075. DOI: 10.1002/14651858.CD004075. pub3. (Meta-analysis)

45. Kulier R, Hofmeyr GJ. Tocolytics for suspected intrapartum fetal distress. Cochrane Database of Systematic Reviews 1998, Issue 2. Art. No.: CD000035. DOI: 10.1002/14651858.CD000035. (Meta-analysis)

46. Egarter CH, Husslein PW, Rayburn WF. Uterine hyperstimulation after low-dose prostaglandin E2 therapy: tocolytic treatment in 181 cases. Am J Obstet Gynecol 1990;163:794–6. (Level II-2)

47. Miyazaki FS, Taylor NA. Saline amnioinfusion for relief of variable or prolonged decelerations. A preliminary report. Am J Obstet Gynecol 1983;146:670–8. (Level III)

48. Hofmeyr GJ. Amnioinfusion for potential or suspected umbilical cord compression in labour. Cochrane Database of Systematic Reviews 1998, Issue 1. Art. No.: CD000013. DOI: 10.1002/14651858.CD000013. (Meta-analysis)

49. Rinehart BK, Terrone DA, Barrow JH, Isler CM, Barrilleaux PS, Roberts WE. Randomized trial of intermittent or continuous amnioinfusion for variable decelerations. Obstet Gynecol 2000;96:571–4. (Level I)

The MEDLINE database, the Cochrane Library, and ACOG's own internal resources and documents were used to conduct a literature search to locate relevant articles published between January 1985 and January 2009. The search was restricted to articles published in the English language. Priority was given to articles reporting results of original research, although review articles and commentaries also were consulted. Abstracts of research presented at symposia and scientific conferences were not considered adequate for inclusion in this document. Guidelines published by organizations or institutions such as the National Institutes of Health and the American College of Obstetricians and Gynecologists were reviewed, and additional studies were located by reviewing bibliographies of identified articles. When reliable research was not available, expert opinions from obstetrician–gynecologists were used.

Studies were reviewed and evaluated for quality according to the method outlined by the U.S. Preventive Services Task Force:

I Evidence obtained from at least one properly designed randomized controlled trial.

II-1 Evidence obtained from well-designed controlled trials without randomization.

II-2 Evidence obtained from well-designed cohort or case–control analytic studies, preferably from more than one center or research group.

II-3 Evidence obtained from multiple time series with or without the intervention. Dramatic results in uncontrolled experiments also could be regarded as this type of evidence.

III Opinions of respected authorities, based on clinical experience, descriptive studies, or reports of expert committees.

Based on the highest level of evidence found in the data, recommendations are provided and graded according to the following categories:

Level A—Recommendations are based on good and consistent scientific evidence.

Level B—Recommendations are based on limited or inconsistent scientific evidence.

Level C—Recommendations are based primarily on consensus and expert opinion.

The American College of Obstetricians and Gynecologists
409 12th Street, SW, PO Box 96920, Washington, DC 20090-6920

Intrapartum fetal heart rate monitoring: nomenclature, interpretation, and general management principles. ACOG Practice Bulletin No. 106. American College of Obstetricians and Gynecologists. Obstet Gynecol 2009;114:192–202.

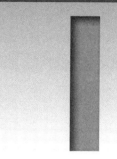

Resuscitation Supplies and Equipment

Neonatal Resuscitation Supplies and Equipment

Suction equipment

Bulb syringe

Mechanical suction and tubing

Suction catheters, 5F or 6F, 8F, 10F, 12F or 14F

8F feeding tube and 20-mL syringe

Meconium aspirator

Bag-and-mask equipment

Device for delivering positive-pressure ventilation, capable of delivering 90% to 100% oxygen

Face masks, newborn and premature sizes (cushioned-rim masks preferred)

Oxygen source

Compressed air source

Oxygen blender to mix oxygen and compressed air with flowmeter (flow rate up to 10 L/min) and tubing

Pulse oximeter and oximeter probe

Intubation equipment

Laryngoscope with straight blades, No. 0 (preterm) and No. 1 (term)

Extra bulbs and batteries for laryngoscope

Endotracheal tubes, 2.5-, 3.0-, 3.5-, 4.0-mm internal diameter (ID)

Stylet (optional)

Scissors

Tape or securing device for endotracheal tube

Alcohol sponges

CO_2 detector or capnograph

Laryngeal mask airway

Medications

Epinephrine 1:10,000 (0.1 mg/mL)—3-mL or 10-mL ampules

Isotonic crystalloid (normal saline or Ringer's lactate) for volume expansion—100 or 250 mL

Dextrose 10%, 250 mL

Normal saline for flushes

Neonatal Resuscitation Supplies and Equipment—*continued*

Umbilical vessel catheterization supplies
Sterile gloves
Scalpel or scissors
Antiseptic prep solution
Umbilical tape
Umbilical catheters, 3.5F, 5F
Three-way stopcock
Syringes, 1, 3, 5, 10, 20, 50 mL
Needles, 25, 21, 18 gauge, or puncture device for needleless system

Miscellaneous
Gloves and appropriate personal protection
Radiant warmer or other heat source
Firm, padded resuscitation surface
Clock with second hand (timer optional)
Warmed linens
Stethoscope (with neonatal head)
Tape, 1/2 or 3/4 inch
Cardiac monitor and electrodes (optional for delivery room)
Oropharyngeal airways (0, 00, and 000 sizes or 30-, 40-, and 50-mm
  lengths)

For very preterm babies
Size 00 laryngoscope blade (optional)
Reclosable, food-grade plastic bag (1-gallon size) or plastic wrap
Chemically activated warming pad (optional)
Transport incubator to maintain baby's temperature during move to
  the nursery

Neonatal Resuscitation Program Quick Pre-resuscitation Checklist

Neonatal Resuscitation Supplies and Equipment at Radiant Warmer

This checklist includes only the most essential supplies and equipment needed at the radiant warmer for most neonatal resuscitations. Tailor this list to meet your unit-specific needs to ensure that supplies and equipment are present and functioning and unit-specific safety checks have been done prior to <u>every</u> birth.

Warm	Preheat warmer Towels or blankets
Clear airway	Bulb syringe 10F or 12F suction catheter attached to wall suction set at 80-100 mm Hg Meconium aspirator
Auscultate	Stethoscope
Oxygenate	Method to give free-flow oxygen (mask, tubing, flow-inflating bag, or T-piece) Gases flowing just prior to birth, 5-10 L/min Blender set per protocol Pulse oximeter probe (detached from oximeter until needed) Pulse oximeter
Ventilate	Positive-pressure ventilation (PPV) device(s) present with term and preterm masks PPV device(s) functioning Connected to air/oxygen source (blender) 8F feeding tube and 20-mL syringe
Intubate	Laryngoscope Size 0 and Size 1 (and size 00, optional) blades with bright light Endotracheal tubes, sizes 2.5, 3.0, 3.5, 4.0 Stylets End tidal CO_2 detector Laryngeal mask airway (size 1) and 5-mL syringe
Medicate	Access to 1:10,000 epinephrine and normal saline Supplies for administering meds and placing emergency umbilical venous catheter Documentation supplies
Thermoregulate	Plastic bag or plastic wrap Chemically activated warming pad Transport incubator ready
Other	

Organizing Resuscitation Supplies and Equipment

It is difficult for members of the resuscitation team to perform well if they cannot find or use necessary equipment. Anxiety increases and tempers flare when resuscitation interventions cannot be performed because of missing or malfunctioning equipment. A comprehensive list of suggested supplies and equipment is found on pages 32-33 of the *Textbook of Neonatal Resuscitation, 6th Edition.* The Quick Pre-resuscitation Checklist (page 380 of this manual and page 34 of the *Textbook of Neonatal Resuscitation, 6th Edition)* lists the most essential supplies and uses the same organizational routine as the Performance Checklist for resuscitation supplies. You may wish to post the Quick Pre-resuscitation Checklist on every radiant warmer to help ensure that all essential resuscitation supplies are present and functioning at every birth.

Many hospitals use an emergency cart system to organize resuscitation supplies. Others use a tackle box, a wall cabinet, or a supply system hanging on a hook. Whatever the system, certain basic principles of organization apply.

Supplies and equipment must be

- **In a predictable location**
  Organize supplies in a similar fashion in every place where neonatal resuscitation occurs in your practice setting. For example, if all labor rooms look alike, the resuscitation equipment should be arranged identically in all those rooms. The nursery or operating room is arranged differently than a labor room, but, if an emergency cart system is common to the labor rooms, it may be wise to keep this commonality in the nursery and operating room as well. Staff will be frustrated if they must learn and remember different locations or systems of organizing supplies all over the unit.

- **Immediately available**
  Have basic supplies in the labor room, not outside the room or down the hall from the delivery suite. Equipment that is basic to all birthing areas includes a warmer, a suction device, towels or blankets for drying the newborn, a device for delivering positive-pressure ventilation, and a system for oxygen delivery. If a system for blended oxygen, pulse oximetry, and medications are located away from the birth area, part of your mock code evaluation should include how quickly these emergency supplies arrive at a neonatal resuscitation.

- **Immediately accessible**

Ensure that staff members know how to break the lock and release the drawers of the emergency cart. The lack of this seemingly simple skill can frustrate resuscitation efforts in a hurry. Equipment kept inside boxes or taped into bags can be difficult to access. Drawer organizers from the office supply store can keep supplies and equipment organized, visible, and easily accessible.

- **Preassembled and ready for use**
  Make the steps of preparing equipment for use as simple as possible. For example,

    - Attach the oxygen reservoir to the self-inflating oxygen bag.
    - Connect the oxygen tubing to the flowmeter on the wall or tank.
    - Attach the most-often-used size of blade to the laryngoscope.
    - Connect the suction catheter and tubing to the wall suction ready for use and keep clean inside the bag.
    - Use a rubber band to wrap the syringe and the saline flush to the box of epinephrine or put all these items inside a reclosable plastic bag.
    - Attach the endotracheal tube and tube-securing device packages together.

- **Immediately visible**
  People under stress can sometimes fail to see an item that is right in front of them. To make supplies visible,

    - Arrange your supply system so that the contents of drawers are clearly marked on the outside of each drawer and clearly visible when you open the drawer. Do not stack different items on top of each other.
    - In bold marker on the package, write the size of items that look alike (such as endotracheal tubes).
    - Use clear bags for small items (such as airways and medication labels) and secure these small items so that they are not loose in a drawer or pocket.
    - Post the neonatal resuscitation wall chart or code cart cards in prominent places on top of your emergency cart, on the wall of the operating room, near the radiant warmer, or on both sides of the radiant warmer itself. While staff should not rely on the NRP flow diagram during resuscitation, it may boost confidence to know it is there. Staff should know the medication doses for resuscitation but can double-check a decision and possibly prevent an error if the medication chart is visible near the emergency medication preparation area.

- **In supply and maintained in working order**
  - Check key pieces of equipment (suction, positive-pressure ventilation device, laryngoscope light, oxygen/air tanks) after each use, prior to every birth, and additionally per hospital protocol.
  - Write the expiration dates of medications and packaged supplies clearly and boldly on the box or package for easy visibility. In locked emergency carts or cabinets, stick a label on the outside with the expiration date of the medication that expires first. This alerts staff to restock medication before the expiration date and saves time checking supplies.
  - Check emergency supplies every 24 hours. If an ancillary department, such as central supply, checks the emergency supplies, ensure that staff members who participate in resuscitations know where these supplies are located. If unit personnel check emergency equipment, rotate this responsibility to acquaint all staff with the contents and location of emergency cabinets or carts.
  - Establish a routine for ordering and restocking supplies before the last one of something is used.
  - Tag equipment in need of repair according to your hospital policy. Take the equipment out of use and replace it immediately.
  - Check or establish your hospital policy for replacing oxygen/air tanks and for routine maintenance of biomedical equipment.

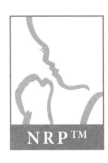

Index